THE
HOLFORD
DIET

THE
HOLFORD
DIET

Lose Fat Fast using the
Revolutionary Fatburner System

PATRICK HOLFORD

PIATKUS

Visit the Piatkus website!

Piatkus publishes a wide range of best-selling fiction and non-fiction, including books on health, mind, body & spirit, sex, self-help, cookery, biography and the paranormal.

If you want to:

- read descriptions of our popular titles
- buy our books over the Internet
- take advantage of our special offers
- enter our monthly competition
- learn more about your favourite Piatkus authors

VISIT OUR WEBSITE AT: www.piatkus.co.uk

First published in Great Britain in 2005 by
Piatkus Books Limited
5 Windmill Street, London W1T 2JA
e-mail: info@piatkus.co.uk

ISBN 0 7499 2543 4

Text design by Paul Saunders
Edited by Barbara Kiser and Andrew Armitage

Typeset by Phoenix Photosetting, Chatham, Kent
Printed and bound in Great Britain by Bookmarque Ltd, Croydon, Surrey

Contents

Appendices

While all the nutrients and dietary changes referred to in this book have been proven safe, those seeking help for specific medical conditions are advised to consult a qualified nutrition therapist, clinical nutritionist, doctor or equivalent health professional. The recommendations given in this book are intended solely as education and information, and should not be taken as medical advice. Neither the authors nor the publisher accept liability for readers who choose to self-prescribe.

All supplements should be kept out of reach of infants and young children.

Acknowledgements

This book has been a continual evolution over the past ten years and I would like to thank both the people who have been involved at every stage, and the many scientists around the world who have contributed to our understanding of weight loss and blood sugar. Most of all, I'd like to thank the thousands of people who have tried my Fatburner approach and volunteered for the trials you'll read about. No doubt this approach will continue to evolve, thanks to your invaluable feedback.

Specifically, I'd like to thank nutritionists Natalie Savona, Deborah Colson and Fiona Macdonald-Joyce (thank you for your excellent recipes!), all trained at the Institute for Optimum Nutrition, and Paul Bedford from the YMCA for his help with the exercise chapters. I would also like to thank Gill, Anna and Barbara at Piatkus for their skilful and patient editing.

Finally, I'd like to thank Gaby, my wife, for being a guinea pig and putting up with my crack-of-dawn lifestyle that gives birth to books!

Guide to abbreviations and measures

Vitamins

1 gram (g) = 1,000 milligrams (mg) = 1,000,000 micrograms (mcg, also written μg)

Most vitamins are measured in milligrams or micrograms. Vitamins A, D and E used to be measured in International Units (iu), a measurement designed to standardise the various forms of these vitamins, which have different potencies.

6 mcg of betacarotene, the vegetable precursor of vitamin A, is, on average, converted into 1mcg of retinol, the animal form of vitamin A. So, 6mcg of betacarotene is called 1mcgRE (RE stands for retinol equivalent). Throughout this book beta-carotene is referred to in mcgRE.

1mcg of retinol (1mcgRE)	= 3.3 iu of vitamin A
1mcgRE of betacarotene	= 6mcg of betacarotene
100iu of vitamin D	= 2.5mcg
100iu of vitamin E	= 67mg

British (imperial)	Metric
1oz	28g
2oz	57g
3oz	85g
4oz	113g
5oz	142g
6oz	170g
7oz	198g
8oz	227g

British (imperial)	Metric	Metric	USA
1 teaspoon (0.17oz)	5ml	5g	1 teaspoon
1 dessertspoon	10ml	10g	2 teaspoons
1 tablespoon (0.5oz)	15ml	14.3g	1 tablespoon
2 tablespoons (1oz)	30ml	28.35g	2 tablespoons
4fl oz	112.5ml		½ cup
1 teacup (8oz)	1 cup (225g)	225ml	
⅘ imperial pint	(16oz)	450ml	2 cups (1 pint)
⅘ imperial quart	900ml		1 quart
⅘ imperial gallon	3.6 litres		1 gallon
1 pound (lb)	454g		1 pound

Conversion sums
Ounces to grams:
Multiply oz figure by 28.3 to get number of g

Grams to ounces:
Multiply g figure by 0.0353 to get number of oz

Ounces to millilitres:
Multiply oz figure by 30 to get number of ml

Calories
Carbohydrate has 3.75 kcals per g
Protein has 4 kcals per g
Fat has 9 kcals per g

In each part of the book, you'll find numbered references. These refer to research papers listed in the References section at the end of each part, and are there for readers who want to study this subject in depth.

Preface

Are you fed up with fat, and the fad diets that claim to vanquish it?

You may have spent years embarking on every weight-loss diet going – cut out entire food groups, followed the culinary habits of far-flung tribes, spent a fortune on 'miracle' foods. But, however wonderful these regimes seemed when you began them, the fact that you picked up this book probably means that none of them gave you what you need: a diet for life.

Chances are, you're still carrying unshed pounds, but that's just for starters. You may also feel gnawingly hungry much of the time, exhausted and beset by cravings. And, above all, fed up with hollow promises and 'sure-fire' methods that are soon unmasked as just another gimmick.

Ten years ago I proposed a way out of this wilderness. *The New Fatburner Diet* pinpointed the secret to successful weight loss and weight control: balancing blood sugar.

Put simply, when your blood sugar is too high you turn the excess into fat, and when your blood sugar is too low, you feel lethargic. So you may grab a sugary, refined snack to boost your energy, only to find that you sink back into exhaustion soon afterwards – while piling on more weight. This pattern of eating can be seriously bad for your health: once a person is obese, their risk for the severe blood-sugar-imbalance diabetes actually increases 77 times. That's the bad news.

But there's good news. You can break out of this vicious circle for ever. And, when you do, the pounds fall off easily, and your energy springs back to optimum levels.

Evolution of an idea

This discovery grew out of a growing conviction that I developed gradually at the Institute for Optimum Nutrition. I founded ION in the mid-1980s with the support and encouragement of the twice Nobel prizewinner Dr Linus Pauling, who famously declared that 'optimum nutrition is the medicine of the future'.

A friend of Einstein's, Pauling was to chemistry what Einstein was to physics. I established ION in the spirit of this remarkable nutritional pioneer. With the ION team, I worked with hundreds of overweight people to find the key to losing weight.

Back then, of course, calorie counting was the sacred cow of weight loss. The dominant belief was that the number of calories you ate, minus what you burned off through exercise, ended up as a wodge of fat around your middle. Diets aimed to cut calories – usually by cutting fat, since fat has the most calories per gram.

But I was seeing something very different – that eating different *kinds* of foods, such as what we call 'low glycemic-load' foods, can lead to more weight loss per calorie than 'high-glycemic-load' foods. At the time, it was sheer heresy.

However, we were right. There are specific foods and food combinations that cause rapid weight loss, and I used this knowledge to devise the Fatburner System. I soon realised that people who balanced their blood sugar not only lost weight – they also kept it off, felt superb and had all the signs of improved health and vigour.

They happily slipped into a new way of eating, but, more importantly, they found that it works for life – the food on offer is so delicious and varied that boredom and hunger are just not an issue. Hundreds of thousands of people followed the system with great success, and numerous scientific trials have validated the initial research.

Today's Holford Diet takes this tried-and-tested method into another dimension. With ongoing advances in nutrition, and feedback from users, it is now a cutting-edge guide to optimal health that's also a breeze to follow. And there are gourmet recipes for everything from snacks to banquets. All this, and weight loss too!

Beyond Atkins

Overall, we owe a lot to the late Dr Atkins, who boldly stated that you could lose more weight by eating a high-protein, high-fat, low-carbohydrate diet. He claimed, as I do, that obesity results from losing blood sugar control. And he knew that the body's 'cleanest' fuel is carbohydrate, which is simply digested down into glucose – the substance your cells run off.

Fat and protein, however, are much harder to metabolise and turn into usable fuel, so Atkins proposed that you'd lose some of the energy or calories they contain as ketones – breakdown chemicals – in the urine. In this way, he said, you could eat more calories and still lose weight.

Atkins was on the right track, but for the wrong reasons, and so was his diet. Despite all the hype, we now know why high-protein diets work. It isn't because fat and protein are so hard to break down for energy that you lose calories by eating them. This theory has been proved wrong.

High-protein diets work for a very simple reason. People actually eat less. You tend to feel much fuller when you eat meat and cheese than when you eat carbohydrates because a high-protein diet does control blood sugar. However, there are some serious problems with this approach, as we'll see. Meanwhile, there is an easier, safer, healthier and tastier way to lose weight – and you'll see results in just 30 days.

On your marks, get reset …

I say 30 days because, if your blood sugar is out of balance (and there's a 95 per cent chance of that if you are overweight), it takes up to 30 days to 'reset' your system to work properly. Then the pounds really fall away – although you'll be losing weight and gaining energy from Day One.

How can you tell whether you've lost control of your blood sugar? Check out this page from the food diary of someone who has.

Woke up tired. Staggered out of bed on remote control to the kettle. Made a strong cup of coffee. Had a piece of toast and jam. Avoided eating anything substantial till lunch to cut down on calories. Got really hungry. Craved some bread, pasta, biscuits. Had a big bowl of tuna pasta for lunch. Wanted something sweet to end the meal. Felt depressed in the afternoon and really lethargic. Had another coffee and some chocolate. Felt better. Got home and had some toast. Meant to go to the gym but felt too tired …

If this sounds like you, let me ask you a few simple questions.

- Do you find it hard to get going in the morning without a cup of tea or coffee, a cigarette or something sweet – cereal or toast with jam?

- Do you crave something sweet after meals?

- Does your energy dip during the day, and do you find yourself craving a stimulant (such as tea, coffee, a cigarette or chocolate) or something sweet?

- Do you feel too tired to exercise?

- Does your mood go up and down?

- Are you gradually gaining weight, and finding it hard to lose, even though you're not noticeably eating more or exercising less?

If you answer 'yes' to any of these questions, the Holford Diet is perfect for you.

It is also radical enough to change the way you eat and live – which might prompt you to ask who I am, and why you should trust what I have to say. The fact is, the kernel of the Holford Diet began as a personal experience that transformed my life long before I even set up ION.

Life study

When I was 19 and studying psychology at York University, I met two extraordinary nutritionists, Brian and Celia Wright. Like Linus Pauling, they had realised that most disease was the result of suboptimum nutrition. At the time I found this hard to swallow, but, being an adventurous spirit, I asked them to devise a diet for me.

So there I was, a university student, eating a virtually wheat-free diet, masses of fruit and vegetables, and taking a daily handful of supplements shipped from the US (they weren't yet available in Britain). A far cry from the usual fish and chips, cigarettes and pints of bitter! My colleagues, friends and family thought I was crazy. But I persisted.

Within two months I had lost a stone in weight, which has never returned; my skin, which had resembled a lunar landscape, cleared up; and my regular migraines virtually vanished. But most noticeable of all was the extra energy. I no longer needed so much sleep, my mind was much sharper and my body full of vitality. I started to investigate this 'optimum nutrition', and I haven't stopped since.

I set up ION, which is an independent, non-profit-making charity with no funding from food, supplement or drug companies, and it has grown into Europe's largest and most respected training school for nutritional therapists. Here are some of the breakthroughs:

- In 1986 I researched zinc and proved that it was Britain's most deficient mineral. Deficiencies can cause bad skin, poor appetite control, depression and even schizophrenia. In those days virtually no one had even heard of zinc, there was no RDA for it, and few supplements contained it.

- In 1988 we ran an experiment, filmed by the BBC's *Horizon* programme and published in the *Lancet*, that proved vitamin supplements could boost children's IQ by a massive 9 per cent. This was a world first.

- In the 1990s we showed that antioxidants reduce cancer, heart disease and Alzheimer's and slow down the ageing process. No one had heard of antioxidants then, but now they're the big buzzword.

- In 1998 I wrote *The Optimum Nutrition Bible*, now translated into 15 languages and sold in 30 countries, with sales approaching a million copies.

- In 1993 I went public as saying that HRT causes breast cancer and advised women to use safer and equally effective natural alternatives. (An estimated 20,000 women in Britain have got breast cancer because of HRT between 1994 and 2004 alone.)

- In 2003 I put the spotlight on homocysteine – an amino acid more important than cholesterol, your blood pressure and even your weight as a gauge of health. It is your single most important health statistic, measuring exactly where you are on the scale from superhealth to heading for an early grave.

In short, I've been walking my talk for 25 years – during which time my weight, size, blood pressure, pulse and cholesterol level haven't gone up a single point.

So, after a quarter of a century at the cutting edge of diet and health – having studied thousands of research trials, tested my theories on myself and on more than 200,000 people, and gained more than a million readers worldwide – I can say with confidence that there is a simple way to lose weight, feel and look great, and stay young. And that is the Holford Diet.

How to use this book

Part One gives you the background, and tells you why this diet is scientifically proven, safer and better for you. It also reveals why it will give you the quickest, safest, easiest and most sustainable weight loss, as well as increased energy and better skin, mood and concentration.

Part Two explains the five key principles of the Holford Diet – which are just as applicable to kids as to adults – and how to discover your good foods and bad foods. Once you've read this you'll understand why the Fatburner System is the state-of-the-art weight-loss and maintenance strategy.

Part Three tells you exactly what you need to do on the Holford Diet, and answers all your practical questions.

Part Four gives you scores of easy, delicious Fatburning recipes and menus to enjoy.

Part Five covers the hidden benefits of the Holford Diet.

Wishing you the best of health, and looking forward to seeing less of you!

Patrick Holford
October 2004

PART ONE

Dieting – The Bottom Line

1

Why the Holford Diet Works

Imagine this.

You've just woken up. You feel full of energy. Your mind is clear. You get up, have a healthy breakfast and, throughout the day, your energy is good, your mood is stable, you're mentally sharp and your concentration is good. You haven't once experienced a single craving. You haven't had energy dips or got cranky and irritable.

But that's just the *inside* story. You also look great. Your weight is more or less where you want it to be. You're well toned. Your skin has a healthy glow. People often comment on how slim and well you look and how young you look for your age. You feel young, both physically and mentally. And this is how you feel every day!

Welcome to the new you. This is not only how you could be, this is how you should be. More importantly, it's how you will be when you follow the Holford Diet. And all it takes to see dramatic differences is 30 days.

I realise that you may have spent the last decade trudging through a succession of diets with nothing to show for it but a slimmed-down bank balance and more fat than you started with. Every bookshop bristles with 'miracle' weight-loss techniques, and 'guaranteed' recipes for everything from longevity to cellulite control. So I know you may be feeling cheated by claims and promises that have never panned out. Why, then, should you believe what I'm saying?

You can be thin *and* healthy

This is why. The Holford Diet works because it is much more than just a way to lose weight. It is a holistic system for attaining optimum health – and a healthy, self-regulating body is naturally slim.

The fact is that many of the people who discover my diet, follow it and write to me reporting substantial weight loss didn't set off to lose weight in the first place. They wanted to be healthy and thought the optimum nutrition approach made sense. And, as their health improved, the pounds dropped off. Optimum health, they found, also means optimum weight.

The body will naturally reach its ideal weight given the chance. You'll eat less if your blood sugar is stable, and your metabolism will be better able to burn off excess weight.

I have yet to see any diet work better in the long run than this approach. I teach doctors, healthcare practitioners and nutritionists all over the world, but none is as slim, energetic and healthy as the thousand nutritionists we have trained at ION – the Institute for Optimum Nutrition.

At ION, decades of work with more than 100,000 volunteers first revealed how overall health determines weight, by showing that overweight is a symptom of a much wider condition. We sometimes call it 'twenty-first-century-itis'.

Exhaustion, moodiness, depression, bloating – twenty-first-century-itis is a response to our polluted, urbanised, speeded-up world, and overweight is a common symptom of it. Could you be suffering from it? Check yourself out by answering the questions below, scoring 1 point for each 'yes' answer.

Are you:

☐ Tired most of the time? (80%)

☐ More than 7lb over your ideal weight, and rising? (74%)

☐ Prone to PMS? (64%)

☐ Suffering from poor memory and concentration? (43%)

☐ Quite often low or depressed? (46%)

☐ Plagued by dry skin, in need of daily moisturisers? (56%)

☐ Having difficulty sleeping? (53%)

☐ Often feeling anxious or stressed? (64%)

☐ Prone to indigestion or bloating after food? (62%)

☐ Often constipated – that is, you rarely go twice a day? (90%)

☐ Suffering from dark circles or bags under your eyes? (54%)

In Britain, the average person ticks seven boxes. The percentages on the right are of people who answered 'yes' in our MyNutrition health and diet survey of over 30,000 people – Britain's largest ever – which we carried out in 2004.

You may have ticked a few boxes yourself. And the reality of being, say, tired all day, uncomfortably overweight and feeling ill is no joke. Remember, though, that all this could change in just 30 days. Your load could be significantly lightened. And three months on the Holford Diet will leave you completely free of these symptoms, as well as up to 2 stone lighter.

A diet for life

The point is that we already know how to cure twenty-first-century-itis, and that is my goal for you. I want you to lose weight fast, keep losing weight until you reach your goal, and maintain your weight once you get there – but always within the context of optimum energy and wellbeing. This is what you can look forward to:

● Within 7 days you will start to lose pounds as quickly as you'll gain energy.

● Within 20 days you'll notice your skin has dramatically improved.

● Within 30 days you'll be starting to feel like a new you.

● And within three months? You will have seriously undamaged your health.

Of course, if you just want to lose weight there are plenty of ways to do it. I've studied them all. I was there with the rise and fall of the F Plan Diet, the Hip & Thigh Diet, the Atkins Diet and many others. I advised Rosemary Conley as I believed her diets were dangerously low in essential fats. I challenged Dr Atkins when the science just didn't seem to stack up.

I know the pros and cons of all of them. I know why high-protein diets work better for some but not for others, and don't work in the long run. I've tested Atkins dieters and I believe that his regime can actually seriously damage health. I know why you can lose weight on low-fat diets, only to end up with dry and wrinkly skin. I know why most diets leave you exhausted. Most of all, I know why the pounds you lose keep coming back!

For me to get excited about a diet that claims to be successful, it must fulfil the following criteria:

It works in both the short and the long term

Instant results may be thrilling, but they're usually not sustained. The body can't burn more than 2lb of actual fat in a week, unless you go into starvation mode. I look for a steady loss of 6 to 10lb a month, or 2 stone (28lb) in three months, or 8 stone (112lb) in a year – if you've got that much to lose – with no rebound weight gain. That said, you can lose up to 6lb of excess water if you're eating foods you've developed an intolerance to. That's why some people lose 7lb in the first week of the Holford Diet.

You never feel hungry

If a diet leaves you feeling famished, you won't stick to it. So from Day One it has to satisfy your appetite. The Holford Diet specifically recommends the foods scientifically proven to satisfy your appetite the best and I'm going to tell you exactly which those foods are.

It's enjoyable

If you can't eat a wide variety of food or have to actively avoid eating certain food groups, a diet will start to feel boring very fast, and it will be neither enjoyable nor sustainable. The framework of my diet, the Fatburner System, allows a cornucopia of delectable foods containing good fats, protein and carbohydrates. You'll be able to eat bread and pasta, mayonnaise, meat – the lot. You'll just pay more attention to quality and the quantity.

It's safe

I'm not interested in helping people lose weight by cheating the body. Sure, you can lose weight with slimming pills, or by cutting out all carbohydrates, but it just isn't good for you and, in the end, crime doesn't pay. The only side effect I want you to experience is added health.

It makes you feel great

If a diet is working with the body's design, not against it, you should start to feel better, with more energy, improved mood and concentration and better skin within days.

There's no rebound weight gain

You can lose weight by massively restricting food intake – but the body thinks it's gone into starvation mode and slows down your metabolism. So, as soon as you start eating enough for your needs, the pounds boomerang back. The same is true with stimulants such as caffeine. They can suppress your appetite so you can lose weight in the short term, but in the end they slow down your metabolism. As you'll see, these can give short-term weight loss, but rebound weight gain.

It's easy to follow

At the end of the day, if a diet becomes as easy and natural as breathing, you'll stick to it for life. So, if the food is delicious, is easy to find and prepare and leaves you satisfied and feeling wonderful, you're far more likely to make it part of your life.

The word from the weight-loss coalface

The Holford Diet scores 10 out of 10 for each of these criteria. But you don't have to take just my word for it. Here are the stories of a handful of the many thousands who have followed the Fatburner System.

Linda H was just 5 foot 2 inches tall, but had gradually expanded sideways in her twenties. She had tried every diet under the sun and finally settled on Weight Watchers, with some success. She had been a member of Weight Watchers for five years and had managed, with much sacrifice, to get down to and maintain a weight of 8 stone 10lb. But she found she couldn't get below this. She wasn't quite at the right weight for her and it was a frustrating impasse. Then she discovered the Fatburner System:

> ❛ On your diet I began to lose weight at once. Within 30 days I came down to 8 stone 4 – a thing I thought impossible! However, I was totally unprepared for the new energy levels. I cannot believe how marvellous I feel – I am no longer tired no matter what I do or how active I am. I have stopped falling asleep at odd moments when I relax. I no longer feel bloated and tired after eating. Your diet has changed my life! ❜

Carol P had been gradually gaining weight, year on year. When she turned 60 she realised her weight was out of control:

> ❛ I felt too fat and it was hard to bend over and tie the laces on my walking boots. I was getting out of breath going up hills and started to worry about that. I decided to do your diet and the exercises. I cut out nearly all wheat, ate mainly oat porridge for breakfast, and cut out biscuits and cakes. I also cut out caffeine, had less alcohol – just the odd glass of wine. I lost 30 pounds steadily over six months. Also, my stomach used to really stick out! It doesn't do that any more. I think wheat was making me bloat. Now I have wheat occasionally, but not every day.
>
> What I liked about your approach is the understanding of the human psyche and the reality of living. You don't have to be a

total puritan and you don't get hungry. If I were hungry, I'd have a piece of fruit. What I needed was a diet for life. I'm not so strict now on the exercise, but still generally follow the dietary principles. I definitely feel a lot better. I like the way my body looks. I have more energy. I feel happy and my mood is more even. I will have no problem staying on this general routine for life. 〕

Wayne P had been gaining almost a stone a year, and was now seriously obese. He realised he had to do something about it:

〔 *As a teenager I was very fit. By the age of 17 I was playing ice hockey for England. When I hit my twenties and went to work I stopped exercising, but kept eating and drinking – curries, lager and takeaways. I reckon I put on close to a stone for every year I was alive. By the age of 33 I was 27 stone 9lb and basically addicted to junk food. I met Patrick when I became a volunteer for ITV's* Tonight with Trevor McDonald, *testing whether junk food was addictive. I started following Patrick's Fatburner System.*

In the first four months I lost 32lb, a little more than 2lb a week, and I'm still losing weight, week by week. I'm still following the Fatburner principles, and I'm not even that strict. I eat more fresh food and less packaged food and snack more on fruit. My downfall is drinking – I still knock back a few lagers and a bottle of wine at the weekends. But I feel better. I have more energy. I feel happier and more comfortable and have gone down two sizes. I'm also becoming more active and my weight is still reducing. 〕

What many people following my diet love most, apart from the inevitable weight loss, are the unexpected dividends. I receive letters like the following on a regular basis:

❝Since following your diet I have totally cured my migraines.❞

❝For eight years I suffered incredibly badly from rheumatoid arthritis. I could barely walk without suffering from pain and exhaustion. Following your advice has enabled me to control arthritis and to lead a full and active life: I am eternally grateful for that.❞

❝I was both surprised and pleased to see a rapid reduction in the wrinkly skin under my eyes.❞

❝Following your diet and supplements my cholesterol has dropped from 6.5 to 5.1. My GP couldn't believe it!❞

❝I used to have constant pain in my knees and joints, could not play golf or walk more than 10 minutes without resting my legs. Since I've been following your advice my discomfort has decreased 95 to 100 per cent. I never would have believed my pain could be reduced by such a large degree, with no return, no matter how much activity in a day or week.❞

❝Within two weeks, I had much more energy. My mood is very positive – no panic or depression. I feel buoyant, energetic and enthusiastic. I haven't had any colds or infections. I'm sleeping much better, my PMS is much better. I experienced no breast tenderness in my last period, and no mood swings or tearfulness.❞

And this is how you should feel all the time. I call it 100 per cent health, and there's no reason why you can't claim it for yourself. You can lose weight and feel great.

You know the definition of insanity? To keep doing the same things and expect different results. And that's what millions are doing – eating the same foods and expecting to feel better and magically shed the excess pounds. But the real magic lies in a very different means to this end.

The science of slimming

Your body has evolved over millions of years to work perfectly with a certain kind of diet. Our ancestors weren't fat because they ate this optimum diet, as do the lucky ones such as the Hunzas in the Himalayas, whose average lifespan is over a hundred and who never get fat or suffer from diabetes, heart disease, cancer, Alzheimer's or any other of the diseases plaguing the twenty-first century. This is, in all its essentials, my diet.

If you follow the Fatburner System, you will lose weight, gain energy, improve your skin, sharpen your mind, balance your mood – and add years to your life, and life to your years. Now let's look at why.

The science behind the Holford Diet is very simple. Your body is designed to burn glucose for energy, which is carried by blood to the cells. Carbohydrates such as grains and fruits are broken down into glucose in the body. But carbohydrates figure hugely in today's typical Western diet, and if you eat too much of them – particularly the refined type – you'll end up with more blood glucose than you need. You'll then store the excess as fat.

If your blood glucose levels are even, you'll have a steady supply of energy and a healthy but balanced appetite. This is the reason you'll have no problem maintaining the right weight. But, if your blood glucose levels are sometimes high, sometimes low, you'll see the beginnings of twenty-first-century-itis. When levels are too high, you'll lay down fat; when they're too low, you'll feel lethargic, and it will be harder to burn fat. A quarter of all people, and nine out of ten people with weight problems, have difficulty keeping their blood sugar level even. The result is exhaustion and overweight.

And this is just the beginning. Obese people are 77 times more at risk of developing diabetes than non-obese people – a statistic that alone tells you how strongly linked weight gain is to blood sugar control.

So the best way of losing weight is to regain blood glucose control, which heralds the return of your body's ability to burn fat. You'll lose weight effortlessly without having to starve, and gain health and vitality at the same time.

The five key principles

The Holford Diet is based on five key principles, which, taken together, form the fastest, safest and most effective way to lose weight and gain health. Each is explained in detail in Part Two, but let's take a look at them now.

1: Balance your blood sugar

This is the crux: once you achieve it, weight loss is inevitable. Keeping your blood sugar balanced depends not only on what you eat, but also on how and when you eat it. In Chapter 7 I'll explain exactly which foods and food combinations stabilise your blood sugar best and help to burn fat. I'll be introducing you to something called the *glycemic load*, or **GL**, of a food. This is a much superior method of measuring a food's suitability than 'carbohydrate points' or the 'glycemic index' (GI).

Put simply, the GI of a food is a *qualitative* measure that tells you whether the carbohydrate it contains is 'fast' or 'slow' releasing. It doesn't tell you, however, how much of the food is carbohydrate. Carbohydrate points or grams of carbohydrate are *quantitative* measures that tell you how much of the food is carbohydrate, but they don't tell you what that carbohydrate does to your blood sugar. The **GL** of a food is the quantity times the quality of its carbohydrate, and that is the best way of telling you how much weight you'll gain if you choose that food.

You may be amazed by some of the foods that have a high-🔵 score. But it's important to know the truth: if you understand why you gain weight, you'll hold the key to losing it. Cornflakes and corn chips, for instance, have a very high 🔵, while ice cream and peanuts do not. One single date has the same effect on your blood sugar and weight as a whole large punnet of strawberries. So be ready for some surprises.

Your goal will be to limit your 🔵 to 40 a day – that's 10 per meal and 5 each for two snacks. So knowing your 🔵 is essential. Just look at this comparison of two typical breakfasts.

Breakfast	🔵		🔵
A bowl of porridge oats (30g)	2	A bowl of cornflakes	21
Half a grated apple	3	A banana	12
A small tub of yoghurt	2	Milk	2
Milk	2		35
	9		

The two may seem broadly similar, but in 🔵 terms they are worlds apart. The Fatburner breakfast on the left will cut your blood glucose load, and your propensity to store fat, by no less than a third. It will push your body's metabolism one giant step towards fatburning and away from fat-storing – and you will feel fuller and more energetic for longer.

And there will be masses to choose from. Part Four is packed with zesty, delicious recipes and menus, including Crunchy Thai Salad, Cod Roasted with Lemon and Garlic, Chicken Tandoori and even Beef Burgers. In case you're wondering, I've done all the adding up of 🔵s for you. You'll find that '🔵 awareness' swiftly becomes second nature; before you know it you'll be doing your own mixing and matching of low-Ⓖ foods at every meal.

You'll note that the fatburning breakfast combines porridge oats and yoghurt. Mixing carbohydrates with proteins is another important way of regulating blood sugar, and again, very easy to master. There's a full discussion in Part Two, but, basically, it means you'll eat low-Ⓖ carbohydrates with good-quality protein – for example, brown basmati rice with organic chicken, wholewheat pasta with wild salmon, or rye toast with scrambled egg.

Fibre plays a starring role, too, because a food's fibre content lowers its Ⓖ. So you'll find plenty of high-fibre choices, from beans to brown rice. Lastly, *when* you eat is very important. Unlike most diets, which are snackless deserts, mine will encourage you to eat two snacks a day along with your three meals.

2: Eat good fats and avoid bad fats

Essential fatty acids (or EFAs) may be a bit of a buzzword these days, but they thoroughly deserve their celebrity status. These are the 'good fats' I've talked about for years, and, although it may seem counterintuitive, there's evidence that eating them can actually help you to lose weight.

The reason is very simple. Your body and brain depend on omega-3 and omega-6 EFAs. In fact, excluding water, one quarter of your brain is made up of omega-3s. So almost nothing works well without them. Your brain can't function, leading to lower IQ, poor memory and a tendency to depression. Your hormones go up the creek, possibly leading to mood swings, PMS, sugar cravings and weight gain. Your skin shrivels, and your heart and arteries suffer.

This is why these fats are called essential. And, since we can't manufacture them ourselves, it's as if our body and brain are designed to seek them out. We literally have an instinct to eat fat. We are instinctively drawn towards the creamy texture of fats, sauces, cheese and cream, and not only this: the body's 'fat sensors' are in your mouth, there to tell you when you've hit nutritional gold. Think about it. If the body needs anything (water, air, essential fats, vitamins) there's always an instinct that makes you crave it. That's why fat-free diets are such a titanic struggle for most of us.

But our need for fats has also spawned a legion of 'bad' fats – fried fat, processed fat in junk food, saturated fats, even 'fake' fats. When you eat EFAs, your body's fat sensors tell the brain that your essential fat needs are satisfied. But, when you eat bad fats, your fat sensors are not satisfied, even though your eyes and taste buds may have been fooled into believing you've eaten the fats that you need. The sensors respond much more strongly to essential fats than to processed or saturated fats. So, if you've packed away a burger and chips or several doughnuts, you'll find yourself craving fats the next day because your body hasn't received what it needed. And you'll keep on craving them until it has.

The Holford Diet gives you exactly the right kind and amount of essential fats, not only to help you stay healthy and glowing (and cellulite-free!), but also to reduce your desire to eat unhealthy fatty foods. But that's not all. The essential fats also tune up your metabolism and help you burn unwanted fat. So it's not true to say that a calorie of *any* fat has the same effect on weight gain. You'll hear the whole story and the latest research in Chapter 8.

3: Eliminate your hidden allergies

We are all unique. Think about your friends. Their appearances may be wildly different. Some will be night owls, others skylarks. They'll have different blood types. A number may be natural carnivores, others natural vegetarians. And most of us have different intolerances or allergies to certain foods, but very few even know it. Weight gain, however, is a common reaction to foods we're intolerant to.

It follows, then, that eliminating the food that you are unknowingly allergic to can lead to highly dramatic weight loss. Lisa M, for instance, lost 5 inches off her waist in three days and 3 stone in three months by discovering and avoiding what she was allergic to.

Rebecca S also lost 3 stone simply by avoiding her food allergies. In her twenties Rebecca had a stable weight, and used to exercise three or four times a week. But in her thirties she started to pile on the pounds. Over three years her weight drifted from 10 stone up to 13 stone and her dress size went up to 16. 'I started feeling tired and lethargic and generally unwell,' she said. 'I didn't have the energy to go to the gym any more. But it seemed the foods I ate were blowing me up, which was why I thought I could have a food allergy.' She decided to test herself for a food allergy, which you can do with a home test kit, involving a pinprick of blood. The results showed that she was reacting to milk, egg white and gluten – the protein found in wheat. Within a week of excluding these foods her skin and mood improved and the weight started to fall away.

Don't think that all allergies are for life. After three months strictly avoiding the foods she'd become allergic to she reintroduced egg whites and then milk to see if there was a reaction. Now she's fine on both foods, but still reacts to wheat. 'I can't tell you how much better I feel. I'm 100 per cent,' she said. 'Eliminating my food allergies has transformed my health. I just wish I'd done it sooner.' Why did she lose so much weight? Because water retention, bloating and puffiness are all common allergic reactions, and they make you feel and look fatter.

This is great news because, once you've singled out and

eliminated the 'bad' foods, you can see really dramatic changes very fast. It's not unusual to lose up to 7lb within three or four days.

Aside from weight gain and bloating, food allergies also cause many other niggling problems – aches and pains, headaches, fatigue, mood swings, annoying skin and digestive conditions. These also go when you identify and avoid what you are allergic to. You'll find out how to pinpoint the 'baddies' lurking in your larder in Chapter 9.

It's reassuring to know that, as in Rebecca's case, most food allergies aren't for life. You can often 'unlearn' your intolerances in as little as three months, which means you can reintroduce previously 'bad' foods back into your diet.

4: Take the right supplements

By now you're probably realising that caloric intake and weight loss are not all that firmly linked. In fact, one of the biggest lies in nutrition today is 'You can lose only weight by eating fewer calories.'

The other is 'You can get all the vitamins and minerals you need from a well-balanced diet.' This is untrue. You simply can't guarantee that the nutrients you need are in your food.

Take vitamin C, which not only protects against degenerative diseases such as cancer, but also helps stabilise your blood sugar and speeds your fatburning. At ION, we've examined more than 500 studies – including the 'gold standard' type, which are known as 'randomised, double-blind, placebo-controlled' – that have led us to conclude that the optimal intake of vitamin C is 1,000mg a day. This is what our jungle-dwelling, fruit-eating ancestors could have got from leaves, berries and fruits.

But how much C is there in a supermarket orange? As much as 116mg and as little as zero. Yes, the 'average' orange contains

60mg of the precious vitamin, but some contain virtually nothing! And, even if your supermarket orange contains 60mg, you'd need to eat 22 of them to achieve 1,000mg.

So I recommend that you supplement 1,000mg of C a day, along with eating vitamin-C-rich foods such as strawberries. You can eat strawberries till the cows come home and never gain weight. (Not all fruits are this useful for fatburning or general health, however, as we'll see.)

There are some 30 vitamins and minerals that are essential for health, and along with vitamin C a number will help you burn fat, too. Essentially, they boost your metabolism, reprogramming your body to turn food into energy rather than fat. For example, the mineral chromium helps to even out appetite and energy dips by stabilising your blood sugar. It's so effective that it's given to diabetics, with amazing results. There are also amino acids and herbs that really can give you the edge when it comes to losing weight. Hydroxy citric acid, or HCA, is a herbal extract from the tamarind plant, which makes it harder for your body to turn glucose into fat. There's another herbal extract from a bean called *Griffonia*, which is naturally high in an amino acid called 5-hydroxytryptophan. Known as 5-HTP, this amino acid has an extraordinary capability to ease excessive appetite and sugar cravings.

These aren't drugs. They're nutrients, and they will help fine-tune your metabolism.

5: Do 15 minutes of exercise a day

If you exercise just to burn calories, quite frankly you might as well just not eat that piece of toast. The real value of exercise is that it helps stabilise your blood sugar levels and reduce your appetite. And the great news is that you don't have to do much to achieve this result – just 15 minutes a day, in fact.

It has been found that people who don't exercise eat more

than people who do a little exercise or just have active jobs. The human body, it seems, needs physical activity to work properly in the way that it needs water or vitamins. Certain kinds of exercise boost the rate at which you burn fat for up to 15 hours afterwards.

That's the immediate effect, but there's a long-term effect too. With the right kind of exercise, you'll put on more muscle and lose fat, and a pound of muscle burns many more calories a day than a pound of fat. So every pound of fat you lose and every pound of muscle you gain increases your body's long-term ability to burn fat.

To kick-start this process, you'll do 15 minutes a day, or 21 minutes five times a week, or 35 minutes three times a week, of the right kind of muscle-building and fatburning exercise. And, fortunately, the fatter and less fit you are right now, the easier it will be to get the same benefits! For example, if you are over-weight and underfit, jogging half a mile slowly can burn 300 calories, while if you are fitter and lighter you'd need to jog a mile.

Following these five principles is easy, and enjoyable – yet they'll revolutionise the way you live, simply because of the way you'll feel and look, day by day. And, if you feel and look great, that's the best motivation for making it a diet for life.

Meanwhile, the dieting industry continues to make money from you by selling quick fixes that are destined to fail. That's what keeps you coming back for more. How many diets have you been on and how many have worked? I want to make sure that the Holford Diet is the last diet you'll ever go on.

2

Why So Many Diets Fail

Dieting can be like negotiating a minefield of misconceptions. Many methods for losing weight have no basis in science whatsoever – so, if your dieting life has been one long string of depressing failed attempts, it's hardly surprising.

Here I'd like to debunk some of these 'methods', and expose them as myths. That way, you'll have the knowledge to prevent a life of yo-yo dieting and long-term health problems.

Myth number 1: You can lose weight only by eating fewer calories or exercising more.

Yes, it is true that you'll lose weight if you eat fewer calories and exercise more. But the real picture is a lot more complex than this.

Take fat. Since fat has 9 calories per gram, compared with approximately 4 per gram for protein and carbohydrate, the most successful original low-calorie diets were low-fat diets. Then the world woke up to the fact that some fats, such as the omega-3 essential fatty acids, are necessary for health. So we realised it wasn't so smart to cut out all the fats from our diets.

Meanwhile, the facts reveal something very puzzling about our calorie consumption.

People are eating less. Calorie consumption has gone down, and fat intake has gone down even more. Yet there's an obesity epidemic. That's a real paradox. At the same time, our consumption of sugar, refined carbohydrates and stimulants such as caffeine has risen. Could that be only down to coincidence?

Let's start with the big picture, using data derived from two government surveys.[1] In the figure below you will see the estimated average calorie intake (from food) of the average person in Britain over the past 15 years.

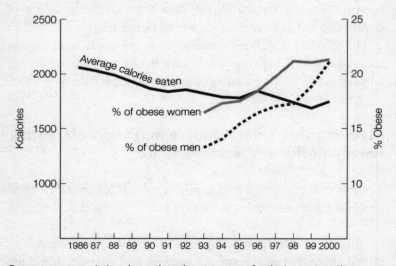

Government statistics show that the amount of calories we eat has steadily decreased over the last 15 years, while the percentage of obese people has steadily increased.

This clearly shows that we're eating fewer calories, not more, while obesity rates have trebled! And this trend runs like a thread throughout the Western world, from America to Australia. Something doesn't quite add up.

In fact, if you look globally, you won't find that calorie intake predicts obesity. For example, in the US – where obesity is epidemic – the average calorie intake is 2,360 kcals. Yet in China, where obesity is exceedingly rare, the average calorie intake is 2,630 kcals!

One possible explanation is exercise. The Chinese lead less sedentary lives than we do. But exercise alone, or lack of it, simply cannot explain why 1,000 people a day are becoming obese in the UK alone. What's more, surveys estimate that women increased their level of physical activity between 1994 and 1998, from 22 to 25 per cent. For men it seems there has been little change.[2]

What's going on? We're not eating more calories. So the crucial element must be not quantity, but quality – and that's the focus of the next big diet myth.

Myth number 2: A calorie is a calorie is a calorie.

High-protein diets tried to prove this wrong, and failed. Recent studies, however, *have* proved that not all calories are the same in relation to weight loss.

Let's start with the figure overleaf, which gives us some essential clues. You can see how our diets have changed in relation to the three main food groups – protein, fat and carbohydrate.

As you can see, our consumption of calories from fat is decreasing, while our calories from protein and especially carbohydrates have gone up. So the culprit in the obesity epidemic we're seeing seems to be not the much-maligned fat, but

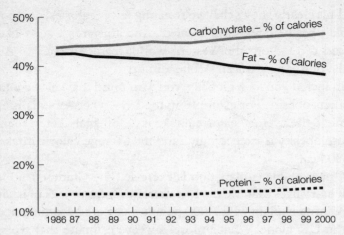

Government statistics show that over the past 15 years we have been eating less and less fat, while carbohydrate intake is on the increase.

carbohydrates (that's sugar, grains, vegetables and fruit) and possibly protein. Only calories from carbohydrates, however, have gone up consistently in line with increasing rates of obesity.

If carbohydrates were to blame, you'd expect countries that eat large amounts of carbohydrates to be the fattest. But that's not a hard and fast rule. Some of the healthiest communities in the world get 55 per cent or more of their calories from carbohydrate. China, where the figure is 70 per cent of calories, is a classic example. So let's go in closer and look at the *kind* of carbohydrates we are eating more of.

In the figure opposite we are looking at the percentage of calories consumed from three kinds of carbohydrates – (added) sugar, starch and fibre, which is indigestible carbohydrate and has no caloric value. Fibre has gone up, which is nothing but good news and, if anything, would reduce weight because it fills you up and you eat less. But what really stands out now is our intake of sugar, which is steadily rising.

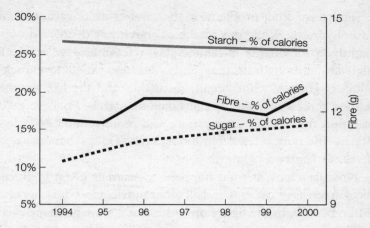

Over the past 15 years our intake of sugar has gone steadily up, while our intake of more complex carbohydrates (starch) has gone down. Fibre intake has also increased.

But it's highly likely that these figures relating to sugar consumption are a gross underestimation. Let's make this real. According to these figures, the average person in Britain eats 22kg (48lb) of sugar a year. Yet according to government sources, 2.3 billion tons of sugar go into the British food supply every year.[3] That amount translates as an average of 38kg (84lb) per person per year, almost double what the government diet survey above shows. This makes a lot more sense because more comprehensive surveys in the US, which tops the world in obesity, show that the annual intake of sugar there has gone from 56kg (124lb) in 1975 to 71kg (157lb) in 1999.

So where is all this sugar lurking? You'd be amazed at the amount not just in cakes and sweets, but in soft drinks, convenience foods, flavoured crisps and other savoury snacks, condiments and many breakfast cereals. Whichever way you slice it, there's obviously an awful lot of hidden sugar being consumed, and your body simply can't cope with it.

There are other problems in the calories we're getting from carbohydrates. While our intake of starch has decreased very slightly, a lot of this is refined 'fast-releasing' – what I call high-**GL** – carbohydrate, that sends your blood sugar level rocketing. Baguettes, white bread, cornflakes and the like are the nasties here. If we had the right data on starch, I believe we'd also find that we are eating more and more refined carbohydrates. And quite a few other foods, such as chips, bananas and dates, also carry a heavy **GL**.

Now let's look at what happens to animals given identical diets in terms of calories and all other nutrients – with only one difference: **GL**. In the figure opposite you'll see what happened to one group of rats. Half were given a high-**GL** diet, the other a low-**GL** diet. They couldn't cheat. They had exactly the same number of calories – and there weren't any sweetshops round the corner.

In this strictly controlled study by one of the world's leading experts on weight loss, Professor Jennie Brand-Miller from the University of Sydney, the low-**GL** 'fatburner' rats gained no weight.[4] But the high-**GL** rats gained weight week on week, and pound on pound. By the end of 32 weeks, the high-**GL** group were not only 16 per cent heavier – they had gained 40 per cent more body fat! A recent study, published in the *Lancet* medical journal, found that mice with a low-**GL** diet lost almost twice the body fat in nine weeks as mice given identical nutrients with high-**GL** carbohydrates instead. The low-**GL** dieters were substantially leaner and slimmer.[5]

Same calories, very different results. Yet this is nothing short of heresy for conventional calorie theorists.

But, you may be asking, does the same thing happen to us? After all, rats and humans don't always respond in a similar way. The answer is yes. Researchers in the human nutrition department at South Africa's University of the Orange Free

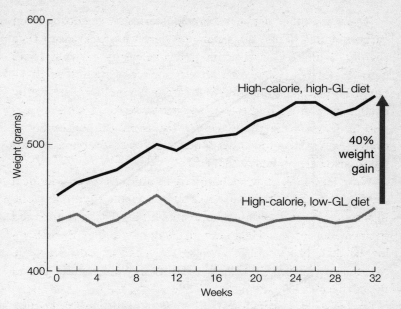

What diet works best? This chart shows weight change on high-🄶🄻 and low-🄶🄻 diets of equal calories and fat/protein/carbohydrate percentage.

State assigned 15 volunteers to a low-🄶🄻 diet and 15 others to a normal calorie-controlled diet for 12 weeks.[6] Both diets contained identical numbers of calories. The two groups then switched diets for 12 more weeks. As you can see from the figure overleaf, during the first 12 weeks both groups lost weight, but those on the low-🄶🄻 diet lost more weight. During the second 12-week period, the group that switched to the low-🄶🄻 diet lost 40 per cent more weight than the group that switched to the normal diet. Yet the caloric content of both diets remained the same.

Despite all this evidence (and there's a lot more), some so-called experts still say 'a calorie is a calorie', as far as weight loss

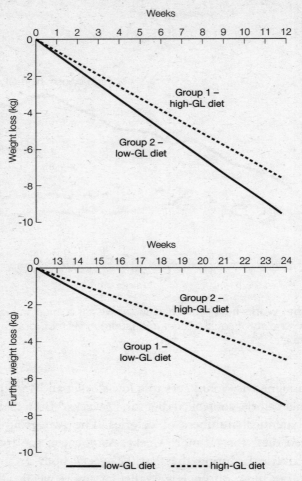

Two groups of overweight women were given a low-calorie diet, with equivalent amounts of protein, fat and carbohydrate. One group ate low-**GL** carbohydrates and the other group ate high-**GL** carbohydrates. Both groups lost weight, but those on the low-**GL** diet lost considerably more weight over 12 weeks. Those on the low-**GL** diet were then switched onto the high-**GL** diet, and vice versa. During the second period of 12 weeks, again, those on the low-**GL** diet lost considerably more weight.

is concerned. Whichever way you look at it, this is simply not true. You can lose weight by changing the quality of what you eat, even if you don't change the quantity. Of course, if you eat fewer calories of lower-Ⓖ foods, that will trigger the most rapid weight loss.

Not only that, we now know that people who eat low-Ⓖ food eat significantly less anyway, as they feel much more satisfied.[7] So, if you eat a low-Ⓖ diet, you not only lose weight, but you tend to want to eat less. It's a double whammy in your favour.

But calories can't just vanish. If two people eat the same number of calories and one, eating the high-Ⓖ diet, stores some of the calories as fat, what happens to the calories in the Fatburner? Here's the real magic. If you are not storing calories as fat you are turning calories into energy. That is why people on the Holford Diet, such as Linda H, say, 'I can't believe how marvellous I feel.' I hear this kind of feedback from Fatburners all the time. You really can and you will lose weight and feel great. This is precisely why the Holford Diet works so amazingly well.

Myth number 3: If you eat a high-protein diet you lose calories in urine, so you shed more weight.

When you're on a high-protein, low-carbohydrate diet, your body switches from using carbohydrates as its primary fuel to using fat and protein instead – including the body's fat reserves. As the body burns fat, ketones – a by-product of the process – are excreted in the urine. This process is called *ketosis*.

Supposedly, since fat and protein constitute a less efficient fuel than carbohydrate, you can eat more. The thinking is that the body will excrete some of the calories of this inefficient fuel as ketones.

Nice theory, but wrong. It is true that people do lose more weight on high-protein diets. But the reason is that they eat less on those diets. And the reason they eat less is that high-protein diets help stabilise blood sugar.

The high-protein-diet camp, led by the late Dr Atkins, were one of the first to say that sugar makes you fat. But their solution was to say that carbohydrates are bad and protein is good, so you should eat a high-protein diet that's very low in carbohydrates. Now, a high-protein meal has a low 🅖🅛, which as we've seen is the key to stabilising blood sugar, which in turn balances our appetite and helps us lose weight. But a meal with some protein and some low-🅖🅛 carbohydrate works in the same way. There is absolutely no need to avoid or massively restrict carbohydrates to lose weight, provided you are eating the right low-🅖🅛 kind, plus protein.

Take a look at the science. There have been two proper weight-loss trials to date published on the Atkins-type high-fat/high-protein diet versus a conventional low-fat diet. The first showed that, after six months, those on the high-fat/high-protein diet had lost 12.7lb, compared with 4lb on the low-fat diet. That's a rather unexciting half-pound a week. However, after 12 months, there was no significant difference.[8]

The other trial showed no real difference in weight loss between the high-protein approach and conventional dieting, with an average weight loss of 10lb after six months.[9] That's less than half a pound a week. Similarly, a review of all the high-protein/low-carbohydrate diet studies done to date concludes, 'Weight loss was principally associated with decreased calorie intake.'[10]

In other words, an Atkins-type diet works, but the results aren't spectacular and are principally due to eating less in general, rather than eating fewer carbohydrates. Moreover, there are problems, and even serious dangers, associated with eating high-protein, low-carbohydrate diets. I go into these in detail in Appendix 3 (see page 453), but here's an overview.

The first problem is ketosis itself. In excess, ketones can be very toxic and in extreme cases ketosis can be fatal. Reports suggest that 58 deaths have been associated with very low-calorie, very high-protein diets. Moreover, recent research has proved that the amount of calories lost through ketosis is negligible. This makes the risk pretty high for diets based on this principle.

The diet promises more than it delivers in other ways. As I've said, I think the switch to ketosis triggers weight loss by stabilising blood sugar, and it's known that ketosis also suppresses appetite. A low-carbohydrate diet also kick-starts weight loss because you use up your short-term stores of glucose, which are stored as glycogen, bound with water. In fact, for every pound of glycogen, you store 3 to 4lb of water. The net result is an immediate weight loss of up to 5lb – just one reason why people claim spectacular short-term weight loss. But it's not sustainable. The glycogen and water will come back, as will your appetite. Many people on high-protein diets lose weight, get bored, then gain it all back.

A diet lacking in carbohydrates such as fruit and green leafy vegetables will leave you deficient in antioxidants and vitamins, unless you are very careful about what you eat, and take supplements. You won't get enough fibre, and could get constipated as a result, which can lead to digestive problems. Additionally, many people feel ill as they go through sugar withdrawal and switch to ketosis. Nausea and tiredness continue for some, making it hard to stick to the diet.

Finally, high-protein diets, especially those based on meat and milk, can be dangerous. They potentially increase the risk of bone and kidney problems, and breast and prostate cancer. And as we've seen, the weight-loss results are little different from those of conventional dieting in the long run. In my opinion the high-protein approach to stabilising your blood sugar, and hence your weight, is certainly not worth the risk.

Myth number 4: Don't eat protein with carbohydrates. These foods fight.

'Food-combining' diets separate protein foods from carbohydrate foods. Nature doesn't. Beans, lentils, nuts and seeds all contain both. And the healthiest nations of the world are the nut, bean and seed eaters.

Despite this, a number of food-combining diets abound, based on the principles of Dr Hay, a physician writing back in the 1930s. He emphasised eating wholefoods and lots of fruit and vegetables; he also advocated eating fruit away from other foods, since, if trapped in the stomach after a steak for example, fruit can ferment. So far, so good.

He also recommended never eating carbohydrate-rich foods with protein-rich foods. So, for example, fish with rice or chicken with potatoes is out. The only study I've seen recommending that overweight or obese people follow this kind of diet showed a 3.5 per cent average body-weight change over 12 weeks. Although subjects in this trial were not advised to eat less or change the kind of food they ate, there was no measure to indicate whether their weight loss was due solely to food-combining or to changes in the quantity or quality of food.[11]

It is now known, however, that combining protein with carbohydrate slows down the release of sugars from a meal to the bloodstream, helps stabilise blood sugar levels and hence helps control weight (see Chapter 7). Since the majority of overweight people have blood sugar problems, it would seem that combining protein with carbohydrate would be better, not worse for you. So, in my book, fish with rice is in, not out. This is the staple diet, along with fruits and vegetables, of many island and coastal people around the world, many of whom are exceedingly healthy and slim.

Dr Hay's approach, if followed strictly, is probably best for those with digestive problems and worst for those with blood sugar problems. I remain to be convinced that the benefits reported by those on food-combining diets aren't largely due to changes in the kind of foods eaten, rather than their non-combination.

Myth number 5: You can't change your metabolism.

Your metabolism is the way in which you turn your food into energy or into storage as fat. We are each programmed to respond differently to the food we eat. This programming is partly inherited: some people's metabolism rapidly turns food into fat, for instance. But your metabolism is primarily down to what you eat and how active you are.

Because of this, you can change both the efficiency of your metabolism and your metabolic rate – the speed at which you burn calories. Crash diets can lower your metabolic rate to half-speed, for instance, while aerobic exercise can increase it ten-fold, and leave it raised for up to 15 hours. By changing the kinds and combinations of food you eat, you can reprogramme yourself to burn fat more rapidly.

And the less fat and the more lean tissue you have, the more calories you burn off just keeping your body alive. In other words, your metabolic rate has increased, and you've changed from fatmaker to Fatburner. This is what a low-ⒼⒾ diet will do for you.

Myth number 6: It's eating fat that makes you fat.

It isn't just fat that makes you fat. All sugar or carbohydrates and all alcohol, as well as all fats, is turned by the body into glucose. (Protein, too, can be turned into glucose, but not so easily.) Glucose, remember, is the fuel our bodies run on, and any excess is turned into fat. So too much fat, protein, carbohydrate or alcohol can lead to fat gain and weight gain.

And, looking at fat alone, it isn't just any old fat that makes you fat. As far as your body is concerned there's a world of difference between, say, 100 calories of saturated fat from meat and 100 calories of essential fat from seeds. Saturated fat can only be burned for energy or stored as body fat. But essential fats – properly known as EFAs or essential fatty acids – are used by the brain, the nerves, the arteries and the skin, and balance your hormones and boost immunity into the bargain. Only if there's any left over does the body burn it or store it. So you are more likely to gain weight eating saturated fat or damaged fat in fried or processed foods than you are eating EFAs.

One big reason for this is that the body craves EFAs, precisely because it needs them to function. This craving means we are drawn to fats in general, and, as we're surrounded by saturated and processed fats the minute we enter the average supermarket, we may well end up eating them. Yet afterwards the body still keeps craving fat – so we eat more fatty foods. But, if you eat EFA-rich food such as fish and seeds, you'll fully satisfy the craving and will end up eating less.

Does eating fat make you fat? Of course it does, in excess, but fat isn't the main culprit. As we saw earlier, the number of calories we eat from fat has dropped, while our intake of sugar has increased dramatically, paralleling the rise in obesity.

Low-fat diets rose out of the belief that fat is the prime culprit in weight gain. But, as with high-protein diets, there are two potential problems with this approach. First, most low-fat diets are high in carbohydrates, so sugar and refined foods replace fatty foods. This encourages a blood sugar problem that, in turn, makes it harder to maintain weight control. For this reason, very low-fat, high-carbohydrate diets can often cause fatigue, mood swings and sugar cravings.

The worst aspect of a low-fat diet, however, is that it cuts out EFAs. Ann Louise Gittleman is the former director of nutrition at the Pritikin Longevity Center in Florida, which emphasised low-fat eating. In her book *Beyond Pritikin*,[12] she notes conditions in people placed on low-fat diets, such as a lack of energy, allergies, yeast problems, mood swings, and dry skin, hair and nails, that she believed were due to the lack of EFAs.

While most of us could do with cutting back on fat, the real emphasis should be on reducing foods rich in saturated fats and devoid of essential fats (meat and dairy produce), and instead eating foods rich in essential fats (seeds, their oils and fish).

Myth number 7: The best way to lose weight fast is to eat far fewer calories.

I'm dead against very low-calorie diets and calorie-counting. It not only encourages obsessive eating – but the maths are patently wrong.

Consider this simple example. A banana is approximately 100 calories, so, if you eat a banana fewer every day for a year, you'd lose 36,500 calories. A pound of body fat is equivalent to around 4,000 calories. That means you'd lose nearly 10lb in the first year, 50lb by the fifth year, and 100lb after 10 years – and vanish completely after 15 years!

The calorie equation for exercise is equally ridiculous. Cycle vigorously for 15 minutes each day and you will lose 10lb in the first year. Quite possibly. But 100lb after 10 years? No chance. However, according to calorie theory, merely a banana every day undoes all that hard work anyway.

According to Dr Michael Colgan, nutritionist to many Olympic athletes, some athletes burn off more than 7,000 calories a day, but eat only 3,500 calories. Going by calorie theory alone, these athletes should have completely disappeared by now.

An investigation by Dr Marian Appelbaum of the Bichat Hospital in Paris, of people living in famine in the Warsaw ghetto during World War One, came up with the same contradiction.[13] With an average calorie intake of 800 calories a day, and a requirement of around 2,500 calories, a deficiency of 1,241,000 calories would have built up over two years. The average body has 30lb of fat, representing 120,000 calories, to dispose of. Even if all the fat were lost, what happened to the other million calories?

If you still believe it's all down to calories, listen to this. *The Sunday Times Magazine* put two similarly overweight people on diets, one on my original Fatburner Diet (approximately 1,500 calories a day), and one on the Cambridge Diet (then 330 calories). The Fatburner volunteer lost more weight after six weeks.

The missing link in the low-calorie approach is metabolism – the process of turning the fuel in food into energy that the body can use, and burning off unwanted fat. As we've seen, people's metabolism can vary considerably. Having a slow metabolism means you'll turn more food into fat. Most obese people have slower rates of metabolism than slim people.

If you start out this way, a low-calorie diet can simply exacerbate the problem. With crash diets below 1,000 calories a day, the body sees this reduction in food as a threat, and slows down the metabolic rate by as much as 45 per cent.[14] According to Dr John Marks from Cambridge University, 'As weight falls, the metabolic rate always falls too.' In the short term you can lose around 7lb of body fluid and, if you're lucky, an absolute maximum of 2lb of body fat a week, which together could account for as much as 10lb in two or three weeks. But the minute you go back to what you were eating before, the fluid returns. And so will the fat, because your metabolic rate has slowed down, meaning that you now need to eat less food to maintain a stable weight.

This 'rebound effect' is good business for mortuaries. A report by the National Institutes of Health, using the findings of a 22-centre study called the Multiple Risk Factor Intervention Trial, showed that among people whose weight showed a wide variability over six to seven years there was a higher death rate.[15] It's also good for food-replacement programmes, whose customers try crash-dieting on average three times a year.

To see how dramatically unpleasant the rebound effect can be, hark back to the *Sunday Times Magazine* trial I mentioned above. Michelle, who was on the Cambridge Diet, said,

> ❛ *The first three days were torturous but from then on it got worse. Walking down the road required serious will: I was constantly exhausted and couldn't concentrate so that my work suffered badly. Weight loss came slowly – I'd expected miracles after reading the publicity boasts – but in the final week it finally plummeted … I blew up like a balloon when I resumed eating, and seemed to retain gallons of water; conversely, 'loose' skin has appeared, creating an underarm bat-wing effect. When I first stopped the diet, irresistible bingeing took over but after six weeks, with the exercise of limbs and discipline, I've managed to limit the damage to a gain of 5 pounds.* ❜

Michelle lost 10lb over the month and gained 5lb in the weeks that followed – making her net weight loss 5lb.

Caroline, on my Fatburner Diet, also lost 10lb in a month. She then put 2lb back on while on holiday. She commented,

> *One of the hardest – but best – things about it was the insistence on giving up coffee and stimulants. I had caffeine-withdrawal headaches for the first few days, but began to feel wonderful after that – alert and fit and thoroughly detoxified, with no more puffy eyes staring back from the bathroom mirror. I regained 2lb while on holiday but will whittle it off by eating sensibly.*

The bottom line is that the body is intelligent. If you try to starve it, it will turn down your metabolic fire. If you work with its natural design you'll burn unwanted fat easily. (By the way, you don't have to give up all stimulants and caffeine-containing drinks on the Holford Diet, but there's no question that it helps speed up weight loss. More on this in Chapter 7.)

However, very low-calorie diets do more than make you feel bad and gain weight afterwards. They can be dangerous, and are now required to provide at least 400 calories and 40g of protein per day for women and 500 calories and 50g of protein per day for men to ensure the dieter's body will not be breaking down muscle tissue or vital organs to meet calorie requirements. They do not encourage the re-education of eating habits. And they leave you very hungry.

The solution in the eyes of the people designing these diets is wheat bran, which fills you up while at the same time supposedly triggering weight loss. But does that make dieters want to stick to the regime? To find out, I put ten people on a 1,000-calorie-a-day diet plus high fibre for three months. Only four lasted the course, with an average weight loss of a measly 3.25lb. The high dropout rate is a reflection of how difficult it is to stick to a low-calorie diet for a long period of time. In another study we put ten slimmers on high-fibre tablets claimed to induce weight loss for a period of three months. Five completed the three months with an average weight loss of 1.5lb. Not very impressive.

However, some special kinds of fibre do assist weight loss and having a high-fibre diet by eating wholefoods – not by adding wheat bran – is definitely good for you. This is explained in Chapter 7.

Myth number 8: Stimulants help you lose weight by reducing your appetite.

It's true that caffeine, nicotine and the body's own adrenalin all help reduce your appetite. They do this by releasing stores of sugar held in your body. So, sure, you can lose weight by just drinking coffee – in the short term.

However, long-term use of stimulants messes up your blood sugar control. When your blood sugar dips, this leads to fatigue, mood swings, anxiety, sugar craving, weight gain and, of course, dependence on stimulants. The best way to control your appetite, and your cravings, is to eat a low-GL diet.

Myth number 9: Slimming pills work.

Every year there is a new pill or potion that claims to do it all for you – starch blockers, fat blockers, appetite suppressants, slimming pills. Avoid them at all costs. You can't cheat the body without paying a price.

Starch blockers inhibit the digestion of carbohydrate. The theory is that if you can't digest it you can't gain weight. But having a whole lot of undigested carbohydrate in the digestive tract is bad news. It feeds the wrong kind of bugs, causing bacterial and yeast infections as well as terrible gas.

Much touted as an answer to weight loss is a supplement called chitosan, sometimes called the fat attractor or fat magnet, which inhibits the digestion of fat. It apparently works because it has a positive charge and attracts fats, which have a negative charge. Once bound together with chitosan, the fat is less likely to be absorbed and passes through the body, so it is claimed, and cholesterol levels decrease.

However, three studies have found no significant differences in either weight or cholesterol levels between people taking chitosan and those taking a placebo. One study involved 30 overweight people who took chitosan or a placebo for 28 days while eating their normal diet. There was no difference in weight or cholesterol.[16] The second study involving 51 obese women found that the chitosan group had slightly greater cholesterol reduction than the placebo group, but no difference in weight loss after eight weeks.[17] Another study, with 68 obese men and women, found no improvement in weight or cholesterol.[18]

Drug companies are also cashing in on the weight-loss market with drugs that stop you from digesting fat. An example is Xenical, the drug name for a chemical called orlistat. This drug does actually work, in the sense that it does reduce fat absorption. The immediate potential side effects are oily spotting, gas with discharge, oily or fatty stools, oily discharge and an inability to control bowel movements. If that doesn't put you off, more worrying are the effects on essential fats, so vital for heart, brain and skin. Since EFAs are probably the most commonly deficient nutrient in the West, the last thing you want is to swallow something that stops you from using the little there is in your diet. Also, it probably isn't a good idea to have undigested fat in your digestive tract.

Some slimming drugs are basically stimulants that suppress appetite and wire you up, inducing anxiety and hyperactivity. Similarly, if you drank 15 cups of coffee a day, it would also work in the short term. In the not-so-long term, stimulants mess up your body's metabolism as well as your physical, mental and emotional health (see also Myth number 8). Even if it sounds 'natural', avoid any herb or supplement whose active ingredient is caffeine – and that includes guarana.

Myth number 10: There's nothing wrong with being overweight.

The health risks associated with weighing more than you should accumulate as soon as you are as little as 7lb overweight. With over half of people in Britain overweight and 20 per cent obese, that's a lot of extra health risks.

And these are serious risks: heart disease, diabetes, kidney problems, osteoporosis, cancer and arthritis. One study showed that about 40 per cent of heart disease in women is linked to overweight, while others connect it to higher risks of breast cancer, arthritis, osteoporosis and other complications.[19] Diabetes is strongly linked to obesity.

In fact, every year obesity causes the premature deaths of 30,000 people, costs Britain's National Health Service £1 billion and is responsible for the loss of more than 20 million working days. According to Dr Susan Jebb of the Dunn Clinical Nutrition Centre in Cambridge in the UK, 'Obesity is a serious medical condition that reduces life expectancy by increasing the risk of many chronic and potentially fatal diseases.'

And with a thousand people becoming obese every day, we need to wake up to the fact that there's a disaster in the making here – but only potentially. It only *looks* like a slippery slope: there is a way out.

Why the Holford Diet works where others fail

You can lose weight on a low-calorie diet, a high-protein diet, a low-carb diet or a no-fat diet. But you are stacking the odds against you. Why? Because ...

- You get short-term weight loss as your body burns its essential store of glycogen – that's 5lb gone, but it all comes back!

- None of these diets satisfies your appetite better than the Holford Diet, so you have to fight hard to stay on them.

- All of these diets are highly restrictive in some way – who wants to live without carbohydrates or fats?

- None of these diets has been shown to trigger as much weight loss in the short term or long term as the Fatburner System.

In a trial comparing the Fatburner System with Unislim – a low-calorie, high-exercise regime, with weekly support meetings – the Fatburner volunteers lost, on average, four times more weight (14lb in three months) than the other dieters. Every single trial by third parties proved highly successful, with many reports of additional benefits besides consistent weight loss, such as 'increased alertness', 'concentration improved', 'no wobbly feeling', 'never felt hungry', 'easy to stick to', 'extra energy', 'thoroughly detoxified'. In these trials, not one person failed to lose weight.

The original Fatburner Diet worked brilliantly, but there's now an even faster, easier and healthier way to chisel away at those unwanted pounds and promote your health and energy every step of the way. The Holford Diet takes about 30 days to 'tune up' your metabolism and stabilise your blood sugar. Once this is achieved, not only will fatburning become much easier, but your weight will become much more stable and less likely to fluctuate with the odd indulgence. Although the diet may mean slightly fewer calories than you are eating now, slightly less fat and slightly more protein, the major emphasis is on quality, and there will be plenty of it – all delicious.

Now let's summarise what *doesn't* work, and find out what does.

- The major cause of the obesity epidemic is an increase in sugar and refined carbohydrate, not an increase in fat.

- Different sources of calories have different effects on weight loss.

- Eating a low-🄶🄻 diet triggers the most rapid weight loss.

- If you eat too few calories your metabolic rate slows down to conserve your fat, so you have to suffer to lose weight and will inevitably develop rebound weight gain.

- High-protein diets stabilise your blood sugar levels and reduce your appetite, but they don't work better than conventional diets and they're not good for you in the long run.

- Low-fat diets are bad for you because the body needs essential fats and keeps craving fats until it gets them.

- The best diet for long-term weight loss is a low-🄶🄻 diet, in which low-🄶🄻 carbohydrates are combined with protein and essential fats – in short, the Holford Diet.

3

The Inside Story on Fat

Losing extra inches is very simple. It's all about keeping your blood sugar even, a balancing act your body is designed to do. All you have to do is create the right environment for this to happen. Most people, probably including you, have unwittingly created a set of circumstances that have led your body to lose this balancing act. The result is roller-coastering blood sugar, energy and weight.

For instance, do you need to kick-start the day with coffee, cigarettes or something sweet? Do you gravitate towards bread, biscuits, pasta and sweet foods? Do you drink caffeinated drinks or alcohol every day? If so, the chances are you have significant dips in blood sugar. Then, when you've satisfied the craving with a big plate of pasta, a cola, a large glass of wine or a couple of pastries, your blood sugar levels shoot up – and you dump the excess as fat.

If you lose blood sugar control, you gain weight, yet feel hungry – and exhausted – a lot of the time. If you can keep your blood sugar level on an even keel, you'll gravitate towards your natural weight, stay there and have a consistently high energy level.

If you have poor blood sugar control you are three times more likely to have difficulty losing weight. That's what we found in our health and diet survey in 2004, when we surveyed 37,000 people using the web-based MyNutrition questionnaire (see page 475 for details on how you can assess your own health using MyNutrition).[20] We also found that when you gain blood sugar control you lose weight.

The question is, how do you regain blood sugar control? To tell you, I need to introduce you to the key players in this drama. First we'll meet the villain – insulin.

Why sugar makes you fat

Carbohydrates are turned into glucose by the body and conveyed through the bloodstream for delivery to cells, where it's used as fuel. The trouble is that glucose is the equivalent of high-octane fuel, and dangerous stuff.

If glucose levels in the blood are too high, it can be very harmful – that's why diabetics can get nerve, eye, kidney and artery damage. So as soon as your blood sugar level shoots beyond a certain level, the body moves quickly to get it out of your blood and, if you don't need it for energy, stores it as fat.

Insulin, a hormone produced by the pancreas, moves the glucose out of your blood. So why is it the villain of this story? The more frequently your blood sugar is raised, the more insulin you produce. The more insulin you produce, the more sugar you dump as fat. As a result, insulin can be thought of as the fat-storing hormone.

But there's more bad news. Having a high insulin level doesn't only encourage your body to turn food into fat: it also

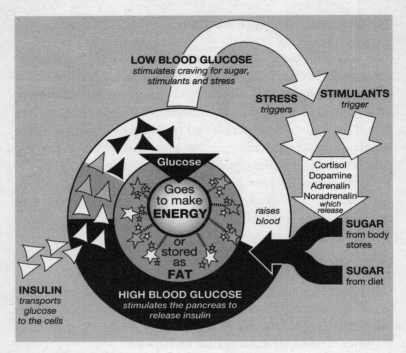

The sugar cycle. Eating sugar increases blood glucose levels. The body releases insulin into the blood to help escort glucose out and into body cells, to make energy or convert into fat. The result is low blood glucose. Either stress, causing more adrenalin, or induced stress, caused by consuming a stimulant such as caffeine, which raises adrenal hormones, causes breakdown of stores of sugar in the liver and muscles, called glycogen, which raises blood sugar levels. Low blood glucose causes stress or cravings for either something sweet or a stimulant.

inhibits the body's breakdown of stored fat. So, once you're fat, you stay fat. If you're overweight, you've probably got elevated insulin levels.

Insulin is implicated in another factor that messes up your blood sugar level – 'insulin resistance'.

In the grip of resistance

Let's say that, during the day, you're snacking or bingeing on sugary foods, drinking several cups of coffee, or smoking a few cigarettes. Every time you get a 'hit' of sugar or a jolt from caffeine or nicotine, your blood sugar peaks. And, if this is happening a lot, more and more insulin will be rushing out to escort the glucose out of your blood as quickly as possible and into your cells. In effect, insulin will be subjecting your cells to a constant cry of 'Open the door!'

Eventually the cells become so bored of hearing the same old message that it's as if they had become deaf to it. So your body has to produce more and more insulin, just as if it were shouting louder and louder to be heard. The end result is that you become insensitive to your own insulin – a condition called *insulin resistance*.

According to Professor Gerald Reaven from Stanford University in California, one of the world's leading experts in blood sugar problems, the majority of obese people and 25 per cent of non-obese people are insulin-resistant.[21]

This means they, and quite likely you, need to produce more insulin to lower blood sugar peaks. So you will eat more carbohydrate before your body says 'Stop!' and then, by the time the insulin does kick in, your blood sugar levels will have plummeted too low, leaving you once again craving something to give you a lift.

When you're in the grip of this vicious cycle, that lift is likely to be something high-GL, such as refined pasta, and, for up to four hours afterwards, insulin resistance will mess up your body's response to it. So you could either suffer from brain fog, sleepiness and low mood after a meal, or cave in to the cravings for something to raise your blood sugar levels once more. Most people choose the latter, either eating more carbohydrate such as pudding, or homing in on a stimulant such as a cup of tea or coffee (more on this later). Meanwhile, with all these inefficient peaks and troughs in blood sugar levels, you're turning the excess glucose to fat and feeling exhausted.

But there's a more insidious downside. Remember, glucose is very damaging, so, as your insulin becomes more ineffectual at getting it out of your bloodstream, you spend more time with too much glucose in your blood. This literally damages your arteries, and paves the way for heart disease.

Diabetes is another direct result. This condition arises when you've become so insulin-resistant that the cells in the pancreas that make insulin become exhausted, and you can't produce enough. So you can't lower your blood sugar level very well, and some actually spills over into the urine (normally, the kidneys filter all glucose out, leaving it in the bloodstream, but even your kidneys have limits). Thus too little insulin is also bad news. As always in the body, it's a balancing act.

The plain truth is that most of us are digging our own graves with a knife and fork. But it doesn't have to be this way. The Holford Diet can literally save your life.

You can measure your own insulin resistance (see page 479 in Resources). Another way to get a measure on where you stand is the questionnaire below.

Are you insulin-resistant?

☐ Are you rarely wide awake within 20 minutes of getting up?

☐ Do you need tea, coffee, a cigarette or something to get you going in the morning?

☐ Do you really like sweet foods?

☐ Do you crave bread, cereal, popcorn or pasta most days?

☐ Do you feel as if you 'need' an alcoholic drink on most days?

☐ Are you overweight and unable to shift the extra pounds?

☐ Do you often have energy slumps during the day or after meals?

☐ Do you often have mood swings or difficulty concentrating?

☐ Do you fall asleep in the early evening or need naps during the day?

☐ Do you avoid exercise because you haven't got the energy?

☐ Do you get dizzy or irritable if you go six hours without food?

☐ Do you often find you overreact to stress?

☐ Do you often get irritable, angry or aggressive unexpectedly?

☐ Is your energy now less than it used to be?

☐ Do you get night sweats or frequent headaches?

☐ Do you ever lie about how much sweet food you have eaten?

☐ Do you ever keep a supply of sweet food close to hand?

☐ Do you ever go out of your way to make sure you have something sweet?

☐ Do you feel you could never give up bread?

☐ Do you think of yourself as addicted to sugar, chocolate or biscuits?

If you answered 'yes' to 10 or more questions, there's a very good chance that you are insulin-resistant, and struggling to keep your blood sugar level even. You are also three times more likely to have trouble losing weight. If you'd like to find out more about insulin resistance, read *The Insulin Factor*, by Antony Haynes, published by Thorsons (2004).

You'll note that I've asked whether you need tea, coffee or cigarettes to kick-start your day. Obviously, these have nothing to do with carbohydrates, so let's take a closer look at the role stimulants play in blood sugar chaos.

How caffeine ties you to the vicious cycle

Let's say you find yourself in an energy trough triggered by low blood sugar. You may not have eaten for a while, or you're experiencing the rebound low blood sugar that happens after a high-ⒼⓁ meal. One of the effects is that your body releases hormones from your adrenal glands, which sit on top of your kidneys in the small of your back. These hormones are adrenalin and cortisol, and, if your blood sugar levels are out of control, they're bad news.

You may have learned about the 'fight-or-flight' mechanism at school. Adrenalin is the driving force behind this response, as it immediately raises your blood sugar level to give you fuel to fight back or run away. While adrenalin doesn't last long in the body, cortisol, another adrenal hormone, sticks around for much longer.

When this kind of thing happened in our prehistoric past, of course, we'd have burned off the extra glucose by either bashing that sabre-toothed tiger on the head, or legging it to the nearest cave. Our hormone levels would then return to normal and all would be well. But the twenty-first-century reality is that we may simply be sitting at our office desk hungry for lunch when adrenalin and cortisol start circulating. And, if we do nothing, they'll keep doing just that, leaving us anxious and stressed.

So what's caffeine got to do with all this? This stimulant also prompts the release of adrenalin and raises blood sugar levels. So, if your levels are low, you may as easily reach for a coffee as for a doughnut.

Even more seductive are the 'treats' that combine sugar with stimulants, such as tea or coffee with sugar, mocha drinks, chocolate or colas. This pairing adds up to a powerful fix. Some people become more addicted to carbohydrates, others more addicted to caffeine, but most are addicted to both. Either way, they further disrupt your blood sugar control, make you more insulin-resistant and keep you in the prison of seesawing weight and energy levels.

The bottom line is that the body's and brain's sensitive mechanisms for keeping your blood sugar in balance simply can't cope with a daily onslaught of sugar and other high-Ⓖ foods and snacks, topped up with stimulants such as caffeine and nicotine. It will respond by turning you into a fatmaker.

But there's good news. It doesn't take long to turn insulin resistance round and recover your fatburning ability. And *glucagon* is central to the process.

Enter glucagon – a Fatburner's best friend

Although it's another hormone produced by the pancreas, glucagon is the hero to insulin's villain. It is, in fact, the Fatburner's best friend, and will get you out of the vicious cycle of seesawing blood glucose levels.

Glucagon enters the picture when your blood glucose levels are very low. It evens your blood glucose level up by telling the

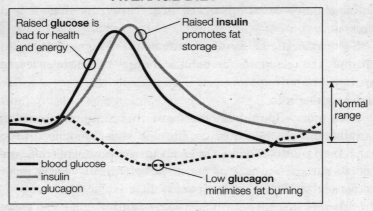

AVERAGE DIET

Raised **glucose** is bad for health and energy

Raised **insulin** promotes fat storage

Normal range

—— blood glucose
—— insulin
▪▪▪▪ glucagon

Low **glucagon** minimises fat burning

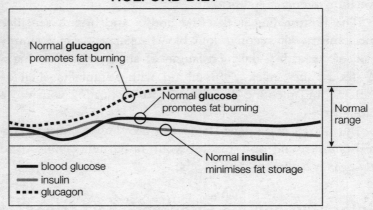

HOLFORD DIET

Normal **glucagon** promotes fat burning

Normal **glucose** promotes fat burning

Normal range

—— blood glucose
—— insulin
▪▪▪▪ glucagon

Normal **insulin** minimises fat storage

Blood sugar balance. When you eat a high-sugar food your blood glucose level shoots up, followed by a release of insulin. Insulin helps turn glucose into fat. When you eat a low-**GL** food your blood glucose level stays more stable, with less insulin release and relatively more glucagon.

body to break down fat and burn it for energy. In the process, glucagon reduces any cravings for something sweet.

If insulin makes you store fat, glucagon makes you burn it. So glucagon is a fatburning hormone. The more glucagon you produce in relation to insulin, the more you are programming yourself to burn fat.

As we've seen, if you eat the kinds of foods or consume stimulants that send your blood sugar rocketing, out pours the insulin and on creeps the fat. But, if you eat the kinds of food that keep your blood glucose level in check, you'll produce only small amounts of insulin and, whenever your energy is low, release glucagon to burn some fat.

The Holford Diet is calculated to maximise glucagon release and minimise insulin release, thus literally reprogramming your metabolism to burn fat.

We've seen the inside story on hormones, sugar and fat. Now let's frame it differently, and look at the dynamics of what stops people losing weight, and how this diet overcomes the obstacles.

- Sugar and refined carbohydrates can turn easily into fat and cause the release of an insulin overload.

- Eventually the body can become more and more resistant to insulin, leading to blood sugar peaks, followed by troughs, which lead to carbohydrate and sugar cravings.

- Insulin resistance is the hallmark of obesity and is present in most overweight people.

- Glucagon counters the effect of insulin and helps stabilise blood sugar levels and reduce appetite, sugar and carbohydrate cravings.

- When your blood sugar level crashes you release adrenal hormones. These further raise your blood sugar. Caffeine has a similar effect and, in the long term, encourages insulin resistance and weight gain.

● The Holford Diet promotes glucagon and reduces insulin resistance, literally reprogramming the body to burn fat.

4

How to Lose Weight For Ever

Losing weight isn't difficult as long as you work *with* your body's design, not *against* it. As you learned in Chapter 2, you can lose weight with 'extreme' diets, very low in fat, very low in carbohydrate or very low in calories. But your body and your mind fight back. Your body will crave all three – fat, protein and carbohydrate – and will signal its lack if you cut them down too far. This kind of diet fails because, in the end, your cravings win.

In fact, long-term studies have shown that 'dieters' gain more weight than non-dieters.[22] As we've seen, this is because just about any short-term extreme diet slows down your metabolism. It's because of this that many diets gradually move you from the unsustainable 'weight-loss' phase to a more sustainable 'weight-maintenance' phase.

The Holford Diet is sustainable from the start because it is scientifically calculated to satisfy your cravings and your appetite from Day One. It's the Rolls-Royce of diets. Your body will love it, and will reward you with a myriad superhealthy side effects – from extra energy to smooth, clear skin.

The trick with the Fatburner System is that there *is* no trick. It doesn't cheat or fool your body. Remember: given the right circumstances, your body will go to its ideal weight – and stay there for ever.

Overweight or underlean?

We've looked at the crucial role hormones play vis-à-vis your blood sugar balance, and how an imbalance leads to weight gain. As you rev up to start the Holford Diet, I'd like you to understand how we actually lose weight, and to have realistic expectations about the results.

Although I will tell you about some rapid, miracle weight-loss results, the truth is that the body limits how quickly it can burn off fat without harming you. Many popular diets cheat the body by kicking off with instant weight loss in the first week or two, but after this you pay the price, not only in how you feel, but in weight gain over the long term.

I don't want this to happen to you. I'm more interested in your reaching your ultimate goal and staying there, even if it takes months, not weeks.

At this point we need to look at how much you weigh, and how much you want to lose. But we won't look at poundage alone: we'll be sorting out the relative percentages of fat and lean.

This is because it's not so much being overweight that's the problem, but being underlean. Your body is made of both fat tissue and lean tissue (muscle and organs). A significantly higher proportion of fat increases health risk, so your body fat percentage is actually more important than overall weight.

Ideally, no more than 15 per cent of a man's body and 22 per cent of a woman's body should be made up of fat. Yet in the West the average man has a body fat percentage of a little over 20, and the average woman's is above 30.

Your body fat percentage is a little harder to measure than your weight. With a little patience and a tape measure, you can work it out roughly using the formula in Appendix 1 (see page 428). Some gyms work it out by making a few body measurements with callipers or with a piece of equipment that measures your electrical resistance. Since fat doesn't conduct electricity, the less 'electric' you are the more fat you've got.

But how can you measure the fat lost as your fatburning capacity really gets going? Fat is relatively light and bulky while protein is hard and heavy. So, as you convert fat into lean muscle, you may lose inches more quickly than you lose pounds. This is good news for several reasons. One is obviously that you'll look better. The other is that, when you follow the Holford Diet, you are giving your lean muscle a tune-up so it is ready to burn your excess fat. Exercise is an essential part of the plan (and remember, it's for only 15 minutes a day), and the more exercise you do the more efficient your muscles will become at fatburning.

So, as the diet progresses, you'll take a simple measurement with a tape measure once a week, as well as getting on the scales.

Measuring your body mass

The next best measurement to know is your body mass index (BMI). To work this out, all you need to know is your weight and height; then look on the chart below. (There's another chart in Appendix 1, on Page 426, that does this for you and shows you the ideal weight range for each height.) If your BMI is between 25 and 30 (Class 1) then you are technically overweight. If it's 30 (Class 2 or 3) or above, you are technically obese.

If you find you are technically obese, it may come as a shock. But you are not alone – the number of overweight and obese people doubled in the 1980s and continued to grow at the same alarming rate in the 1990s. In some parts of the US, as many as 50 per cent of women are now obese. By the end of this book you'll understand why. And you will have in hand the best way out of the trap – for ever.

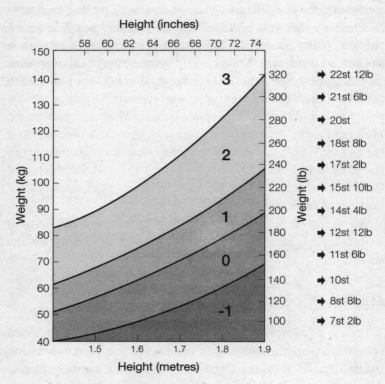

Class 3 – severely obese
Class 2 – obese
Class 1 – overweight
Class 0 – desirable weight
Class –1 – underweight

Are you overweight?

If you are in Class 1, 2 or 3, then your risk for certain diseases, such as diabetes, is much higher. Weight-related diseases account for about as much of the total healthcare cost as the nation's cancer therapy or treatment of heart disease. The closer to your ideal weight you are, the healthier you are and less risk you have of life-threatening and debilitating diseases.

Statistics show that, if you're over 50, it may be better to be a little on the heavier side of the BMI range of 'desirable weight'.[23] Having a BMI below 23 has been associated with an increased death rate. This is partly because very sick people can lose a lot of weight. But if you are healthy, a BMI of around 20 to 24 is probably the best, whatever your age.

> ## TOP TIP
>
> Measure your waist. It's the best predictor of insulin resistance. Measure your girth one inch below your belly button. For women, this should be less than 34 inches, for men less than 40 inches. Hip and thigh weight gain is much less harmful for your overall health.

A pound of fat

Go to the butcher and ask for a pound of fat. It's about the size of this book. Now imagine losing twice that amount of fat a week! Sound good? Read on.

The most you can easily lose in a week, without starvation, is between 1 and 2lb of fat. If you follow my recommendations strictly you'll lose, on average, 2lb of fat a week for the first month. If you follow the general principles loosely, you'll probably lose a pound of fat a week. So, if you're 24lb overweight, and you decide to take on board what I've said in essence, you'll lose this weight in 24 weeks – six months, more or less.

Ian W from Coventry is a typical example:

> ❲ *I bought your book last year in an effort to lose weight. Whilst I was not exactly fat, I was certainly not happy with my size and felt miserable all the time. I tried to stick to the essence of what was in the book. My weight dropped around 1½ stone (21lb) over six months and is currently stable. I can now come home from work and feel OK and the evening is mine to do with as I please. I would recommend your approach to anyone for life in general but remember, there is no need for obsession, all you have to do is choose the better option all the time.* ❳

Linda H is a 48-year-old mother of two. For years, she'd tried to lose weight by dieting and painstakingly counting calories. But it was only when she switched to the Fatburner System that the weight came off and her overall energy and health improved. Here's what she has to say:

> ❲ *At 130 pounds and 5 feet 2 inches, I'd tried to diet for six years. I hoped that, if I was very strict, I might get down to 124 pounds, but this never happened. Finally, I decided to try the diet as a 'quick fix' for 30 days before I went on vacation. For a month, I followed all the recommendations (except I ate even larger portions than recommended). Amazingly, I lost my craving for sweets! Before starting to eat this way, I'd crave sweets about four times a week, and would binge on cakes, sweets and biscuits. This has completely ended. It's as if I've educated my taste buds into a far healthier eating regimen. The best part? I lost 13 pounds!*
>
> *I quickly decided to continue eating this way for the rest of my life. Not just because of the weight loss, but because of how wonderful*

I felt. For instance, an unexpected benefit was that the redness, or rosacea, I'd always noticed on my face, which I thought was a result of ageing, disappeared. My energy also increased, so much that I realised I hadn't understood how tired and run-down I was before. I thought being tired was just a normal part of life!

Because I continued following the regimen, for the first time in two years I returned from vacation the same weight as when I left. After the first 30 days, I allowed myself wine on weekends and my weight still remained steady. Today, I have dessert about once a week, but my weight still remains steady. Since my blood sugar levels are stable, one dessert a week is enough. Best of all, it is now a way of life to say 'no' to dessert – not an effort or sacrifice. ❞

Both Linda and Ian achieved their goals easily and are still slim today and experiencing all the health benefits of my diet.

No 'miracle' weight loss

Linda lost 13lb in 30 days, which is actually a bit more than the maximum average I predict. But, as the weight dropped off, she was never hungry, and her energy levels began to soar. She lost the excess pounds without taxing her body in any way.

Don't be lured by diets that claim amazing weight loss in a couple of weeks. We all feel desperate sometimes – to fit into that outfit, to look good on the beach, just to feel right striding to work. However, you don't want to add insult to injury. Being overweight isn't much fun, and it's bad for our health, but crash diets get rid of a lot of weight that isn't fat, and most of it comes right back afterwards. Let me explain why.

We've seen how the body runs on glucose. It's the equivalent of four-star petrol, and it's why athletes rely on glucose drinks, not protein or fat, when they're practising endurance sports. Your body aims to use a lot of this immediately to power your cells, and you've seen how the excess is laid down as fat.

But, before that happens, excess glucose is first put into short-term storage in the liver and muscles in a form known as *glycogen*. It's only when stores of glycogen are full up that glucose is converted into fat and laid down for long-term storage. If you have insulin resistance this will happen fast, and the excess fat will be dumped most readily around the belly. So carrying a lot of fat around the middle is a sure sign of insulin resistance.

Conversely, when you run out of glucose the body breaks glycogen back down into glucose. When glycogen stores are used up, the body burns fat into sugar to stock them up. If it

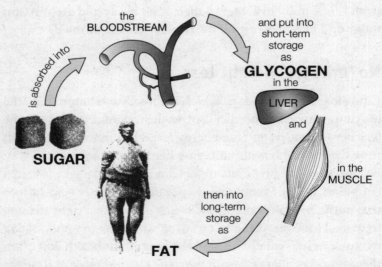

How the body stores energy as fat. The body runs on sugar (glucose), and converts any extra into glycogen, which is stored in muscles and the liver. If glycogen stores are full the body can convert glucose into fat, our long-term energy storage.

has to, the body can also turn protein into sugar and burn this instead. That's why people on starvation diets lose muscle and possibly even damage body organs.

How losing fast is losing out

Each unit of glucose your body puts into storage as glycogen is bound together with three units of water. So, if you run out of glucose and start burning glycogen, you lose water. This is how you can get short-term rapid weight loss on a very low-calorie diet, say below 1,000 calories a day, or on a very low-carbohydrate diet. Since the maximum amount of glycogen in short-term storage in the body is 1kg or 2lb, you could lose a maximum of 8lb – but in reality you'd be more likely to lose 4lb. That's why, when you complete the first week of a diet with great gusto and enthusiasm, you may well be rewarded with a 4lb weight loss. That's 1lb of fat and 3lb of water.

However, the sad truth is that, when you start eating enough for your energy needs again, the glycogen and water stores are replenished, and the water weight comes back.

So the measure of a diet that's actually burning fat is not what happens when you starve yourself during the first week and temporarily run out of glycogen. Instead, it's a regular week-by-week loss of around 1 to 2lb, not sudden weight loss over two weeks.

Look at the two charts overleaf. The top one shows the average weight loss, week by week, of a group of nine dieters on a regular low-calorie diet. In the first week there's 3lb lost, in the second 2lb. Things are looking good – 5lb in two weeks. But most of this is water. By Week 4 there's no loss and, presumably as willpower wanes, the volunteers start eating what they need to eat for energy, restoring glycogen and, with that, back comes the water. The end result: an average of 2lb lost in 12 weeks.

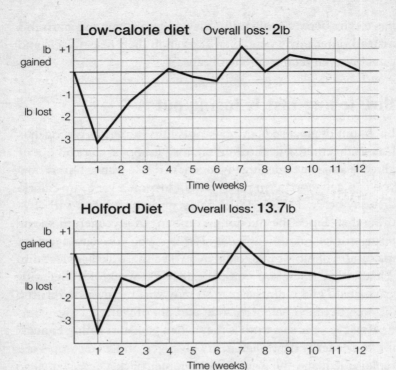

Weight loss on a low-calorie diet versus Holford Diet[24]

The bottom graph shows the results of seven Holford dieters. Once again, there's a sudden weight loss in the first week, but then it settles in at an average of a pound a week. After 12 weeks, the average weight loss is 13.7lb. This pattern of weight loss indicates fatburning – and where there's fatburning, there's long-term, maintained weight loss.

And it is better not to lose weight faster than this. Ultimately, the amount lost will be about 1 to 2 stone (up to 28lb) over three months. Weight loss of over 2lb a week will not all be fat loss. The body simply cannot burn off fat that fast. Of course, most of us want to lose 14lb in a week, despite having taken a year to put it on!

A good target during the first 30 days is to lose 6lb in weight. You'll probably lose more, but it's better to set yourself up for success. Even a weight loss of 1lb a week, maintained over a year, equals over 50lb.

And this can be achieved, without any suffering, on my diet. After all, Rome wasn't unbuilt in a day.

... with one exception

There is, however, one way you can instantly lose weight and never put it back. It's by avoiding a food you are allergic to. One in three people has specific food intolerances, and some of these cause excessive weight gain – probably by triggering excessive fluid retention. Unlike the water that's stored with glycogen, which will come back once you stop starving yourself, this is *excess* water that the body lets go of when you avoid the foods you are intolerant to.

I remember my first overweight patient, Mary, who had struggled with her weight for years. I advised her to cut out wheat, and within two days she had lost 7lb! I'm going to tell you how to discover whether you are allergic to certain foods and what to replace them with in Chapter 9.

This step is one of the five simple principles of my diet, which I introduced in Chapter 1. If you want to lose weight for ever and turn yourself from a fatmaker into a Fatburner, these form the essential framework for your new life:

1. Eat no more than 40 Ⓖ of carbohydrate foods a day (I'll show you how easy this is), with protein.

2. Eat essential omega-3 and -6 fats, and no saturated, processed or fried fats.

3. Find the foods you're allergic to, and avoid them.

4. Take the right supplements.

5. Do the equivalent of 15 minutes' exercise a day.

Remember, you're unique

These principles work well for just about everybody – but it's important to remember that you're unique. For one thing, how much you need to eat will vary depending on how tall you are and how much exercise you do. If you are over 6 feet tall or under 5 feet 4 inches, or exercise an hour or more five or more days a week, you'll need to adjust the Holford Diet according to your needs. The principles, however, remain the same.

There's another factor: some people do better on more protein and less carbohydrate than others. Thanks to the excellent research of Dr Peter D'Adamo, author of *Eat Right for Your Blood Type*, we now know that people with type O blood generally function better on more animal protein, while people with type A blood function better on more carbohydrate and vegetable protein.

If you are blood type O, or simply want to experiment with how you feel eating a little more protein and less carbohydrate, you can do so on the Holford Diet by adding 5g of protein a day and subtracting 5 ⒼⓁ. I will make it crystal clear how you do this in practice. It's much simpler than it sounds – you don't need a calculator!

In summary:

- You cannot lose more than 2lb of actual fat a week unless you are starving yourself or running for England.

- The body loses around 4lb in water on a very low-calorie or very low-carbohydrate diet when you deplete your body's glycogen stores – but this inevitably comes back.

- You can lose 7lb or more fast – and permanently – if you avoid foods you are allergic to.

- Losing inches is more important than losing pounds. Gaining lean body mass and losing fat, measured as your body fat percentage, is the real goal.

- The body will naturally gravitate to its own ideal weight if you give it the right balance and kinds of protein, fat and carbohydrate.

5

Why Fatburning Is Easy

The Holford Diet is the state of the art of keeping you satisfied. For a decade, I've been researching exactly what keeps you replete – not only which foods, but which foods in combination, and when to eat them.

And you'll be eating plenty of them. If all you've ever heard about weight loss is calorie-cutting, this may make you wary. But eating little and often of low-ⓖⓛ foods will reduce, not increase, the number of calories you consume. And it will be easy and brilliantly satisfying, because you've got three meals and two substantial snacks a day, and no cravings brought on by low blood sugar.

Even better, the process will kick in fast. Most people's blood sugar begins to even out within seven days of starting the Holford Diet, and within 30 days you will no longer be insulin-resistant – you'll be reprogrammed to burn fat. That's why I call this a 30-day diet.

Parts Two and Three of this book will get down to the nitty-gritty of the diet. This overview will show you how you can move from being a fatmaker to a Fatburner with real ease.

Seven days to stop cravings

When you're on Day One of the diet, chances are you'll feel fantastic right from the start. But, for a few, it may take a few days for that feeling to kick in. This initial hiccup is simply the effect of simultaneously launching out on a new diet and deciding to go cold turkey on caffeine.

Doing it like this is the quickest way to start the fatburning process, but it does mean that people who drink a lot of coffee or cola, or eat a fair amount of chocolate or sugary snacks, will experience a withdrawal phase. A few people may feel a bit rough for the first three days, and a very small minority can feel bad for the entire first week. The blood sugar dips that go with withdrawal can make you feel sleepy, mentally foggy, anxious, moody or tired, or spark cravings and headaches.

If you find yourself experiencing any of these sensations, be aware that it's all down to resistance. The more insulin, glucagon, adrenalin and cortisol you've been forcing your body to produce, the more resistant it becomes to their 'fine-tuning' effects. In Chapter 3 I explained about insulin resistance, but you also can become adrenalin-resistant. Remember that stimulants such as coffee can kick-start the release of adrenalin. If you're downing four or five cups a day or more, you can become increasingly deaf to your own adrenalin. You might even find it tough to get out of bed in the morning. You can't hear your own inner adrenalin alarm because you've developed adrenalin resistance.

On the Holford Diet, it takes only a few days to overcome resistance – on three delicious meals and two snacks a day. I'm also going to be asking you to call in the cavalry – special supplements that work wonders for stabilising blood sugar and appetite.

If you feel you're very addicted to caffeine or chocolate, however, it is probably best to give yourself two weeks to give it all up before you actually start the diet. You'll see how to do that in Parts Two and Three.

You'll eat less without trying

After seven days you'll find that your desire to eat high-Ⓖ foods will rapidly fall away. You won't get the blood sugar dips after meals that lead you to crave the wrong foods. Even though I don't want you to try to eat less, you will naturally do so. Britain's first Fatburner said this: 'I lost three stone and never felt hungry. I know I'll never go back to eating like I used to.'

Dr David Ludwig of the Department of Medicine at the Children's Hospital in Boston, Massachusetts, decided to put this to the test. He gave children one of two breakfast cereals. One was a low-Ⓖ cereal made from unadulterated oat flakes. The other was a processed 'instant oatmeal' that sounded good but actually had a high Ⓖ. Both groups of kids ate the identical calorie amount of each cereal and also had a calorie-identical lunch. In the afternoon and evening they were free to eat as they chose. The children on the low-Ⓖ diet ate 47 per cent fewer calories in the afternoon – they just weren't hungry.

The same thing will happen to you. That is why Fatburner dieters say that 'as far as hunger is concerned it's an easy diet to stick to' (*She* magazine).

The way it works

To get an idea of how the diet tackles hunger, first imagine a plate. Now divide it in half. In any main meal, one of those halves can be chosen from almost a hundred vegetables.

Divide the other half in half. One quarter is protein – fish, chicken, lamb or vegetarian proteins such as tofu or beans.

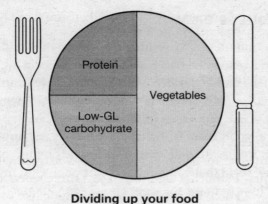

Dividing up your food

Later I'll give you portion sizes of, say, a piece of chicken or a piece of fish.

The remaining quarter is a low-🄖🄛 carbohydrate food serving, equivalent to 10 🄖🄛. This could be bread, potatoes, pasta or any other of the foods that so many high-protein diets forbid. They're firmly part of the Holford Diet, but the serving size will vary depending on the 🄖🄛 of that carbohydrate. For instance, you can eat twice as much boiled as baked potato, or even more sweetcorn. You can eat twice as much whole rye bread as white wheat bread. You can eat twice as much wholemeal spaghetti as French fries. Very soon you'll learn which low-🄖🄛 foods fill you up the best.

This is a sketch of a main meal. You'll roughly follow the same rules for your other two meals, allowing 10 🄖🄛 per meal – and don't forget, there are two substantial snacks a day, at 5 🄖🄛 each. So the 🄖🄛 limit for each day is 40, because that's the maximum possible for fatburning.

Eating out is easy

I travel around the world, visiting an average of 30 cities in any given year. I've learned that I can follow this diet in every country anywhere in the world. Sure, some countries and types of food are easier than others. It's harder in the US, where more people are obese, and easier in Thailand, where most people are skinny. The good news is that there are Thai restaurants, Chinese restaurants, Indian restaurants and many others all around the world that cater perfectly for people on my diet. I'll show you how to make the right choices in Chapter 19.

Effortless shopping

You may have encountered diets for which you had to buy foods by mail order, or hunt out exotic substances in specialist shops. Everything on my diet can be bought in the supermarket – including the organic foods I recommend – or, failing that, in a common-or-garden health-food shop. Granted, you may be throwing a few things you've never cooked before into the trolley, but I can guarantee it's all going to be delicious – and may even become a culinary adventure. As it's a diet for life, it will never be dull.

Veggie heaven

The diet is a cinch for vegetarians. There's a vast and tasty array of vegetables and good, slow-releasing carbohydrates, as well as recipes for preparing them. On the protein front, vegetarians will just need to ensure they're eating the optimal amount for the diet to work.

Tofu, which comes in a number of delicious forms, features in a number of recipes, or can be substituted for fish or chicken in others. Beans and lentils figure large in the Holford Diet, as they are key to regulating blood sugar. Other vegetarian protein options – Quorn, soya mince, yoghurt, cottage cheese, eggs – are all well represented. So there's no shunting of vegetarian needs to the sidelines, which can happen with some high-protein diets.

No forbidden foods

Never say never. So I'm not going to tell you never to eat chocolate, bread, pasta or potatoes. But I *am* going to tell you how much of these foods you can eat to keep within your 40- Ⓖ limit for the day. How you do that is up to you.

Let me give you an example. Below are four snacks. Each equals 5 Ⓖ. The choice is yours.

Strawberries	1 large punnet
Apple	1 small apple
Peanuts	2 small packets
Chocolate	Less than a quarter of a bar
Oatcake	2 oatcakes with third of a tub of hummus

Many people, myself included, like their diets cut and dried. For that reason I have divided carbohydrate foods into low, medium and high. As you can see, high-Ⓖ foods such as chocolate aren't much fun because you can't eat much of them. Low-Ⓖ foods are the best value because they'll fill you up and stop food cravings.

So my advice is to eat mainly low-Ⓖ foods and food combinations, with occasional medium-Ⓖ foods. High-Ⓖ foods are probably more frustrating than they're worth. All in all, that's certainly the fastest way to lose weight and gain energy.

And gaining energy is only one of the beneficial side effects of fatburning. In the next chapter we get a taster of many more.

- The Holford Diet reduces your appetite because it stabilises your blood sugar levels so you don't get hungry.

- Sugar cravings take no more than seven days to cure. After that, you'll find that your food cravings will virtually vanish.

- As long as you don't exceed 40 🅖🅛 a day you can eat anything. However, you can eat much more of the best low-🅖🅛 foods so you won't go hungry. Either way, you lose weight.

6

Better by Design

With most diets, you will probably experience side effects when you've been following the regime for some time. On very high-protein diets, these may be constipation or bad breath. On low-fat diets, they can include problems with skin or hair.

The only side effects you'll get on the Holford Diet are extra energy, better memory, clearer skin and resistance to degenerative diseases such as diabetes and cancer.

As I said at the start, weight loss itself is simply a side effect of optimum nutrition – the only kind the Holford Diet offers. Balancing your blood sugar and ensuring you're getting all the right nutrients will leave you in optimum health, slim, mentally fit and glowing with vitality.

Here's what you can expect:

- An end to fatigue. You'll never experience that weakened, lowered state that can creep up on you when you follow some low-calorie diets. Instead, you will wake up alert and clear-eyed – and, even better, get through the day without any energy slumps or exhaustion. This is the effect of cutting right back on stimulants and sugar, eating a low-Ⓖ diet, and supplementing nutrients known to boost energy.

- Younger, smoother skin. You'll discover the six secrets of having great skin, such as eating the right kinds of fruits (berries are tops), vegetables and omega-3 fats.

- A lowered homocysteine level. Having a high level of this toxic amino acid in the blood can indicate a real vulnerability to many degenerative diseases, from cancer to heart disease. The Holford Diet encourages the best defence: lots of green, leafy vegetables, supplemented with B vitamins and crucial minerals.

- No more blues. Being fat can be depressing, and it's now known that overweight people have lower levels of the 'happy' brain chemical serotonin. A low-Ⓖ diet emphasising high-quality carbohydrates will help you beat the blues by raising serotonin levels – and, of course, helping you shift the weight.

- A sharper mind. A diet rich in omega-3s, vitamins C and E and the nutrients and practices that will help balance blood sugar – such as the Holford Diet – will banish mental 'fogs', muzziness and poor memory, and significantly reduce any risk of developing Alzheimer's.

- Freedom from stress. Long-term stress causes too much of the hormone cortisol to circulate in the body, and cortisol can damage the brain. But cutting out sugar and stimulants can swiftly lower stress levels, and give your brain a chance to recover and rebuild itself.

- Lowered risk of disease. The Holford Diet, with its emphasis on balancing blood sugar, can clearly reduce your risk of getting diabetes. But it can also significantly decrease your risk of developing heart disease or strokes, cancer and arthritis.

We'll be looking at all these side benefits in detail in Part Five. For now, get set for the full lowdown on the Holford Diet's five simple principles.

References: Part One

1 MAFF National Food Survey, HMSO (1996); L. Henderson et al., 'The National Diet and Nutrition Survey', Trading Standards Office (2003); Department of Health, 'Health Survey for England' (data relating to 1995–2002), http://www.publications.doh.gov.uk/stats/trends1.htm

2 Health Survey for England, National Centre for Social Research (1998)

3 Department of Environment, Food and Rural Affairs (DEFRA) data on http://www.defra.gov.uk/farm/arable/sugar/sugar05.htm#consumption

4 J. Brand-Miller et al., 'Glycemic Index and Obesity', *American Journal of Clinical Nutrition* (2002), Vol 76 (suppl.), 281S–5S

5 D.B. Pawlak, J.A. Kushner, D.S. Ludwig, 'Effects of dietary glycaemic index on adiposity, glucose homoeostasis, and plasma lipids in animals', *Lancet* Vol 364 (9436) (August 2004), pp.778–85

6 M. Slabber et al., 'Effects of a low-insulin-response, energy restricted diet on weight loss and plasma insulin concentrations in hyperinsulinemic obese females', *American Journal of Clinical Nutrition* (1994), Vol 60(1), pp. 48–53

7 D. S. Ludwig, 'The Glycemic Index', *Journal of the American Medical Association*, Vol 287(18) (2002), pp. 2414–23

8 F. F. Samaha et al., 'A low-carbohydrate as compared with a low-fat diet in severe obesity', *New England Journal of Medicine*, Vol 348(21), pp. 2074–81

9 G. D. Foster et al., 'A randomized trial of a low-carbohydrate diet for obesity', *New England Journal of Medicine*, Vol 348(21) (2003), pp. 2082–90

10 D. M. Bravata et al., 'Efficacy and safety of low-carbohydrate diets: a systematic review', *Journal of the American Medical Association*, Vol 289(14) (2003), pp. 1837–50

11 H. Hull, 'The Effect of Food Combining on Weight Loss', ION research project (1997)

12 A. L. Gittleman, *Beyond Pritikin*, Bantam (1996), revised

13 M. Appelbaum, 'Influences of level of energy intake on energy expenditure in man', reported in *Dieting Makes You Fat*, G. Cannon and H. Einzig, Simon and Schuster (1985)

14 R. Leibel et al., 'Changes in energy expenditure resulting from altered body weight', *New England Journal of Medicine*, Vol 332 (1995), pp. 621–8

15 M. and A. Wynn, 'How dieting can damage your health', *Which? Way to Health* (February 1995), pp. 22–4

16 M. H. Pitler et al., 'Randomized, double-blind trial of chitosan for body weight reduction', *European Journal of Clinical Nutrition*, Vol 53 (1999), pp. 379–81

17 E. Wuolijoki et al., 'Decrease in serum LDL cholesterol with microcrystalline chitosan', *Methods and Findings in Experimental and Clinical Pharmacology*, Vol 21(5) (1999), pp. 357–61.

18 S. C. Ho et al., 'In the absence of dietary surveillance, chitosan does not reduce plasma lipids or obesity in hypercholesterolaemic obese Asian subjects', *Singapore Medical Journal*, Vol 42 (2001), pp. 6–10

19 W. McArdle, *Medical Aspects of Clinical Nutrition*, Keats (1983)

20 P. Holford et al., ONUK Survey, (2004), Institute of Optimum Nutrition, London, www.ion.ac.uk

21 G. Reaven, 'Role of Insulin Resistance in Human Disease', *Diabetes*, Vol 37 (1988), pp. 1595–1607

22 *Pediatrics*, Vol 112(4) (2003), pp. 900–6

23 Wynn (op. cit.)

24 P. Maconaghie, 'A comparison of the metabolic diet with the Unislim diet for inducing weight loss', ION (1988)

PART TWO

Five Simple Principles

7

Step 1: Balance Your Blood Sugar

We've seen how the key to losing weight and increasing energy is stabilising your blood sugar and insulin response to food. Now I'm going to explain the dynamics of this process so it's crystal-clear why you are following the rules of this diet. The principles are remarkably simple, and this way of eating will become part of your daily routine very quickly.

There are four ways to stabilise your blood sugar:

- reduce the total amount of carbohydrates in your diet;
- choose low-glycemic-load (ⒼⓁ) carbohydrates;
- combine carbohydrates with protein; and
- cut back on stimulants and stress.

Sounds great, you're thinking, but how do I put it all into practice?

The lowdown on carbohydrates

I'm going to make it really easy. As far as carbohydrates are concerned there are only two rules:

Rule 1: Eat no more than 40 ⑬ a day.

Rule 2: At main meals, eat low-⑬ carbohydrates with protein-rich foods.

We've had a look at ⑬ in Part One. If a food is high-⑬, such as white bread, it will contain a lot of fast-releasing carbohydrate that will contribute to seesawing blood sugar and all the ills we've seen it leading to, such as weight gain, lethargy and insulin resistance. (Note that the figure of 40 ⑬ a day refers to what we *eat*; there's an extra of allowance of 5 ⑬ for drinks, or desserts and sweets, discussed in Part Three.)

Everything I'm going to tell you in this chapter is designed to reverse this process, stabilise your blood sugar, lower your insulin release, make you more responsive to the insulin you produce and turn you into a high-energy Fatburner. You'll feel better and the pounds will fall away. It's a win–win situation for you and your body.

So low-⑬ eating is vital for health. Now we need to find out more about this crucial scoring system.

What determines ⑬?

How a food is processed, prepared or cooked is a key element in the ⑬ of a food, and therefore in what it will do to your blood sugar.

In the figure opposite, you can see how blood sugar levels, followed by insulin, rise and fall after you eat spaghetti. As the blood glucose level rises the body produces insulin, and down it comes again.

The figure on page 92 shows what happens when you eat white bread. Notice that the blood sugar level not only peaks twice as high as with the pasta, but it also dips much lower. It's the peaks that damage your arteries, making them less respon-

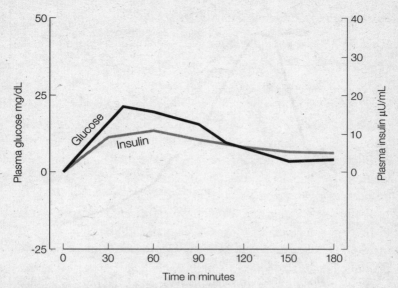

Glycemic response: spaghetti. Within 40 minutes of a person's eating spaghetti blood sugar levels are at a maximum. The body releases insulin to help get the glucose out of the blood and into body cells. Two hours later both blood glucose and insulin levels have returned to normal.

sive to insulin, and the troughs that leave you tired, sleepy and craving carbohydrates or stimulants. Again, you can see a massive increase in insulin release. In fact, compared with levels for spaghetti, four times as much insulin was produced in the first two hours after eating that bread!

What's fascinating is that this particular bread and spaghetti were made from the same flour, using the same amount.[1] So the only difference is in the processing. Bread rises when you feed yeast with sugar, and it is then baked for some time. Pasta is just wheat, and perhaps some egg. It has no yeast or sugar and it isn't cooked so long.

It's obvious that this small difference in preparation makes a big difference in blood sugar response, and hence in how

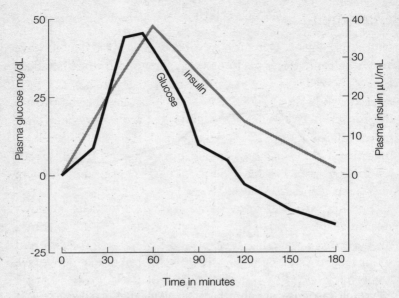

Glycemic response: bread. Within 40 minutes of a person's eating bread blood sugar levels are almost double those seen with spaghetti. The body produces more than three times as much insulin to bring blood glucose levels under control. The body overreacts and blood glucose goes to low, leading to strong cravings for something sweet or a stimulant such as caffeine peaking three hours later.

much weight you put on. That's why I recommend that you eat very little bread, but you certainly don't need to give up pasta, especially if it's wholewheat as opposed to refined.

Harking back to Rule 2, above, it's also important *how* you eat your low-ⒼⓁ carbs. I'm going to recommend that you eat some fat and protein with your carbohydrate because this will lessen its low-ⒼⓁ score even further.

We'll be looking at the kinds of combinations that work best to lower your blood sugar in a while. But, for now, let's stick to the ⒼⓁ scenario, exploring which carbohydrates you can eat lots of and which you should probably avoid.

Enter the GI

It was the discovery that even quite similar foods could have very different effects on blood sugar that led to the classification of foods as slow- or fast-releasing carbohydrates. The fast-releasing foods include white bread, which as we saw above are like rocket fuel, releasing their glucose in a sudden burst. They give a quick shot of energy with a rapid burnout. Slow-releasing carbohydrates such as wholewheat spaghetti supply steadier energy over a longer period of time, and thus help in balancing blood sugar levels.

But how do you know what is fast- and what is slow-releasing? This is where the GI – the glycemic index – comes in. The GI is a scale that compares the levels to which different foods raise your blood sugar with the effect of pure glucose (see below). It is also key in determining a food's **GL**.

To discover a food's GI, a portion of it providing 50g of carbohydrate is eaten, and the effect on the person's blood sugar over a three-hour period is compared with the effect

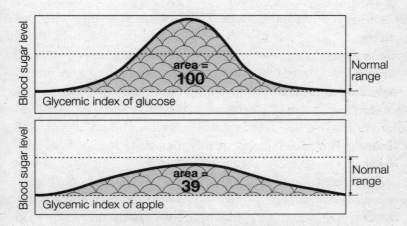

Measuring the glycemic index of a food

of eating 50g of the 'reference' food, glucose. Glucose is the fastest-releasing carbohydrate, because it requires no digestion.

In the diagram on page 93, the curve created by eating 50g of glucose is given a value of 100. If another food raises blood sugar level significantly, and for some time, the area under the curve made by glucose is bigger. Conversely, if a food hardly raises blood glucose levels at all, and only for a short time, the area under the curve is smaller. The amount of food tested obviously affects how high the blood sugar level will go.

Below you can see the GI for a variety of foods. As a general rule, a high GI score indicates the ones to avoid; a low GI score, the ones to eat.

As you can see, apples and oats are slow-releasing, while raisins and puffed-rice cereal are fast.

Glycemic index of common foods

Sugars		**Kiwi fruit**	53
Maltose	105	Banana	52
Glucose	100	Grapes	46
Honey	55	Orange	42
Sucrose (sugar)	68	Strawberries	40
Lactose	46	Raspberries	40
Fructose (fruit sugar)	19	Plum	39
Xylitol	8	Apple	38
		Pear	38
Fruit		Grapefruit	25
Dates	103	Cherries	22
Watermelon	72		
Pineapple	59	**Grains and grain products**	
Melon	65	French baguette	95
Raisins	64	White rice	72

Bagel	72
Wholemeal bread	71
White bread	70
Crumpet	69
Ryvita	64
Pastry	59
Basmati rice	58
Wholegrain rye bread	58
Brown basmati long-grain rice	47
Brown rice	55
Instant noodles	47
Wholegrain wheat bread	46
White spaghetti	40
Wholemeal spaghetti	37
Barley	26

Cereals

Puffed rice	82
Cornflakes	81
Shredded wheat	75
Weetabix	70
Kellogg's Special K	69
Porridge oats	58
Muesli	55
Kellogg's All-Bran	42

Pulses

Baked beans	48
Chickpeas	42
Black-eyed beans	42
Haricot beans	38
Butter beans	36
Lentils	29
Kidney beans	28
Soya beans	14

Dairy products/substitutes

Ice cream	61
Yoghurt	36
Skimmed milk	32
Whole milk	27

Vegetables

Parsnip (cooked)	97
Potato (baked)	85
French fries	75
Beetroot (cooked)	64
Sweet potato	61
Potato (new, boiled)	57
Sweetcorn	54
Peas	48
Carrot	47

Snacks and drinks

Lucozade	95
Jellybeans	80
Fanta	68
Squash (diluted)	66
Corn chips	63
Muesli bar	61
Potato crisps	54
Orange juice	50
Mars Bar	49
Chocolate bar	49
Apple juice	40
Peanuts	14

So much for GI. But what's the inside story on what makes one food fast-releasing and another slow? There are two main factors.

The first is how 'complex' the carbohydrate is. Below is a diagram of the chemical structure of glucose, regular white sugar and oats. You don't need to be a scientist to see that oats are more complex than sugar and sugar is more complex than glucose. All it means it that there's more *to* them.

Since the body can use only glucose for fuel, the sugar pictured – sucrose – has to be chopped in two to release the glucose. When you eat sugar, an enzyme released in the gut does this job for you and before long the glucose is whizzing around your bloodstream.

Oats are more complex than glucose. Oats need digesting into single glucose units, which takes time and slows down the release of its sugars. This sugar, which is a molecule of glucose and fructose, is slower in turn than a glucose molecule, which needs no digesting and directly enters the bloodstream.

The carbohydrate in oats, however, needs a lot of digesting into smaller and smaller units in the digestive tract before the glucose is released into the blood. This takes longer, so you don't get such a massive and immediate blood sugar rise.

Cooking some foods affects the release rate by 'pre-digesting' the carbs they contain. That's why the more you cook a carbohydrate food the faster-releasing it gets. Take potatoes. A baked potato, with a GI score of 85, is worse than a boiled potato, which has a GI of 57. Oats, however, are an exception. There's little difference between porridge and oat flakes eaten cold. This is largely because the cooking time is very short – you are really rehydrating rather than cooking.

Another factor that slows down the release of carbohydrate in food is fibre. Fibre is an indigestible carbohydrate, and generally, the more fibre a food contains, the slower is the breakdown of carbohydrate. This is doubly true for foods that contain soluble fibre such as oats. (We'll be looking at fibre in more depth below.)

Sugars – and sugars

And there's one more important thing you need to know. Not all simple sugars raise your blood sugar level. In the diagram overleaf you can see the chemical structure of lactose (milk sugar), sucrose (white sugar) and maltose (grain sugar or malt). The body can use only glucose for energy. So, once the glucose is removed from lactose you're left with galactose, and once the glucose is removed from sucrose you're left with fructose. What happens to fructose and galactose, shown in grey? The answer is they go to your liver, where they can be converted into glucose. But this takes time, so they're classed as slow-releasing.

Now look at the GI score of glucose, sucrose and fructose on page 94. As you would expect, glucose is the fastest (100),

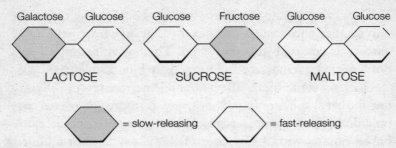

Galactose Glucose   Glucose Fructose   Glucose Glucose

LACTOSE   SUCROSE   MALTOSE

= slow-releasing   = fast-releasing

Lactose (milk sugar) versus sucrose (white sugar) versus maltose (grain sugar or malt). Galactose and fructose (shown in grey) are slow-releasing sugars while glucose is fast. Hence lactose and sucrose are much slower-releasing than maltose, a grain sugar (malt) which is quickly digested into two glucose molecules.

fructose the slowest (19) and sucrose – a combination of glucose and fructose – is in the middle (68). You'll also notice that maltose is as fast as glucose, and honey isn't far off, at 55. That's because 'malt', the sugar, is naturally present in grains and artificially added to things such as cereals and breads – as malted wheat, for example. As you can see from the figure above, malt is just two glucose molecules. It needs virtually no digestion. Most honey is basically glucose (also called dextrose, or grape sugar since it's also found in grapes), especially commercial honey which is heated to clean out impurities and make it easier to pack into jars.

Now have a look at dairy products. You'd expect things such as ice cream to be high-GI. But it isn't that high. It scores 61. This is because lactose is quite slow-releasing. (Be aware, though, that poor-quality ice creams have added glucose.) Milk and yoghurt score lower still (27–36).

Looking at fruits, even these can be fast- or slow-releasing. Not all contain fructose. Dates, for example, contain mainly glucose. Grapes and bananas are also high, while apples and

berries are mainly fructose. Even better than fructose is a natural sugar called *xylitol*, which is particularly high in plums.
This is the reason plums have a low GI score. Xylitol has less
than half the GI score of fructose and a tenth of the GI score
of sugar, and is highly preferable to any artificial sweetener.
Hence 10 teaspoons of xylitol, which tastes just as good, has the
same effect on your blood sugar as one teaspoon of regular
sugar. I use only xylitol as a sweetener and never use sugar.

The GI score of a food is very useful, but there's one problem. Compare carrots with chocolate, or watermelon with
French fries. Why do they have such similar scores? Aren't carrots supposed to be good for you? You'd absolutely right. Aside
from the vitamins and other important nutrients they contain,
a carrot or a slice of watermelon contains comparatively little
carbohydrate. In fact, you'd have to eat two large carrots to get
the same amount of carbohydrate, and the same effect on your
weight, as four pieces of chocolate. The chances are you'll eat
a lot more than four pieces of chocolate and a lot less than two
carrots. Similarly, watermelon has a high GI score but a low
ⒼⓁ. This kind of inconsistency is why the GI is a bit misleading.

It's the ⒼⓁ that counts

This is where ⒼⓁ comes in – the best way of telling how much
weight you'll gain from a food. It's a simple calculation, taking
into account both the amount of carbohydrate in a food (the
quantity) and its GI (the quality).

To get a food's ⒼⓁ, you just multiply its GI by the amount of
carbohydrate it contains (the exact formula is given in
Appendix 2). The result will tell you exactly what a given serving of a food does to your blood sugar. I've worked out the ⒼⓁ
of literally hundreds of foods for you and you can find my ⒼⓁ
index on pages 434–50.

The chart below shows a number of high- and low-Ⓖ foods. The Ⓖ of the quantities listed is 10 Ⓖ – so, for example, two entire punnets of strawberries have the same Ⓖ as two dates.

Ⓖ scores of common foods

Low-Ⓖ foods	High-Ⓖ foods
4 small cans tomato juice	1 small can cranberry juice drink
2 slices wholegrain rye bread	1 slice white bread
2 large punnets of strawberries	2 dates
Large bowl peanuts	Packet of crisps
Carton orange juice	Glass of Lucozade
3 bowls muesli (sugar-free)	1 bowl cornflakes

As the golden rule of the Holford Diet is to eat no more than 40 Ⓖ a day, it's obvious that if you choose high-Ⓖ foods you won't be eating much. You could lose weight this way, but that's not what I want you to do.

It's infinitely more satisfying for you to eat low-Ⓖ carbohydrates. You'll be able to eat more, experiment with the recipes more and generally enjoy your food (remember how that feels?). Let me make this real for you by showing you, on the chart opposite, a typical day in a Fatburner's diet versus a typical diet. Ⓖs are shown for each food.

Take a good look at the food on the left. Imagine you ate that breakfast, rather than the one on the right. It would definitely be more filling, wouldn't it? But it's not just that: by eating it, you'd have cut your propensity to turn glucose into fat by almost a third! The great news about eating the Ⓖ way is that you can actually eat more food *and* lose more weight. And it's all delicious.

Holford daily diet	GL	Average daily diet	GL
Breakfast		*Breakfast*	
A bowl of porridge (30g)	2	A bowl of cornflakes	21
Half a grated apple	3	Banana	12
Small tub of yoghurt	2	Milk	2
Milk	2		35
	9		
a.m. snack		*a.m. snack*	
Punnet of strawberries	1	Mars Bar	26
Lunch		*Lunch*	
Substantial tuna salad,		Tuna salad baguette	15
3 oatcakes	11		
p.m. snack		*p.m. snack*	
Pear + handful of peanuts	4	packet of crisps	11
Dinner		*Dinner*	
Tomato soup, salmon,		Pizza with parmesan	
sweetcorn and green beans	12	cheese and tomato	
		sauce, plus salad	23
GOOD DAY TOTAL GL	37	**BAD DAY TOTAL GL**	110

Let's see what that means in real terms. All the meals below
have identical GL scores, and identical effects on your blood
sugar.

For breakfast you could have:

Either	*Or*
Scrambled egg on rye toast	Fruit and yoghurt smoothie

As a snack you could have:

Either	*Or*
Hummus with crudités	Oatcakes with peanut butter

For lunch or dinner you could have:

Either	*Or*
Trout with puy lentils and roasted tomatoes	Chicken fajitas with salsa and salad

It doesn't look much like hard work, does it? And this is a mere taster. I'm going to give you many mouthwatering recipes and menus ranging from the simple to the elegant, all designed to keep you going at 40 Ⓖ a day. Between these and your own 'freestyle' choices using the complete GL food chart on pages 434–50, you'll soon learn which carbohydrates to go for, while your body unlearns how to store glucose as fat.

Before we run through the best low-Ⓖ foods, I'd like to explain in depth the two important qualities of food that lower Ⓖ: fibre, and combining protein with carbohydrate.

The fibre factor

There's one kind of carbohydrate that's neither slow- nor fast-releasing. This is fibre – all the parts of plants that digestive enzymes cannot break down (although some is digested by bacteria in the colon). While it can't be digested, it does serve a purpose. When you eat a food high in fibre, it tends to slow down the release of sugars in the food. And that, as far as weight control is concerned, is good news.

High-fibre diets are definitely recommended for a variety of general health reasons. People who eat more fibre don't usually suffer from constipation, and have a lower risk of getting bowel cancer, diabetes or certain kinds of bowel disease. As it is a natural constituent of fruits, vegetables, lentils, beans and wholegrains, there should be no need to add extra fibre if you're eating these foods. Fibre is calorie-free and there is little doubt that a diet high in naturally occurring fibre is more filling. After all, which would you find easier to eat: two biscuits, or a pound of carrots?

One of the main reasons why high-fibre foods are more satisfying is that fibre absorbs water, so they become bulkier in the gut. About 10 litres of digestive juices are released every day into the digestive tract, so a food's capability for absorbing this water would make a big difference to how bulky the food would become. Wheat fibre, as in bran, is not very absorbent compared with some vegetable fibres. Placed in water, it will swell to 10 times its original volume. The fibre from the Japanese konjac plant, however, swells to 100 times its volume! Konjac fibre is given to diabetics in Japan because it helps stabilise blood sugar by 'slow-releasing' any eaten carbohydrates.

Soluble or insoluble?

There are two primary kinds of fibre in food: soluble and insoluble. Many foods contain both. Insoluble fibre bulks up faecal content and can 'brush' the gut like a broom, preventing constipation. Soluble fibre is different, dissolving in the gut to form a jelly-like substance. This kind of fibre slows down the release of glucose into the bloodstream.

Whole cereal grains contain both kinds of fibre and will slow down glucose release the most, whereas ground fibre (as is found in wholemeal bread) has little effect. Fruit and vegetable juices are devoid of fibre, and that's why the sugars they contain are so fast-releasing.

The soluble fibre found in beans, lentils and oats is particularly effective at slowing down the digestion of food and thus the blood sugar response. Insoluble fibre makes you feel full immediately after eating, while soluble fibre reduces appetite nine or more hours later. This could be down to its effect on glucose in the bloodstream, but, whatever the case, it makes food more satisfying in the longer term.[2] There are quite a few different kinds of fibre in these two categories, but suffice to say that it's important to eat unprocessed wholefoods to get the most fibre you possibly can.

King of fibres

Of the fibres in grains, oat fibre is the best at controlling blood sugar and is therefore included in the Holford Diet.[3] Some sources of soluble fibre used therapeutically to help with digestion, diabetes and weight loss are even better, however. These include psyllium husks (available from health-food shops) and konjac fibre, which I mentioned above (available by mail order – see pages 479–80 in Resources). The konjac plant is rich in a soluble fibre called glucomannan, and this has been found to be the most effective at controlling blood sugar.

As such, it's a brilliant aid for healthy weight loss. Two studies, one in Japan[4] and one in the US,[5] reported an additional 1lb weight loss a week when patients took 3g of glucomannan a day. At ION, we decided to put glucomannan to the test by giving 3g a day to 10 overweight people over a three-month period.[6] None made any apparent change to their diet or exercise regime. Nine completed the trial, with an average weight loss of 6lb 10oz each, thus confirming the usefulness of this unique fibre.

> ### TOP TIP
>
> Taking 5g (3 capsules) of konjac extract before each meal can halve the ⑥ score and fill you up so you eat less. Always take them with a large glass of water. The glucomannan it contains is at least 50 times more effective than bran.

Be aware that, thanks to a quirk in a new food law, glucomannan is no longer allowed to be sold in the UK. However, konjac root extract is. Konjac extract contains about 60 per cent glucomannan, so a daily intake of 5g would be equivalent to 3g of glucomannan.

The power of protein

We've concentrated primarily on carbohydrates so far. But you'll be eating proteins and fats as well, and the balance of these with carbohydrates in each meal makes a big difference to blood sugar balance and fatburning efficiency.

Barry Sears, author of *Enter the Zone*, first made it widely known that combining protein-rich foods with slow-releasing carbohydrates helps to programme you to burn fat. Remember how high insulin is bad news, and high glucagon (discussed earlier on pages 59–61) is good news as far as fatburning is concerned? Well, protein foods tend to trigger a small and equal release of both insulin and glucagons – which happens to be the ideal. Carbohydrates, especially fast-releasing carbohydrates such as cakes and sweets, trigger a substantial release of insulin with little or no glucagon response. Eating fat has little direct effect on either insulin or glucagon. The relative effects of each combination are shown overleaf:

Effects of protein, carbohydrate and fat on insulin and glucagon

Food eaten	Insulin level	Glucagon level
Carbohydrate only	+++++	No change
Protein only	++	++
Fat only	No change	No change
Carbohydrate and fat	++++	No change
Protein and fat	++	++
High protein and low-🄶🄻 carbohydrate	++	+
High-🄶🄻 carbohydrate and low protein	++++++++	+
Low-🄶🄻 carbohydrate and medium protein	+++	++

From this research, you can see that the best three combinations are protein only, or protein and fat, or low-🄶🄻 carbohydrates and medium-protein. As we've seen, the trouble with a high-protein and fat diet is that it isn't good for your health. It's also very restrictive. That's why the best all-round diet for consistent and easily maintained weight loss, with the lowest boredom factor, is to eat low-🄶🄻 carbohydrates, plus protein. It's great for your health and equally effective for your waistline.

How much protein?

Very high-protein diets have proved effective in weight control, partly because they help to hinder the body in its turning of food into fat and also because you eat less on them. But a lot of the weight loss is water. This is partly because when you starve the body of glucose it breaks down stores of glucose called glycogen, which is stored with water. The other reason is that, when you eat too much protein without enough carbohydrates, ketones are produced. These are toxic, and the body tries hard to get rid of them in urine, which contributes to the fluid weight loss. But any pounds of water lost will come back.

While we all need something in the region of 40g of protein a day, eating above 80g a day over the long term will boost your risk of developing osteoporosis, because protein is acidic and can deplete the bones of calcium. It also stresses the kidneys. If the protein source is beef or dairy produce, this may increase risk of breast or prostate cancer. Also, if a person chooses meat as their main source of protein, their diet will inevitably become high in saturated fat, potentially increasing the risk of heart disease. There's not much point being thin and dead!

Best ratio for fatburning

On a short-term basis, such as 30 days up to three months, increasing your protein intake to between 60 and 75g a day and focusing on fish, chicken and vegetarian sources can help restore blood sugar control[7] and boost fatburning. For this reason the Holford Diet provides a greater proportion of calories from protein than the average diet – 25 per cent of calories over a norm of 17 per cent – to control blood sugar balance and reduce insulin resistance. After that period, the protein percentage drops to 20 per cent of calories to maintain fatburning. Once you've reached your goal and need only to maintain your weight and blood sugar balance over the long term, the ideal amount of protein would be 15 to 20 per cent of calories.

But you won't have to mess about with calorie-counting, as this isn't that kind of diet. So exactly what all this means in terms of the food you eat is explained simply and clearly in Part Three. I'll tell you exactly what to do. For now, check out the table overleaf showing the ideal balance of proteins, carbs and fats.

The perfect balance

	Protein	Carbohydrate	Fat
Average diet	17%	48%	35%
Holford Diet (first 30 days up to three months)	25%	50%	25%
Holford Diet (maintenance)	15–20%	55–60%	25%

Since we all need to eat some protein, some carbohydrates and the right kind of fats, the best combination is to eat low-ⒼⓁ carbohydrate foods that are also rich in protein. Beans and lentils are an example. People who live in countries whose diets contain these are consistently thinner and healthier.

The easiest and healthiest way to achieve this perfect balance is to eat the equivalent of 60g of protein and 120g of low-ⒼⓁ carbohydrate in a day, and to divide it evenly between each meal, that is, 20g of protein and roughly 40g of carbohydrate, at breakfast, lunch and dinner. You needn't worry too much about the maths: the recipes will do this for you. (Details on the quantity and quality of fats to be eaten are given in the next chapter.) Roughly two-thirds of your carbohydrates need to come from vegetables and fruit and one-third from things such as grains and more 'starchy' vegetables.

The simplest way to visualise your meals, as far as lunch and dinner are concerned, is to eat any one of the protein-rich foods shown below, with an equivalent-sized serving of any carbohydrate-rich food, plus two servings of vegetables. Remember the plate model from page 79?

To maximise fatburning, you will probably be eating more protein-rich foods in relation to carbohydrate-rich foods than you are used to, as well as more fresh fruit and veg. The amount of carbohydrate or protein provided by non-starchy vegetables (broccoli, kale, cabbage, peas, spinach, carrots and so on) is small, so these can be eaten relatively freely on the Holford Diet. Aim, too, for two pieces of low-🟢 fruit a day.

Fatburning food combinations

(A more comprehensive list of foods is given on pages 215–21.)

Here are a few examples:

PROTEIN	CARBOHYDRATE	VEGETABLES
Poached salmon	on brown basmati rice	with a green salad
Marinated tofu	on wholewheat pasta	with steam-fried vegetables
Grilled chicken breast	with boiled new potatoes	with steamed runner beans
Cottage cheese	on oatcakes/rye bread	with broccoli and tomato salad

The Holford Diet snacks are also great protein/carb combinations. For instance, eating a few almonds or pumpkin seeds, high in essential fats and protein, at the same time as low-🟢 fruit can further slow the effect of fruit sugar on your blood sugar. But remember: fruits such as apples and strawberries have a low 🟢, so you are already doing brilliantly.

For breakfast, you can achieve the right balance and amount of protein and low-🟢 carbohydrate by, for example, eating a cup of oat flakes with some seeds, some berries and either skimmed milk or soya milk, if you're allergic to milk.

Above all, don't worry about having to calculate all this – the lowdown in Part Three and menus and recipes in Part Four make it remarkably easy.

We've now looked in depth at how to pinpoint the best carbohydrates, and how to combine them, for the most efficient fatburning. But what if you, like millions of others, are in the grip of caffeine and chocolate? Dealing with these very twenty-first-century addictions is essential to balancing your blood sugar – and, as you'll see, surprisingly painless.

Are you addicted to sugar or stimulants?

Ever had an 'I'd kill for a muffin' moment? Or perhaps it was a double espresso, a bar of chocolate, even a piece of toast. Whatever the object of your desire, the urge to get at it probably felt overwhelming. Yet this is a perfectly normal reaction to a blood sugar low.

It is virtually impossible to resist temptation when you're in the middle of a blood sugar crash. One of the reasons sugar is so addictive is that it can cause a release of the body's own 'feel-good' chemicals, opioids and dopamine.

Animals can become addicted to sugar and show all the tell-tale withdrawal symptoms, including the shakes, when deprived, according to research by Dr Bartley Hoebel at Princeton University in the US. This is because the more you overstimulate the release of dopamine, the more insensitive you become to its effects. In a sense you are becoming 'dopamine-resistant' or addicted to your body's own natural highs. This, in turn, upsets your blood sugar levels and ability to control your weight.

Dr Candace Pert, research professor in the physiology and biophysics department at Georgetown University Medical Center in Washington, DC, says, 'I consider sugar to be a drug, a highly purified plant product that can become addictive. Relying on an artificial form of glucose – sugar – to give us a quick pick-me-up is analogous to, if not as dangerous as, shooting heroin.'[8] Dr Pert is among the chief scientists who discovered the central role endorphins play in addiction. There's certainly plenty of research out there to support her view.[9]

Sugar and high-Ⓖ carbs aren't the only culprits in the case. Stimulants, too, promote the brain's 'feelgood' chemicals. Remember the effect of our inbuilt fight-or-flight mechanism? It's as if we humans have a 'fifth gear' for emergencies.

In times of stress, the adrenal glands release a combination of hormones, including dopamine and adrenalin, that break down stores of glucose and raise your blood sugar levels, tapping into your energy reserves to provide instant fuel to deal with the apparent danger. Of course, today's 'emergencies' have nothing to do with woolly mammoths on the rampage but take place mainly inside our heads – overdrafts, relationships, parking tickets and so on. But we still produce adrenalin, and that still raises blood sugar levels.

Stimulants have the same effect, stirring up adrenalin and dopamine. So consuming nicotine or caffeine in colas, coffee, tea, cigarettes and chocolate, added to the stresses of twenty-first-century life, can seriously mess with your blood sugar.

So why do we do it? It's simply because millions of us are caught in the vicious cycle of blood sugar highs and lows already, and feel exhausted much of the time. Stimulants seem to promise instant energy – while, of course, making the problem worse.

We may be eating fast-releasing carbohydrates, devoid of vitamins and minerals. We may be drinking two or three coffees before noon just to deal with our morning weariness. We 'learn' how to cope with the rebound blood sugar low after a meal by having a coffee. If we haven't eaten for two hours, we go for another coffee. And, when we drag ourselves home after a hard day's work, we may be drinking still more just to stay awake.

You may feel that coffee, which speeds up the metabolism, is not only keeping you going but helping with weight loss. The irony is that in the not-so-long term it contributes to weight gain by fuelling blood sugar imbalance. According to research from Holland by Dr Paul Smits and colleagues at the University of Nijmegen, a single shot of caffeine can raise adrenalin fivefold, thus raising blood glucose, and decrease insulin sensitivity by 15 per cent. This means you become more resistant to insulin and more likely to turn glucose into fat.[10]

A cup of chaos

Stimulants are addictive. That's why you need more and more to keep you going. Before long, one cup of coffee and the odd cigarette becomes six or more lattes, mochaccinos or filter coffees and a pack of cigarettes. By the time you reach this stage, you can't even get going in the morning without a stimulant. The combination of coffee, tea or nicotine with stress, high-GI foods and sugar means you lose your blood sugar control and wake up each morning with low blood sugar levels and not enough adrenalin to kick-start your day. So you adopt one of two strategies:

● You reluctantly crawl out of bed on remote control and head for the kettle, make yourself a strong cup of tea or coffee, light up a cigarette or have some fast-releasing sugar in the form of toast, with some sugar on it called jam. Up go your blood sugar and adrenalin levels and you start to feel normal.

Or ...

● You lie in bed and start to think about all the things that have gone wrong, could go wrong, will go wrong. You start to worry about everything you've got to do, haven't done and should have done. About 10 minutes of this gets enough adrenalin pumping to get you out of bed.

One of the most seductive aspects of coffee is that it actually seems to make you feel better, more energised and alert. But, wondered Dr Peter Rogers, a psychologist at Bristol University, does coffee actually increase your energy and mental performance, or just relieve the symptoms of withdrawal? When he researched this he found that, after that sacred morning cup of coffee, coffee drinkers don't feel any better than people who never drink coffee. Coffee drinkers just feel better than they did when they woke up.[11] In other words, drinking coffee relieves the symptoms of withdrawal from coffee. And in the middle sits Starbucks, and all the other coffee franchises, making a buck or two! It's addictive.

Caffeine blocks the receptors for a brain chemical called *adenosine*, whose function is to stop the release of the motivating neurotransmitters dopamine and adrenalin. With less adenosine activity, levels of dopamine and adrenalin increase, as does alertness and motivation. Peak concentration occurs 30 to 60 minutes after you down that cup.

The more caffeine you consume, the more your body and brain become insensitive to their own natural stimulants, dopamine and adrenalin. You then need more stimulants to feel normal, and keep pushing the body to produce more dopamine and adrenalin. The net result is adrenal exhaustion – an inability to produce these important chemicals of motivation and communication. Apathy, depression, exhaustion and an inability to cope set in.

Coffee isn't, of course, the only source of caffeine. There's as much in a strong cup of tea as a regular cup of coffee. Caffeine is also the active ingredient in most colas and energy drinks such as Red Bull, which sold more than 100 million cans in 2003 alone. Chocolate and green tea also contain caffeine, although in much smaller amounts. Have a look at the chart overleaf.

How much caffeine?

Product	Caffeine content
Coca-Cola Classic 350ml (12fl oz)	46mg
Diet Coke 350ml (12fl oz)	46mg
Red Bull	80mg
Hot cocoa 150ml (5fl oz)	10mg
Coffee, instant 150ml (5fl oz)	40–105mg
Coffee, espresso, cappuccino, latte	30–50mg
Coffee, filter 150ml (5fl oz)	110–150mg
Coffee, Starbucks (grande)	500mg
Decaffeinated coffee 150ml (5fl oz)	0.3mg
Tea 150ml (5fl oz)	20–100mg
Green tea (5 fl oz)	20–30mg
Chocolate cake (1 slice)	20–30mg
Bittersweet chocolate 28g (1oz)	5–35mg
Pro Plus	50mg
PEP	30mg

And, if you add sugar to your coffee or drink a lot of cola, you'll exacerbate the effect of the caffeine on your blood sugar balance, and end up piling on even more weight.

That's why I recommend you cut right back on stimulants, including sugar, right at the start of the diet. If the very thought fills you with dread, and leaves you wildly wondering how you'll get to work without that morning cup, it's pretty certain you're addicted. But by quitting you'll be trading a dispiriting round of fatigue and sudden jolts to the system for feeling energetic all day, every day.

Before you panic, let me say that this is not for life. What I'm asking you to do is go cold turkey: give up stimulants and sugar when you start on the diet and supplement programme, and stay off them completely for at least two weeks to a month. This will kick-start your metabolism. After that, you can reintroduce them in moderation if you want to.

Of course, the reason we react with horror to the thought of stopping stimulants is that we 'know' we'll feel terrible without them. We know this for a fact because it's the very symptoms of withdrawal – feeling tired, grumpy and foggy-headed – that make that cup of tea or cappuccino seem like manna from heaven. But, ten minutes later, you want another one.

Once your blood sugar and adrenalin levels are back to normal, however, you can take or leave these stimulants.

So if you follow the Holford Diet and take the supplements I recommend, going cold turkey may well turn out to be much easier than you thought. Nine out of ten people say, two weeks later, that they feel so good they just don't need stimulants any more. With their energy levels soaring, they just don't need the endless jolts to the system that used to punctuate their days.

The first step is to get real about your use of stimulants. This means completing the 'stimulant inventory' overleaf, for a week. Write down what you consume every day, and then add up your total at the end of the week. Be honest!

	Unit	Sun	Mon	Tue	Wed	Thu	Fri	Sat
Green tea	2 cups							
Tea	1 cup							
Coffee	1 cup							
Cola or caffeinated drinks	1 can							
Caffeine pills such as No-Doz, Excedrin, Dexatrim	1 pill							
Chocolate	2oz/57g (approx 1 bar)							

	Unit	Sun	Mon	Tue	Wed	Thu	Fri	Sat
Alcohol (units) Glass of wine is 1 Bottle of beer is ½ Shot of spirit is 1	unit							
Added sugar	1 tsp/5g							
Hidden sugar (see sugar content on ingredients list)	1 tsp/5g							
Cigarettes	1 cigarette							

Add up your total number of 'units'. The ideal is 5 or fewer per week. If you are having more than ten stimulant units a week, this is going to have an effect on your energy and weight.

Eating slow-releasing energy foods and taking energy-stabilising vitamins and minerals, which we'll be investigating in Part Three, will give you even energy levels, and the need for stimulants will evaporate. You'll look back on those bleary-eyed mornings and exhausted afternoons with wonder. As one Fat-burner volunteer quoted earlier said, 'One of the hardest, but best things about it was the insistence on giving up coffee and stimulants.' (She also lost 10lb in a month.)

Kicking the habit

How does the Holford Diet help you quit? Since all stimulants affect blood sugar levels, you can keep yours even by always having something substantial for breakfast, such as an oat-based, not too refined cereal; unsweetened live yoghurt with apple, ground sesame seeds and wheat germ; or an egg. You can snack frequently on fresh fruit, and twice a day add in a small handful of nuts or seeds.

Eating a highly alkaline-forming diet can reduce cravings for cigarettes and alcohol, so eat plenty of low-🄶🄻 fruit and fresh vegetables. These high-fibre foods also help to keep your blood sugar levels even, and you on an even keel. The worst thing you can do is go for hours without eating – but this isn't something I would ever recommend, anyway.

In this way, going cold turkey at the same time as starting the diet will simply not be the nightmare you imagine. I realise that giving up cigarettes might be a little more difficult than tossing out the beer, wine or coffee, but even that process will be significantly smoothed once your blood sugar steadies.

My diet will help stabilise your blood sugar and reduce your cravings. Meanwhile, let's look at the culprits.

Coffee contains three stimulants – caffeine, theobromine and theophylline. Although caffeine is the strongest, theophylline is known to disturb normal sleep patterns and theobromine has an effect similar to caffeine's, although it is present in much smaller amounts in coffee. So decaffeinated coffee isn't exactly stimulant-free.

As a nutritionist, I have seen many people cleared of minor health problems such as tiredness and headaches just by their cutting out their two or three coffees a day. After you quit, you may get withdrawal symptoms for up to three days. These reflect how addicted you've become. If you begin to feel perky and your health improves afterwards, that's a good indication that you're better off without coffee – and, in any case, I recommend having it only as a very occasional treat. The most popular alternatives are Teeccino, Caro Extra or Bambu (made with roasted chicory and malted barley), dandelion coffee (from Symingtons or Lanes) or herbal teas.

Tea is the great British addiction. As we've seen, a strong cup of tea contains as much caffeine as a weak cup of coffee and it is certainly addictive. Tea also contains tannin, which interferes with the absorption of vital minerals such as iron and zinc. Particularly addictive is Earl Grey tea, which contains an extra stimulant, bergamot. If you find you drink more than the occasional weak cuppa, it's time to stop. The best-tasting alternatives are Rooibosch tea (red bush tea) with milk, and herbal or fruit teas.

Chocolate bars are usually full of sugar, and cocoa, the active ingredient, provides significant quantities of the stimulant theobromine, also found in coffee. The action of theobromine is similar to caffeine's, though not as strong. Chocolate also contains small amounts of caffeine. So with an array of stimulants, plenty of sugar and a truly delicious taste and 'mouth feel', it's all too easy to become a chocoholic. If you stop eating it for a couple of weeks, and substitute fruit, and healthy 'sweets' from health-food shops that are sugar-free and the like, you will find yourself losing the craving.

Cola and **'energy' drinks** contain anything from 46 to 80mg of caffeine per can, as we saw in the chart above. These drinks are also often high in sugar and colourings and their net stimulant effect can be considerable. Check the ingredients list and stay away from drinks containing caffeine and chemical additives or colourings.

Cigarettes raise blood sugar levels by acting as a mild stimulant to the central nervous system. There is also evidence that smoking is linked to an increase in insulin resistance. In addition to disturbing blood sugar balance, cigarette smoking drains the body of vital nutrients and contributes to numerous other diseases such as cancer and heart disease. So, needless to say, cigarettes are a big no-no. If you are addicted to smoking, I can't recommend highly enough the benefits of quitting. Not only will it lower your risk of getting certain kinds of cancer and other diseases, but also it keeps you looking younger and feeling much better overall.

For confirmed smokers, I generally recommend stabilising blood sugar first with the diet. This will make quitting easier. Also, you will not get the rebound weight gain that often happens if you haven't solved the underlying issue for every smoker, which is blood sugar imbalance. I also recommend increasing your daily exercise during the time you quit smoking, which further boosts your metabolism and stops any rebound weight gain.

There are now a number of successful methods for quitting. On my website, you'll find a 'How to Quit Smoking' link. Following these steps will dramatically decrease your symptoms of withdrawal and increase your chances of success (see www.patrickholford.com and enter 'quit smoking' in the search box).

Alcohol is not strictly a stimulant, but is chemically very similar to sugar, and potentially very addictive. It's also high in calories. Drinking can suppress appetite but lead to cravings for more alcohol, so you can end up quaffing empty calories with no nutritional value. Worse, alcohol also destroys or prevents the absorption of many nutrients, including vitamins C and B complex, calcium, magnesium and zinc.

Alcohol can also make you fat. It's the most rapidly absorbed sugar, with one-fifth being absorbed directly through the stomach. It takes almost two hours to use up 10g of alcohol – the amount in half a pint of beer. It can be rapidly turned to fat by the action of insulin. With chronic use it converts into fat rather than glucose or glycogen and is stored in the liver. Alcohol also interferes with the liver's ability to break down amino acids and turn them into glucose when blood sugar levels are too low.

So, in this sense, alcohol messes up blood sugar and fat control, and regular drinkers tend to put on weight. Habitual drinking can damage the liver, leading to even further inability to control both blood sugar levels and weight. You'll achieve the best results on the Holford Diet by having no more than three small drinks a week, and preferably none at all for the first two weeks to a month.

The stress connection

Sugar and stimulants may not be the only factors playing merry hell with your blood sugar. Serious stress has a very similar effect. If you think you are suffering from it, you're not alone. Many people wake up in a state of anxiety, arrive at work stressed out from commuting, have to contend with a lot of stress at work and go home in a state of near-collapse. Unfortunately, a life of non-stop twenty-first-century stress takes its toll on your body's chemistry.

We've seen how stimulants trigger the release of adrenalin and cortisol, which prepare the body for action. Stress does this too. The flood of glucose this then releases for our use stimulates, in its turn, yet more hormones to take the glucose out of circulation. While adrenalin works fast and is gone fast, cortisol lingers. If you're stressed for weeks at a time, your cortisol level stays high, and this is bad news. High cortisol levels, the hallmark of the overstressed, make you even more insulin-resistant and even more prone to put on weight. Let me explain why.

Insulin puts glucose into storage, whereas adrenalin and cortisol rapidly raise the glucose supply to cells for fight or flight – partly by blocking insulin's fat-storing effect. That sounds like good news, at least in the short term. And it is. That's why high stress and stimulants, such as coffee, can keep you thin. But when the effect of insulin is blocked, the body simply produces more – and the more it produces, the more insulin-resistant you become. So, over the long term, stress can actually lead to weight gain.

How stressed are you?

Take a look at the symptoms below. If they sound familiar to you, then you know what I'm talking about. They suggest adrenal stress overload.

- finding it hard to get up in the morning
- feeling tired all the time

- craving certain foods
- anger, irritability, aggressiveness
- mood swings
- restlessness
- energy slump during the day
- regular feelings of weakness
- apathy
- depression
- feeling cold all the time

In a survey of patients visiting ION, 54 per cent had a high stress rating at their initial assessment. After six months of improved nutrition, substituting slow-releasing carbohydrates for sugar and stimulants, that figure had dropped to 28 per cent.

The amazing thing is that if you balance your blood sugar, it not only affects your weight, but also has wide-reaching benefits for your health, your mood and your ability to deal with the inevitable challenges of life. When you're stressed, even molehills seem like mountains. When your energy levels are good and your mind is clear, life immediately smoothes out and calms down. As Fatburner volunteers from *She* magazine agreed, 'Increased alertness was a significant benefit. By the third day, everybody felt well – alert on rising, and three of us (including me) were bounding about full of the joys of spring.'

The only way out of the prison of stress, sugar and stimulants is to reduce or avoid all forms of concentrated sweetness, tea, coffee, alcohol and cigarettes, and start eating foods that help to keep your blood sugar level stable. By changing to the right foods, backed up with specific nutritional supplements, most people feel an amazing improvement in energy within days.

That's why I recommend that you:

- avoid regular tea and coffee;

- stop eating chocolate (you can have some after two weeks to a month!);

- quit smoking;

- avoid regular alcohol and reduce your overall intake to three small glasses a week; and

- do what you can to avoid continuously high stress levels.

Remember, the very best way is to have *nothing* stimulating when you start the diet. That includes decaf coffee (the continuing taste of coffee doesn't help you break the habit).

After that, but *only if you have to*, you can drink the occasional cup of weak tea. But coffee, as I've indicated, pretty much has to go. Soon you'll find you can sail past coffee bars with not even a twinge of longing – and with a lot more energy than in the days you were chained to a cup.

As far as sugar is concerned, you'll have to be on the lookout. It comes in many disguises. Peruse food labels for glucose, dextrose and sucrose. Honey is also best avoided for those first two weeks. Fructose (fruit sugar) is somewhat better, but, even so, the emphasis over these two weeks is to get the sweetness you need by having wholefoods, such as fruit, instead of sugar on cereals or in desserts.

It's also a good idea to start cutting down the overall sweetness of what you eat. For example, you can add water to juice. Three oranges may have gone into a large glass of the juice. Would you eat that many whole fruits at one go? Even though oranges contain mainly fructose, there's *a lot* of it in pure juice. Dilute it by a third. You'll soon get used to it. After two weeks, you'll find your craving for sweetness is fading – and overall, you'll find it easy to keep going on the Holford Diet.

- Avoid sugar in its many disguises and foods that contain fast-releasing carbohydrates with a high-Ⓖ score (above 10 per serving).

- Eat foods that contain low-Ⓖ carbohydrates (below 10 per serving).

- Eat no more than 40 Ⓖ a day.

- Eat low-Ⓖ carbohydrates *with* protein-rich foods.

- Eat whole, unadulterated foods high in soluble fibre (beans, lentils, oats).

- Consider supplementing with konjac extract for the glucomannan it contains.

- Cut back on stimulants right at the start of the diet.

- Do what you can to avoid continuously high stress levels.

Part Three shows you how to do all this.

8

Step 2: Eat Good Fats and Avoid Bad Fats

It may seem counterintuitive, but some kinds of fats boost fat-burning. These are the essential fatty acids, or EFAs. So entrenched have we become in fat phobia and the promotion of low-fat diets that the role of EFAs in helping you to burn fat has gone largely unnoticed.

The original idea was that, since 1g of fat gives more calories (9 kcals) than 1g of protein or carbohydrate (approximately 4 kcals), the quickest way to cut calories was to cut fat. Theoretically, this should have been the best way to lose weight, if you believe conventional calorie theory. We now know this isn't true. Low-ⓖⓛ diets work better than low-fat diets, and the ⓖⓛ of your diet predicts weight gain much more accurately than the fat content of your diet.[12]

Go fish

But then we discovered there were essential fats (polyunsaturates) and non-essential fats (saturates). When you eat 100g of saturated fat, all your body can do is burn it for energy or store it as fat. On the other hand, when you eat 100g of the polyunsaturated fats from seeds, their oils or fatty fish, the brain and nerves use them, and they boost immunity, balance hormones, reduce inflammation and promote healthy skin. Only if there's any left will the body use EFAs for energy or to store as fat. In other words, one calorie of saturated fat has an entirely different effect on the body in terms of weight control and health than one calorie of polyunsaturated fat.

And it gets even better. Since you need essential fats, it should come as no surprise to find out that we have 'fat receptors' in the mouth. These register whether or not you've eaten what you need. We humans crave fat in the same way we crave sugar or protein. However, only when you eat the right fat – the essential kind – does your body stop craving that smooth, creamy texture. Not only are you satisfied, but you've just consumed a very special substance.

The omega-3 EFAs, found in flax and pumpkin seeds and oily coldwater fish such as mackerel, herring, salmon and tuna, keep extra weight at bay in a number of ways. They help make hormone-like substances called *prostaglandins* which help to control metabolism and fatburning. They also help to control and limit the potential damage of insulin resistance, by calming down the inflammatory effects of bursts of high glucose in the blood, which damages the arteries.

The omega-6 EFAs, found in hot-climate seeds such as sunflower and sesame, have similar benefits to the omega-3s, and are especially good for the skin and maintaining hormone balance, for example in combating PMS, but not so important for the brain.

The fat in meat and dairy produce, which is saturated fat, simply doesn't come near EFAs in the health stakes. (Luckily, the Holford Diet helps you reduce the amount of protein – and fat – you get from meat and dairy foods.) Worst of all fats, however, are the kind you find in processed and junk food or in deep-fried foods. These are called trans-fats and hydrogenated fats.

There is, however, an 'in-between' fat: mono-unsaturated, or omega-9, fat. Olive oil is a particularly rich source. While this is nowhere near as good for you as food sources of the omega-3 fats, it is also nowhere near as bad for you as saturated fat or trans-fats. A number of studies have found that if people switch from saturated to mono-unsaturated fats, this helps to stabilise blood sugar levels, improve insulin resistance and control diabetes.[13,14] This is good news, and a step in the right direction for fatburning.

My diet emphasises omega-rich foods and avoids trans-, hydrogenated and saturated fats as much as possible. Below you'll see the common food sources of these different kinds of fats. (Please note that most foods contain a mixture of fats, so some appear more than once, as they're rich in several kinds.)

Fat family	Good dietary sources
Omega-3 family	Fish, especially salmon, mackerel, herring, tuna and sardines; flax seeds, pumpkin seeds and walnuts; and their oils
Omega-6 family	Sunflower, sesame and pumpkin seeds and their oils; also safflower oil, corn oil, soya oil
Omega-9 family	Olive oil, almonds, walnuts
Saturated fat	Meat, dairy produce and most eggs (chicken fed flax seeds have more omega-3 fats in their eggs)
Trans- and hydrogenated fats	Deep-fried food, burned or browned fat, margarines, most processed meats (such as hamburgers, sausages), and most vegetarian meat substitutes (such as vegesausages)

As you can see from the figure below, modern times have seen big changes in our fat intake. From 1900 to 2000 there was a massive increase in overall fat intake – although we have started to eat less since the late 1980s – as well as a big increase in saturated fat and a decrease in the best fat of all, omega-3s. Consumption of the essential omega-6 fat has gone up, reflecting the switch from butter to margarine. However, this is slightly misleading because a lot of this 'polyunsaturated vegetable oil', which is what you find on the label, has been processed or

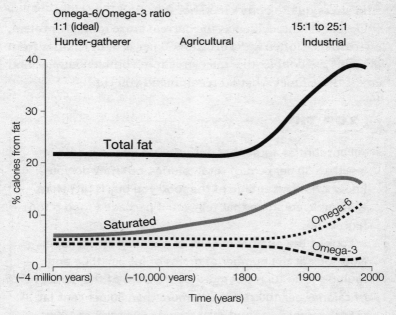

How fat intake has changed. In modern times total fat intake has increased. Saturated fat intake has increased, although it is now levelling off. Omega-6 fat intake has increased but this is slightly misleading because much of it is 'hydrogenated' vegetable oils, which act like saturated fats. Consumption of omega-3 fats, in fish and seeds, have gone down, leading to widespread deficiency.

Leaf and Weber, American Journal of Clinical Nutrition *1987*

'hydrogenated' in such a way that it's as bad for you as saturated fat, if not worse. More on this in a minute.

Say no to saturated fat

To lose weight, it is definitely desirable to cut down on saturated fat. Nowadays even the average child consumes over 700lb of saturated fat, the equivalent of 1,314 packets of lard, between the ages of 6 and 16. Eating excess fat is associated with obesity,[15] heart disease, cancer and diabetes, and it puts extra stress on the body's metabolism.

Despite all this evidence, the current craze for high-protein, low-carb diets often kicks off with 60 per cent of calories from fat! This is double the mainstream recommendations and almost three times what I'd recommend you eat.

TOP TIP

All authorities agree that our total fat intake should be less than 30 per cent of total calories, but how do you know what percentage of the food you buy is fat? Here is a simple equation that tells you if packaged food is too high in fat.

Look at the number of calories per 100g on the label. Now look at the number of grams of fat per 100g and multiply it by 10. Is this more than a third of the number of calories per 100g? If so, it's more than 30 per cent fat.

For example, yoghurt may provide 60 kcals per 100g. The fat content per 100g is 3.5g. Multiply by 10, giving you 35. Divide 35 by 60 (0.58). This means that more than 50 per cent of the calories in this yoghurt comes from fat.

Try this simple formula when you next go shopping.

Hydrogenated – the 'H' word

Just as bad for you as saturated fats are polyunsaturated fats that have been processed, fried or damaged. Remember, the essential fats are polyunsaturated fats, but once they are messed around they're as bad for you as saturated fats, if not worse. When the molecules of these essential fats are altered by food processing (called *hydrogenation*) or frying, they can no longer benefit the body and are called trans-fats. Frying or heating can also make them rancid or oxidised, which means they can set up a chain reaction of oxidation in the body, damaging body cells. Foods rich in trans-fats include:

- French fries
- hamburgers
- deep-fried fish burgers
- deep-fried chicken nuggets
- confectionery
- chocolate bars
- potato and corn chips/crisps
- biscuits
- doughnuts
- margarine
- mayonnaise
- most salad dressings

Unfortunately, many vegetarian processed foods are also high in these hydrogenated fats. Check the label on the vegeburger or vegetarian sausage packets. If the label includes 'partially hydrogenated vegetable oils', don't buy it.

Say yes to omega-3 fats

Most of us are deficient in omega-3s already. But, as we've seen, eating them is vital for health – hence the 'essential' in 'essential fatty acid'. And of course they carry a host of healthy benefits, not least of which is their ability to boost fatburning.

Let's take a closer look at how they help in this respect. In the figure below you can see how the body can make three kinds of prostaglandin – PG1, 2 and 3. PG1 and 3 are good for fatburning. PG2 is not. While omega-3 fats can make only the good PG3, the omega-6 fats can produce either the good PG1 or the bad PG2. People producing a lot of insulin because of blood sugar imbalance tend to produce more PG2. But there's a way to counteract this. Eating more omega-3s, which provide eicosapentaenoic acid or EPA, will help in turning their omega-6 fats into PG1.

I've listed a few of the health benefits of eating omega-3 fats. But there are even more. They reduce the risk of heart disease and of dying from a sudden heart attack by 50 per cent[16], and

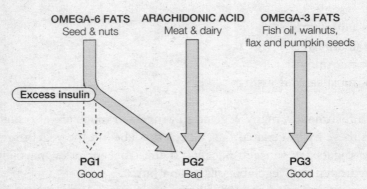

Too much insulin, a consequence of insulin resistance, encourages the formation of prostaglandins that promote inflammation, pain and swelling. Increased intake of omega-3 fats has the opposite effect, reducing pain and inflammation.

also halve your risk of ever suffering from Alzheimer's disease.[17] The moral of this story is that omega-3s are one of your best friends, not just for fatburning but for overall health. The Holford Diet specifically includes these essential fats in one of four ways:

BREAKFAST – A dessertspoon of seeds (half pumpkin, half flax is excellent, or you can mix in some sesame and sunflower too) with your breakfast cereal, yoghurt or Get Up & Go (see page 480 in Resources).

SNACKS – A dessertspoon of pumpkin seeds with fruit.

MAIN MEALS –A small serving of oily fish *or* a dessertspoon of pumpkin seeds on salad.

SALAD DRESSINGS – A dessertspoon of seed oil.

To achieve enough essential fats you need to pick *two* of any of these options each day.

I realise that, if you've spent years avoiding fat like the plague, this routine might jar at first. Yet the truth is that these essential fats clear up dry skin, stimulate your metabolism, boost brain function, protect your heart and strengthen your immune system. So in addition to losing weight more efficiently, you'll find that your skin and hair look better than ever, and that your mind and body are in great working order – with a little help from the omegas.

> ### TOP TIP
>
> A great way to cut calories is to have a substantial breakfast and dinner and a light snack lunch, with two small mid-morning and mid-afternoon snacks.

The quantity of fat in the Holford Diet, which amounts to a quarter of overall calories, is lower than that in the average diet, which provides about 35 per cent of calories as fat. But the biggest difference between the norm and the Holford Diet is not in the *quantity* but in the *quality* of fat. Eating in this way means that less than a third of the fat you eat is saturated, compared with two-thirds, as in the average diet.

The recipes in Part Four will take care of all this for you. The way you cook foods is also important. The best method is actually leaving the food raw, but steaming, boiling, poaching, steam-frying, baking and grilling are all good too, in that order of preference. Avoid all deep-fried food and, as much as possible, anything fried.

- Eat foods high in the essential omega-3 and omega-6 fats, with an emphasis on omega-3 fats from fish, flax and pumpkin seeds and their oils.

- Avoid foods high in saturated, hydrogenated or processed fats.

- Avoid fried, burned or browned food.

Part Three shows you how you do all this.

9

Step 3: Eliminate Your Hidden Allergies

Not all the weight you want to lose is fat. You might be holding as much a stone of extra fluid, or even more, without knowing it. And it could all be down to a food allergy.

One in three people has hidden food allergies, which cause the weight to pile on. If you are one of them, I'd like to help you find out what your bad foods are and which foods to eat instead. I'd also like to show you how to 'desensitise' yourself to foods you're allergic to so you can eat them once more. This normally takes about three months.

Rebecca S is a case in point. In her twenties Rebecca had stable weight and good skin, and used to exercise three or four times a week. But in her thirties she started to pile on the pounds. Over three years her weight drifted from 10 stone up to 13 stone and her dress size went up to 16. She also developed itchy patches on her face and had a lot of colds and sinus trouble. She didn't exercise because she didn't feel good.

'I started feeling tired and lethargic and generally unwell,' she said. 'I didn't have the energy to go to the gym any more.'

For breakfast she'd have toast, then a main meal of meat and potatoes with gravy for lunch, and a sandwich for dinner. 'But it seemed like the foods I ate were blowing me up, which is why I thought I could have a food allergy.' She decided to test herself for a food allergy, which nowadays you can do with a home test kit, involving a pinprick of blood. The results showed that she was reacting to milk, egg white and gluten – the protein found in wheat, barley and rye. Within a week of excluding these foods she found that her skin and mood improved and the weight started to fall away. After six months she had lost 3 stone.

After three months of strictly avoiding the foods she'd become allergic to, she reintroduced egg whites and then milk to see if there was a reaction. Now she's fine on both foods, but still reacts to wheat.

'I can't tell you how much better I feel. I'm 100 per cent,' she said. 'It has transformed my health. Having the food intolerance test has been the best thing I've done. I wish I'd done it sooner.' In the end, she shed all the weight she'd gained during the previous three years.

But first, let's explore why losing control of water balance can cause considerable weight gain and see whether this may be part of your problem.

Water retention, allergies and bingeing

More than two-thirds of your body is water. If you dehydrate the body by not drinking enough water or by drinking lots of coffee or tea, which are diuretic and cause a loss of body fluid, you could lose weight. But this is neither healthy nor lasting weight loss.

Another way to lose water is to eat very few calories or very little carbohydrate. Then, as we've seen, the body will use up your glycogen, which is stored with water – and thus you'll lose water too. However, this weight too will come piling back on, unless you wish to live your entire life on a high-protein, low-carb diet, or a very low-calorie diet, guzzling coffee, dehydrating and ageing rapidly. It is excess body fat, not water, that is associated with the long-term problem of obesity.

Just in case you wondered, drinking plenty of water doesn't lead to weight gain (unless you were seriously dehydrated in the first place). In fact, the opposite is true. The more water you drink, the less likely you are to be overweight, according to the MyNutrition survey we conducted on 37,000 people.

It's a good idea to drink, at the very least, a litre of water every day because it helps the body to eliminate toxins released from fatty tissue as you burn it up. It also helps to dilute the bloodstream to prevent an overconcentration of sugar or protein. (This is why you become thirsty after eating a large dinner or sweets.) Some people have reported tremendous weight loss and health improvements simply by drinking 2 litres of water a day. I recommend you drink the equivalent of eight glasses of water every day, which includes any hot drinks such as herbal teas.

TOP TIP

Press the tip of your finger into the inside of your shinbone. Does your finger make a dent? If it does, you are probably waterlogged.

However, the body can sometimes retain too much water, creating unnecessary weight gain. This is not a consequence of drinking too much, but indicates instead a loss of the body's ability to control water balance, leading to oedema or water retention. Breast tenderness, experienced by many women before their periods, is caused by water retention. In fact, you can easily gain 7 to 14lb in body weight this way – and lose it in as little as 48 hours if you eliminate the cause.

Are you waterlogged?

☐ Does your face look puffy, especially around the eyes?

☐ Does your abdomen, on pressing, feel waterlogged and bloated?

☐ Do your arms feel puffy rather than like pure fat and muscle?

☐ Do your ankles ever swell up?

☐ Do your fingers ever swell up so it's hard to get your rings off?

☐ Do you have dry skin or dandruff?

☐ Do you ever experience sudden fluctuations in your weight?

☐ Do you suffer from breast tenderness?

☐ Are you prone to allergies?

If you answer 'yes' to three or more of the questions above, chances are that water retention is partly to blame for your weight problem. There are four reasons why retention of excess fluid in the body can occur, the most common of which is allergy. But let's look at the other three culprits first.

Are you fat-deficient?

The first of these is fat deficiency. Of course, for many people 'fat' is a dirty word. Yet, as we learned in Chapter 8, you can't live without essential fats.

Have you ever wondered how the body could possibly be something like two-thirds water? How do we keep it all in? The answer is fat. The body holds its water within cells encased in a membrane that's made mainly of essential fats. If you lack them in your diet, you lose the ability to maintain the right water balance. Your skin dries up and you may get dandruffy and sweaty. At the same time, your cells become waterlogged and you look puffy and gain weight.

As we've seen, essential fats are used in the body to make hormone-like substances called prostaglandins, which help control the body's water balance. In women, these fats also balance hormones throughout the menstrual cycle. Without them, the body is more likely to retain excess fluid, especially pre-menstrually or during the menopause. So one way that consuming enough essential fats can help you to lose weight is through water loss, if you're suffering from water retention.

Are you sugarlogged?

You'll also retain excess fluid if your diet is full of sugar. There are two reasons for this. First, every molecule of sugar holds water wherever it is in the body and in whatever form it is in – glucose, glycogen or fat. If a person is 'sugarlogged' from eating too much sugar, they'll retain excess fluid. While it is good to maintain proper glycogen stores, there is no need to have excess fat or excess circulating glucose. By balancing your blood sugar you also help to prevent excess weight being stored as water.

Secondly, too much sugar and too much insulin lead to sodium (salt) retention. Normally the kidneys get rid of the right amount of sodium. However, when you lose control of your blood sugar, the kidneys don't filter out enough, so your body's sodium levels rise. Salt attracts water, and gradually your whole body becomes a little more waterlogged. In due course blood sugar problems can lead to kidney problems, including kidney-stone formation. This is one of the reasons why high-protein diets, which also tax the kidneys, are not advisable for those with blood sugar problems.

How are your kidneys?

Your kidneys filter your blood and decide how much water to keep in your system and how much to excrete. This filtration happens through over a million clusters of tiny blood-vessel masses known as *glomeruli*, which collectively create a surface area about the size of your living room. Through the glomeruli you filter about 48 gallons (218 litres) of blood every day. Your ability to do this decreases with age so, especially if you are over 50, your kidneys may not be working 100 per cent. This needn't be a problem, but there is a point at which it becomes one.

One of the telltale signs of decreasing kidney function is swollen ankles, especially after you've drunk a lot. This means the kidneys can't work fast enough to get rid of the excess fluid. One of the major reasons kidney function decreases is continual damage caused by peaks in blood sugar. The glucose damages the glomeruli. That's why people with diabetes are especially prone to kidney problems. If you do suspect you have poor kidney function it's best to get this checked by your doctor and stay away from high-protein diets (see page 453).

Another way you can give your kidneys a break, and help reduce excess water retention, is to take in more potassium and magnesium and less sodium. On average, a person in Britain is eating at least 10g of sodium a day, which is at least 10 times more than we need. The worst-offending foods are meat and processed foods.

Potassium and the mineral magnesium, both very abundant in fruits and vegetables, help balance out sodium in the body. Potassium works together with sodium in maintaining water balance and proper nerve and muscle impulses. The more sodium you eat the more potassium you need, and few of us eat enough of the latter. Fruits, vegetables and wholegrains are rich in potassium. You need five servings of fruits and vegetables a day to get the right amount of it. Magnesium also helps balance hormones and helps solve premenstrual problems, especially breast tenderness.

A high-meat diet tends to be high in sodium, while a high-plant-based diet, with more vegetarian food, tends to be high in potassium and low in sodium. The Holford Diet is therefore naturally low in salt.

Salt content of foods

Food	Amount	Sodium contained (g)
Bacon	2 slices	2g
Typical pizza	Large slice	1.5g
Sandwich	1 – ready-made	1.2g
Cornflakes	1 bowl	1g
Cheddar cheese	30g – a sandwich	0.5g
Packet soups	1 serving	1g or more
Crisps	100g	2.7g
Bread	100g	1.3g
Burger and bun	1	1–2g
Sausages	100g (3)	5g

Not all salts are created equal

Much sodium is 'hidden' in the form of baking powder, brine or monosodium glutamate. As we've seen, the net result of too much sodium is water retention and weight gain, and possibly high blood pressure and muscle cramps. While there is no 'need' to add salt since there's more than enough in natural foods, not all salts are created equal.

	Sodium	Potassium	Magnesium	Other trace minerals
Solo	41%	41%	17%	√
LoSalt	33%	66%	0	0
Sea salt	<99%	0.2%	<1%	√
Table salt	<100%	0	0	0

Table salt, the stuff you might sprinkle on your dinner, is pure sodium chloride. Sea salt isn't much better on the sodium front, although it does have tiny amounts of other beneficial minerals. LoSalt is OK on the sodium front, but doesn't taste great.

My favourite is Solo sea salt, which has also been shown actually to lower high blood pressure, according to research published in the *British Medical Journal*.[18] Since blood pressure and water retention are caused by the same dynamics, it's a good bet that Solo salt will reduce the risk of water retention, and hence weight gain. This is because it has 60 per cent less sodium and much more of the beneficial minerals potassium and magnesium.

Also check the foods you buy. Most processed foods use sodium chloride. But some 'low sodium' foods have switched to Solo, such as Percy Dalton's peanuts, NutriBread and Asda's own-brand foods.

The run-down on reducing water retention

In a nutshell, what you have to do to reduce the risk of excess water retention is:

- balance your blood sugar;

- eat five servings of fruits and vegetables every day;

- eat seeds (rich in essential fats, plus magnesium and potassium);

- eat wholefoods and wholegrains such as beans, lentils, brown rice and brown bread;

- eat more oily fish (rich in essential fats) and less meat;

- don't add salt to your food, unless it's Solo sea salt;

- choose 'low sodium' processed foods; and

- drink the equivalent of eight glasses of water, including herbal teas, a day.

This alone may cause you to lose weight if water retention is part of your problem. But the real gold, in terms of weight loss, is to find out which foods you are allergic to and stay off them.

Is a hidden allergy leaving you waterlogged?

The most common reason for weight gain caused by fluid retention is allergy. The word 'allergy' simply means an intolerance that causes a reaction in the immune system.

Your body is like a tube. The digestive tract, which has a surface area the size of a small football field, is the gateway between the outside world and your body. It's guarded ferociously by your immune system. If a substance that isn't on the guest list, so to speak, tries to gatecrash and get through your digestive tract and into the bloodstream, your immune system goes haywire.

But why does it lead to waterlogging and weight gain? The reason is twofold. First, histamine, the stuff that makes you sneeze when it's in your nose, makes tiny blood vessels called capillaries more 'leaky'. This allows the immune system's army of white blood cells to move into the battlefield. At the same time, more fluid passes into your tissues. If this is happening several times a day, you literally become waterlogged. Allergic reactions also mess up the balance of prostaglandins, hormone-like substances made from essential fats, and this too can lead to water retention as well as abdominal bloating.

Take the case of Joanne M, who is 36. She didn't have just weight to lose, but girth.

I used to stand in front of the mirror, grab a handful of my tummy – and despair. After a big meal I looked five months pregnant! It wasn't just my weight, which hovered around 11 stone, it was the bloating (I'd gone up to a size 16) and the physical symptoms. I'd have to undo my trousers every time I had a big meal and I was often constipated.

When I was in my late teens, I was diagnosed with irritable bowel syndrome [IBS]. Instead of looking for the cause, doctors simply prescribed drugs to ease the symptoms. Reading up about the problem, I got the impression a high-fibre diet would help the constipation and stop my tummy bloating. But my health regime of wholemeal bread, baked potatoes and beans was actually making it worse.

I felt exhausted all the time and usually fell asleep by 9.30 in the evening. My husband Steve kept telling me I had to do something about it. So in September 2002 I sent away for a food-intolerance blood test. The results told me I was sensitive to all dairy products, yeast, salmon, trout, haricot beans and string beans. Within a week I was going to the loo every two days (instead of weekly), my tummy was gone and I was down to a size 12. My lethargy was caused by the yeasty foods I ate. I've gone from 11 stone 2lb to 9 stone 3lb and look so much trimmer now.

The more often you are reacting allergically, the more resistant you become to insulin. This is because the body releases masses of immune messengers called *cytokines* to deal with the allergy, and cytokines make you less responsive to insulin. Also, repeated allergic reactions mean that more garbage ends up in your bloodstream as your immune cells fight off the invaders.

All this has to be cleaned up by your liver, your body's detoxifying organ. Eventually, the liver's detox capacity gets overloaded. When this happens, your body dumps the toxins in the least harmful place – your fat cells. The more intoxicated your fat cells become, the more weight you gain and the harder it becomes to shift those extra pounds. This is why people with allergies find it harder and harder to lose weight. Also, this continual process of over-intoxication can turn a mild allergy into something more severe.

Many people don't find out about their allergies until it's really obvious. Lori D, for instance, didn't think about testing herself for allergies until she nearly died at the age of 54 simply from drinking a glass of pineapple juice.

I was 8 and a half stone until 10 years ago when I suddenly went up to 15 stone and size 20. One fateful evening I had a sore throat and drank a litre of pineapple juice throughout the night. By morning my throat had closed up, I could hardly breathe and I'd turned purple. I drove to my GP, where I collapsed on the step.

Because of this I decided to have proper food tests done, which proved that I was intolerant not only to milk and yeast, but also to pineapple, cranberry and kidney beans. Now I've cut out those foods, I feel really good. My once stubby fingers are now slim and I've lost more than half a stone in two weeks. Knowing I'm food-intolerant helps as it makes me think about what I should be eating and helps me stick to my diet. ❯

Discovering whether you're allergic

Allergies can be responsible for many symptoms, especially digestive problems, from bloating to constipation, and diarrhoea to abdominal cramps. These are almost always accompanied by mental and physical symptoms, such as mood changes, chronic tiredness, depression, increased appetite, sleepiness after meals, inability to concentrate and a host of minor ailments from itches and rashes to asthma and sinus problems. Check yourself out with the questionnaire below.

Your instant allergy check

☐ Can you gain weight in hours?

☐ Do you get bloated after eating?

☐ Do you suffer from diarrhoea or constipation?

☐ Do you suffer from abdominal pain?

☐ Do you sometimes get really sleepy after eating?

☐ Do you suffer from hay fever?

☐ Do you suffer from rashes, itches, asthma or shortness of breath?

☐ Do you suffer from water retention (see the 'Are you waterlogged?' questionnaire on page 138)?

☐ Do you suffer from headaches?

☐ Do you suffer from other aches or pains, from time to time, possibly after certain foods?

☐ Do you get better on holidays abroad, when your diet is completely different?

Any 'yes' answer to these questions means there's a real possibility that you have an allergy. If you score four or more 'yes's it's pretty much guaranteed.

> ### TOP TIP
>
> Do you get bloated after eating and have to undo a button or two? If so, the chances are you are eating something you are allergic to.

As we've seen, bloating, pain, diarrhoea and constipation are often indicators of an allergy. Lisa M is a classic case. She had suffered for six years with abdominal bloating before she worked out it might be an allergy.

❝ My bloating was so bad that my boyfriend David measured round my waist and found I'd ballooned by 5 inches in one day. Anything I ate seemed to go straight through me – but despite that, I remained 5 stone overweight. My doctor reckoned my body had gone into starvation mode, making the most of anything I fed it because of my tummy upsets. ❞

Lisa then took a food-intolerance test, which revealed she was sensitive to eggs, milk, wheat, yeast, rye and beef. 'I'd been practically living on these foods,' she said. 'I had eggs for breakfast most days, and for lunch I'd often choose cottage cheese and egg sandwiches, thinking they were a healthy option. Little did I know I was poisoning myself.'

Within three days of dropping the culprit foods, Lisa began to feel much better. 'I've now gone six months without a tummy upset and I've lost nearly 3 stone!' she said. 'I feel like I have my life back.'

Pinpointing the allergen

It may seem odd, but more often than not the foods a person is allergic to are those they really crave. If you're craving and eating something frequently, as though you're mildly addicted, there is a chance you're allergic to that food. Through my work with a number of allergic and overweight clients, it became clear to me that they were bingeing only on certain food groups. When they were instructed to eat as much as they liked of anything *except* the suspected allergen (the food provoking an allergic reaction), they often ceased bingeing. And when they avoided the allergen completely, they often lost 3 to 4lb and occasionally as much as 7lb, almost overnight.

This sort of short-term weight loss can only be the result of excess fluid retention, and nothing to do with fat. You can't burn *one* pound of fat in 24 hours, even if you are starving – and much less, seven!

One of the physical symptoms of an allergic reaction can be a sudden fluctuation in blood sugar level which, in turn, affects appetite. So could allergic reactions trigger bingeing? In honesty, nobody has a definite answer to this question, but my observations of a number of clients certainly show that sometimes allergies do play a role in overweight problems, and there's a one-in-three chance they play a role in yours.

There are two ways to find out what you are allergic to. The first we could call 'educated trial and error'. You need to avoid suspect foods for 14 days and note what happens by taking the pulse test, explained below.

The pulse test

Most people are free of symptoms within 14 days of avoiding an allergy-provoking food. And most will react on reintroducing the food within 48 hours, although some may have a reaction delayed by up to 10 days. Delayed reactions are much harder to test. For some, symptoms improve considerably when they leave out offending foods. For others, noticeable changes are slight.

One simple way to help identify possible suspects is the pulse test. The pulse test demands that you avoid all suspect foods for 14 days, then reintroduce them one by one, with a 48-hour gap between each item to be tested. Take your resting pulse, sitting down, before you eat the food, then take it again after 10 minutes, 30 minutes and 60 minutes. Mark all this down on a chart like the one on page 151. If you have a marked increase in pulse rate of more than 10 points, or have any symptoms of ill health within 24 hours including immediate weight gain, bloating, fatigue, headaches or joint aches, for example, avoid the food and wait 24 hours before testing the next food.

continues ▶

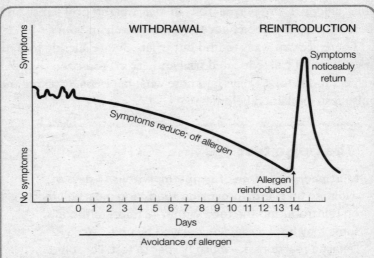

The avoidance/reintroduction test for allergies. If you avoid a food you are allergic to you may notice an improvement in how you feel within 14 days. If you then reintroduce the food you may notice a return of symptoms.

While day-to-day changes in symptoms are hard to pin down to specific causes, avoidance of suspect foods for 14 days often lessens symptoms, which then increase significantly on reintroduction. So you'll be able to pinpoint which foods or drinks make you worse. It is very important to observe symptoms accurately because you may have preconceived ideas about what you do or don't react to, perhaps because of what somebody has told you, or because you dread being allergic to certain foods that you're addicted to.

(If you have ever had a severe or life-threatening allergic reaction I recommend you do this avoidance/reintroduction test *only* under the supervision of a suitably qualified practitioner.)

Suspect food	Pulse Before 10 mins	Pulse and symptoms 30 mins	60 mins
Milk	_____	_____	_____
Yeast	_____	_____	_____
Egg	_____	_____	_____
Wheat	_____	_____	_____
_____	_____	_____	_____
_____	_____	_____	_____

IgG allergy testing – the gold standard

Because the body sometimes delays its allergic reaction to a food, avoidance/reintroduction tests don't always pick it up. This happens because you may not suspect the food, and so not test it. Or you may suspect only one food, yet be allergic to a range of them, so you'll continue to have a background of allergic reactions and may thus have difficulty losing weight.

The best and truly accurate way to find out what you are allergic to is to have what's called a Quantitative IgG ELISA test. This is the gold standard of allergy testing. 'Quantitative' means the test shows not only whether you are allergic, but also how strong your allergic reaction is. Many of us live quite healthily with minor allergies. But stronger allergies can create all sorts of problems, including weight gain. ELISA is the technology used. You don't need to know all the details but, trust me, it's the most accurate system and it's used by almost all the best allergy laboratories in the world.

To convey why it's so good, I need to explain a bit about the human immune system.

Your immune system can produce tailor-made weapons that latch onto specific substances to help escort them out of your body. They are like bouncers on the lookout for troublemakers. The bouncers are called *immunoglobulins,* or Ig for short. There are different types. The real heavies are called IgE, although most allergies involve IgG reactions. IgE reactions tend to be more immediate and severe – like Lori's reaction to pineapple. However, most 'hidden' allergies that may be insidiously causing weight gain are IgG-based. In an ideal world you test for both, but I normally start by testing a person for IgG sensitivity to food.

All that's needed for testing is a pinprick of blood, which is absorbed into a tiny tube and sent to a laboratory. The lab then sends back an accurate read-out of exactly what you are allergic to. Your body doesn't lie. Either you have IgG bouncers tagged for wheat (for example) or you don't. Your diluted blood is introduced to a panel of liquid food 'testers', and if you've got IgG for that food, a reaction takes place.

There are a number of laboratories that do IgG testing (see pages 477–9 in Resources), and one that offers a handy test kit you can use at home. YorkTest have devised a clever procedure that involves a painless pinprick device and an absorbent material that you place against the pinprick. This material is then sent to the laboratory for testing (see pages 478–9).

The good news about IgG-based allergies is that if you avoid the offending food strictly for three to six months, the body forgets that it is allergic to it. The reason is that there will no longer be any IgG antibodies to that food in your system. This doesn't hold for IgE-based reactions, however.

To give you an example, I have an IgE allergy to milk. I react within 15 minutes. Even if I avoid dairy products for a year, I still react if I consume it. I used to have an IgG to wheat. I avoided it for three months and now I no longer react. In my case, weight gain wasn't the problem: it was migraine headaches. I had them every other week from the age of six until I was twenty, until I discovered that wheat and milk were triggering them.

Fenton R, like me, had regular headaches, sinusitis and fatigue and had been plagued by acid indigestion for 20 years. He was also gaining weight year on year. Doctors were unable to help him, suggesting he drank too much fizzy pop and should exercise more. And indigestion tablets helped for only about 20 minutes before the problem returned with redoubled force.

He decided to have a food-intolerance test. The results came back showing he was intolerant of eggs, cow's milk, yeast and wheat. He took all the rogue foods out of his diet, for example by switching to soya milk, and within two days the indigestion began to ease. Now it has gone completely, along with all the other health problems that had dogged him – including an excess 2 stone in weight.

It feels as though a shroud has been lifted from me. Not only have I lost the weight, I have 100 per cent more energy. It used to be an effort to go up the stairs. I used to get headaches most days, and they have gone. I used to get sinus twinges almost every day, and they have cleared up. I used to sweat a lot, and thought I was just a sweaty person. But now I can walk and run and just don't sweat. My skin used to be cold all the time but now it's nice and warm. I feel more relaxed as well. It had got to the stage where I couldn't even think clearly, but now I can do so again.

The usual suspects

The ten most common foods or food groups that people are allergic to are shown in the box overleaf, in order. Of all these foods, by far the most common allergy-provoking substances are cow's milk, followed by yeast, eggs and wheat. This doesn't necessarily means that these foods are bad for you. It just depends whether or not you are allergic to them.

The Top Ten common food allergies

cow's milk
yeast
eggs
wheat
gliadin grains
oats
nuts
beans
white fish
shellfish

Cow's milk

This provides the most common food allergy. It's present in most cheeses, cream, yoghurt and butter and is hidden in all sorts of food; sometimes it's called 'casein', which is milk protein.

Logically, its status as an allergen isn't surprising, since it is a highly specific food, containing all sorts of hormones designed for the first few months of a calf's life. It's also a relatively recent addition to the human diet. Our ancestors, after all, weren't milking buffaloes. Approximately 75 per cent of people (25 per cent of people of Caucasian origin and 80 per cent of Asian, Native American or African origin) stop producing lactase, the enzyme that's needed to digest milk sugar, once they've been weaned. Is nature trying to tell us something? However, it's not the lactose, the sugar in milk, that causes the allergic reaction. It's the protein.

If you react to cow's milk it doesn't necessarily mean you will react to goat's milk or sheep's milk. However, many people do react to all dairy products. Because of this you'll find that there is very little dairy in the recipes in Part Four. In most cases, if you strictly avoid your allergy-provoking foods for three months, your body can 'unlearn' the allergy. So it doesn't have to be a life sentence.

There are many alternatives to dairy now, including soya and quinoa 'milks'. Try them out and find one you like. Use the ⑥ chart on pages 434–50 for your guide to quantity.

Yeast

After milk, yeast is the second most common culprit in allergies. Yeast is not only in bread as baker's yeast, it's also in beer and, to a lesser extent, wine. If you have been allergy-tested, you'll know whether you are allergic to brewer's or baker's yeast. Most people who are allergic to yeast at all are allergic to both. Beer and lager are fermented with brewer's yeast. If you've noticed that you feel worse after beer or wine than after spirits – the 'cleanest' being vodka – then you may be yeast-sensitive. Does this mean you can't drink? Not at all. Just stick to spirits and champagne! Champagne is made by a double-fermentation process that means there's much less yeast in it.

(A word about alcohol. As well as causing allergies in some, alcohol irritates the digestive tract, making it more permeable to undigested food proteins. This increases your chances of developing an allergic reaction to anything, and it's why some people feel worst when they both eat foods they are allergic to and drink alcohol. For example, you might be mildly allergic to wheat and milk and feel fine after either. But when you have both, plus alcohol, you don't feel great.)

Some people think they are allergic to wheat because they feel worse after eating bread. If you've noticed this – perhaps feeling sluggish, tired or blocked up – but feel fine after pasta, you may not be allergic to wheat, but to the yeast in the bread.

Take Janette B, who is 45. Noticing her weight creeping up, Janette didn't link it with food sensitivity:

> *Over seven years my weight soared by 3 stone to 13 and a half stone and although I was a member of a slimming club, stuck strictly to a low-calorie diet and took regular exercise, I could never lose more than about a stone.*

Not only was Janette heavier than before, but also she felt constantly tired and uncomfortably bloated after meals, particularly when she'd eaten bread. 'I was so frustrated by my weight and so fed up with feeling exhausted that I decided to have a food-intolerance test,' she said. The results showed she was intolerant of yeast and milk and also sensitive to corn and soya, as well as haricot and kidney beans. Simply by avoiding her 'bad' foods, Janette lost 2 stone in 5 months!

If you're allergic to yeast, you've got to be on the lookout for hidden yeast in stock cubes and processed food. As the Holford Diet features wholefoods and fresh ingredients, and avoids yeasted breads, this should be far less of a problem for you. I also recommend using yeast-free vegetable stock cubes by Marigold.

Eggs

Some people are allergic to egg white, but not egg yolk. If you are sensitive to eggs, when you come to reintroduce them, it's best to start by reintroducing egg yolk. If you don't react within five days, then reintroduce egg white. Eggs are in quite a lot of processed foods and bakery items, so check the label carefully.

Wheat, gliadin grains and oats

This is the grain that more people react to than any other. It contains gluten, a sticky protein also found in rye, barley and oats. Gluten sensitivity occurs in about one in a hundred people,[19] but is medically diagnosed in fewer than one in a thousand. However, it is a specific type of gluten, called *gliadin*, which most people react to. The only way to know for sure exactly what you are allergic to is to have a food-intolerance test. If you have had an allergy test you'll know whether you are gluten-, gliadin- or wheat-sensitive.

If you are gluten-sensitive, then you cannot eat wheat, rye, barley or oats. Excellent alternatives are rice, quinoa, buckwheat, millet and corn (although some gluten-sensitive people do react to corn). Quinoa and millet cook in 15 minutes, in much the same way as rice. From the 🇬🇱 point of view, quinoa is the best. These days, you can find rice, corn and buckwheat breads and pastas in bigger supermarkets and good health-food stores.

However, there's no gliadin in oats. If you are gliadin-sensitive, then you can eat oats, but not wheat, rye or barley.

If you are only wheat-sensitive, it's relatively easy. Just eat rye, barley or oats. For example, you can eat rye bread, oatcakes and oat-flake cereals, but not Weetabix or wheat bread.

In the big scheme of things wheat's prominence as an allergen shouldn't be surprising. Grains are the second most recent addition into the human diet, and weren't eaten by hunter-gatherers. They have been eaten by farmers for something like the last 10,000 years, but only in certain parts of the world. For example, no gluten grain naturally grows in North America, so Native Americans have been exposed to gluten for only about the last 200 years at most.

A worrying trend in the US, where 'low-carb' diets are the craze, is to remove the carbohydrates from wheat products so you're eating just the protein portion. As this is principally gluten, it's a recipe for disaster for anyone with a hidden gluten allergy.

Nuts and beans

These are part of the same food family, along with fruit pips. In essence, they're all seeds. The most common individual allergens in this group are, in descending order, cashews, Brazil nuts, almonds, peanuts, haricot beans and soya beans. You can react to one and no others, but if you do react to a member of this family there's a greater chance that you'll react to another member of the pip/bean/nut family. Coffee, from the coffee bean, and chocolate, from the cocoa bean, are also members of this family.

White fish and shellfish

This is another major allergen, but most people who are allergic to it react to white fish, not oily fish – such as salmon, mackerel and herring, which are so rich in omega-3s. If you're also allergic to those kinds, have a tablespoon of ground seeds with breakfast every day (see page 206), together with a good-quality supplement, to keep your essential fatty acids topped up.

Shellfish allergies are very common, with prawns and abalone two of the worst villains. You may be allergic to mussels, scallops, whelks, oysters and squid, which are all molluscs, or to lobsters, crayfish, prawns and shrimps, which are all crustaceans. Octopus is in a world of its own! Be careful here, though. If you're allergic to squid but not to octopus, be aware that some people sell squid as octopus to make a bigger profit, because they can buy it more cheaply.

If you suffer from food allergies, you don't have to feel deprived on the Holford Diet. It is always sensible to vary your diet as much as possible, and the menu plans and recipes in Chapters 27 and 28 are designed to include a wide range of ingredients. Such a varied diet, together with the introduction of exciting new foods such as quinoa, soya products and lesser-used legumes such as flageolet and cannellini beans, ensures that there is plenty to tempt your taste buds, even if you do have to avoid certain items.

When you have an allergy test, the best laboratories give you clear instructions on what not to eat and what you can eat, as well as giving you the backup of a nutritionist to answer any of your questions. By avoiding foods that cause symptoms, you will probably find improvements in your health that you didn't ever imagine. I can't count the times I've heard people say, 'I didn't even know I could feel this good.' The Holford Diet and supplements will also help to reduce your allergic potential further.

After three months of abstaining from the allergen, you may then find that you can tolerate it in small periodic 'doses'. For some people the allergy disappears completely. Others have to be careful about certain foods for life. Once you have more than a sneaking suspicion that you are allergic, it is best to have an allergy test.

- Find out if you are allergic to something you're eating and avoid it. You can do an avoidance/reintroduction test but, quite frankly, it's better to have a proper quantitative IgG ELISA test.

- After three months you can reintroduce the foods you tested positive for, although ideally not eating them every day.

- Even if you are not allergic to it, reduce the amount of cow's milk you eat and drink, substituting goat's cheeses, soya produce and the like.

- Even if you are not allergic to it, reduce the amount of wheat you eat, substituting other grains such as oats, rye and rice.

- Limit alcohol. Ideally drink no more than three small glasses of wine, half-pints of beer or lager, or measures of spirit a week.

- Drink the equivalent of eight glasses of water a day.

Part Three shows you how you do all this.

10

Step 4: Take the Right Supplements

So far you've learned that by changing the quality of the big guys – fats, carbohydrates and proteins – you can lose weight because your body's metabolism finally starts working properly. Now, I'd like to take a look at the little guys: vitamins and minerals.

Your body's daily functions depend on a myriad chemical reactions which, in turn, depend on vitamins and minerals. Your fatburning capability, for instance, relies on your getting optimal amounts of certain micronutrients. For example, to make insulin you need zinc and vitamin B6. Insulin's ability to control blood sugar levels is helped by the mineral chromium. To turn glucose into energy, rather than fat, you need B vitamins, magnesium and vitamin C. And to burn fat you need all these, plus the B vitamin biotin.

No doubt you've heard the mantra 'As long as you eat a balanced diet you get all the vitamins and minerals you need' from someone, sometime. As I've said, this is the greatest lie in nutrition today. Why? Because there's only a slim chance that your diet meets even the full range of RDAs – and also because it all hangs on your definition of 'need' as well as what you want from life.

RDAs, or *recommended daily allowances,* of vitamins and minerals are in any case misleading at best. Governments the world over have worked these out by starting from the bottom – that is, looking merely at preventing the obvious vitamin-deficiency diseases. These range from scurvy (vitamin C deficiency) and beriberi (vitamin B1) to pellagra (niacin). But, as we learn more and more about the health-promoting properties of vitamins and minerals, RDAs have crept up and up. In the UK, for instance, the RDA for vitamin C has moved up from 30mg to 45mg to 60mg, and in the US it's now 85mg.

The problems with RDAs go further than this, though. They are mere averages, and you are far from average. You are unique. According to Dr Roger Williams, a pioneer in nutrition who discovered vitamin B5 (pantothenic acid) and helped discover folic acid, even twins with identical genes can have twentyfold differences in their nutritional needs![20] Where you live, how much exercise you get, your gender and your genes can easily alter your needs for various nutrients by a factor of ten. That's why I call the RDAs 'ridiculous dietary arbitraries'. So, if you are happy with average poor health, go for the RDAs.

Optimum nutrition, maximum weight loss

Let's say, though, that you want the most out of life. You want to be the right weight and stay there, and you see your health not just as an absence of ill health, but as total wellbeing. If this is you, you need *optimum* nutrition.

At ION, we worked out micronutrient needs by starting from the top. We sought the intake of a vitamin that would promote optimal health, not just prevent scurvy. We asked the question 'What amount of vitamin X equates to the maximum possible wellbeing and the smallest possible risk of disease?' For the past 20 years, we've been investigating the effects of vitamins, minerals and essential fats on weight, IQ, memory, mood, energy, immunity, infections, lifespan, pregnancy and disease risk. From this we established the ODAs, or *optimum daily allowances*. These are the amounts of nutrients that will tune up your body's metabolism, making it easier for you to lose weight, and keep it off for good.

Have a look at the chart overleaf. You'll notice that the ODAs are often 10 times the RDAs. You'll also see what the average diet provides – and what you could be achieving if you were eating a healthier diet, with plenty of wholefoods, fruit and vegetables. But there's still a shortfall between what we've researched as optimum and what you are likely to get in food.

And that's where supplements come in. They make up the difference – the difference between how you feel now and how you *could* feel if you were optimally nourished, losing weight steadily and feeling fantastic.

Turning glucose into fuel, not fat

To understand how vitamins and minerals help with the crucial job of fatburning, let's take a close look at what happens to glucose in the body.

The brain, muscles, liver, skin, immune system, heart and arteries are all simply a collection of cells that do different jobs for the body, whether it's digesting, thinking or moving. The fuel that keeps them going is, as we've found, glucose. So maintaining an even level of blood sugar – the cells' fuel reserve – is the first step in making energy.

Within each of our 30 trillion or so cells exist tiny energy factories called *mitochondria*. These turn glucose into another chemical, *pyruvic acid*, a process that releases a small amount

NUTRIENTS	RDA	100% RDA				ODA
Vitamin A (mcg)	800	900▶	1500▶		‹Shortfall 1000▶	2,500
Vitamin D (mcg)	5	4▶	7▶		‹Shortfall 4▶	11
Vitamin E (mg)	10	14▶	50▶		‹Shortfall 250▶	300
Vitamin C (mg)	60	100▶	200▶		‹Shortfall 1800▶	2,000
Vitamin B1 (mg)	1.4	2▶	5▶		‹Shortfall 30▶	35
Vitamin B2 (mg)	1.6	2.18▶	5▶		‹Shortfall 30▶	35
Vitamin B3 (mg)	18	39.6▶	50▶	‹Shortfall 35▶		85
Vitamin B5 (mg)	6	2.175▶	20▶		‹Shortfall 80▶	100
Vitamin B6 (mg)	2	3.1▶	5▶		‹Shortfall 70▶	75
Folic Acid (mcg)	200	325.5▶	400▶		‹Shortfall 400▶	800
Vitamin B12 (mcg)	1	5.95▶	10▶		‹Shortfall 15▶	25
Biotin (mcg)	150	36.50▶	120▶		‹Shortfall 105▶	225

GLA* (Omega-6) (mg)	–	20▶	40▶		‹Shortfall 110▶	150
EPA/DHA* (Omega-3) (mg)	–	60▶	100▶		‹Shortfall 600▶	700

Calcium (mg)	800	(800:good diet)▶	912.5▶	‹Shortfall 200▶		1,000
Iron (mg)	14	12.8▶	15▶		‹Shortfall 5▶	20
Magnesium (mg)	300	272▶	350▶		‹Shortfall 150▶	500
Zinc (mg)	15	9.3▶ 10▶			‹Shortfall 10▶	20
Iodine (mcg)	150	193.5▶	240▶	‹Shortfall 60▶		300
Selenium (mcg)*	–	40▶	50▶		‹Shortfall 50▶	100
Chromium (mcg)*	–	50▶	75▶		‹Shortfall 50▶	125
Manganese (mcg)*	–	3▶	6▶		‹Shortfall 4▶	10

Key

■ Average diet
□ Good diet

RDA = Recommended daily allowance
ODA = Optimum daily allowance (diet plus supplements)
* items marked with an asterisk have no RDA

RDAs versus ODAs and dietary intakes. This chart shows the differences between the RDA, our average intake, and our ideal intake. The grey amounts are the levels we could reach if we ate a good variety of fruit and vegetables daily – i.e. a good diet.

Using vitamin C as an example, the RDA is 60mg. The average intake is 100mg. If you eat plenty of fruit and vegetables you could achieve 200mg. The optimal intake is somewhere between 1,000 and 3,000mg. The ODA is set at the mid-point of 2,000mg. The shortfall between a good diet (200mg) and the ODA (2,000 mg) is 1,800mg. This is the kind of level worth supplementing.

of energy, which can be used by the cell to carry out its work. If there isn't enough oxygen around while this is happening, a by-product called *lactic acid* builds up. That's why, when you do strenuous exercise after a relatively sedentary period, your muscles ache the next day. The more you exercise, developing larger muscles, the less strain you put on them and the more oxygen they can use. This is what aerobic exercise is all about – providing muscle cells with enough oxygen so they can work properly.

Next, pyruvic acid is turned into *acetyl-coenzyme A*, or AcoA. This substance is perhaps the most vital in fuelling our body, because if you're starved of glucose, as when for example a marathon runner 'hits the wall', you can break down fat or protein to make AcoA and use this for energy. But, because this method is relatively inefficient, your body prefers to rely on carbohydrates, and glucose, for fuel.

From this point on, oxygen is needed every step of the way. AcoA enters a series of chemical reactions known as the *Krebs cycle* (named after its discoverer, Ernst Krebs). During this, hydrogen molecules split off, meet oxygen – and *bang*! Energy is released. In fact over 90 per cent of all our energy is derived from this final stage. The waste products from this process are carbon dioxide (which we exhale), water (which goes to form urine) and heat. That's why you get hot when you exercise. Muscle cells make lots of energy, creating heat.

Best vitamins for fatburning

Complex carbohydrates and oxygen are only half the story. All these chemical reactions are carefully controlled by enzymes, which are themselves dependent on no fewer than nine vitamins and six minerals (see figure overleaf). Any shortage of these critical catalysts and your energy factories, the

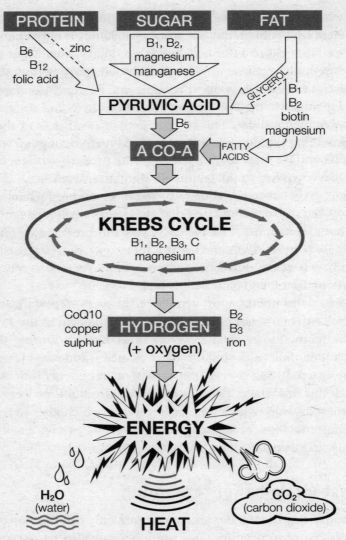

Turning food into energy. The glucose we eat is converted within our cells to release and give us energy. This is done by enzymes that, in turn, depend on vitamins and minerals. Consuming enough vitamins and minerals helps turn food into energy instead of fat.

mitochondria, go out of tune. The result is inefficient energy production, a loss of stamina, and highs and lows – or just lows. These lead to cravings. And whatever your body can't turn into energy easily, it turns into fat. So part of the weight-control equation is making energy efficiently.

The important vitamins here are the B-complex vitamins, a family of eight different substances. Every one is essential for making energy. Glucose can't be turned into pyruvic acid without B1 and B2 (niacin). AcoA won't work properly without B1, B2, B3 and, most important of all, B5 (pantothenic acid). The Krebs cycle needs B1, B2 and B3 to do its job properly, along with vitamin C. Fats and proteins can't be used to make energy without B1, B2, B6, B12, folic acid or biotin.

It used to be thought that as long as you ate a reasonable diet you'd get enough B vitamins. But studies have shown that, over the long term, slight deficiencies – which are all too easy to develop – result in depletion of these vitamins within cells. The results can be serious. Early warning signs are poor skin condition, anxiety, depression, mental confusion and irritability, fatigue and excessive weight in particular. Health and diet surveys, including our own, consistently show that people who take multivitamins containing B vitamins are less overweight.

Most people's diets fall short of the optimal requirements for these vital vitamins, and few even achieve the basic RDAs. In one ION study a group of 82 volunteers, many of whom already had a 'well-balanced diet', were assessed to calculate their optimal nutritional needs.[21] All 82 were given extra B vitamins in supplement form, often in doses 20 times that of the RDAs. After six months, 79 per cent of participants reported a definite improvement in energy, 61 per cent felt physically fitter and 60 per cent had noticed an improvement in their mental alertness and memory.

Being water-soluble and extremely sensitive to heat, B vitamins are easily lost when foods are boiled. The best natural sources are therefore fresh fruit, raw vegetables and wheat germ. Seeds, nuts and wholegrains contain reasonable amounts, as do meat, fish, eggs and dairy produce. But these levels are reduced when the food is cooked or stored for a long time.

As well as eating these foods – and Part Three will give you the details – I strongly recommend that you use a high-strength multivitamin supplement to guarantee an optimal intake of all the B vitamins, plus at least 1,000mg of vitamin C.

Best minerals for fatburning

The minerals iron, calcium, magnesium, chromium and zinc are also vital for making energy. Calcium and magnesium are perhaps the most important because all muscle cells need an adequate supply of these to be able to contract and relax. A shortage of magnesium, which is very common in people who don't eat a lot of fruit or vegetables, often results in cramps, as muscles are unable to relax. Magnesium is involved in 75 per cent of the enzymes in your body[22] – and it is absolutely vital for blood sugar control and burning carbohydrate for energy, rather than storing it as fat. While most diets provide enough calcium, few provide enough magnesium. Good multivitamins will give you an additional 150mg of magnesium and calcium. It is well worth taking a supplement.

Zinc, together with vitamin B6, is needed to make the enzymes that digest food.[23] They are also essential in the production of insulin. A lack of zinc disturbs appetite control and causes a loss of taste or smell, a combination that often leads to overeating of meat, cheese and other strong-tasting foods. Zinc deficiency is very widespread. The optimal intake is 20mg a day, while the average intake is 9mg.

It's well worth correcting this shortfall by taking a daily multivitamin/mineral that gives you 10mg of zinc, as well as eating zinc-rich foods such as seeds and 'seed' foods, meaning anything you could plant in the ground that would grow. This includes beans, lentils and peas. Broccoli, including the 'Tenderstem' variety, are also good sources. And oysters are the very best. If you ate an oyster a day, you wouldn't need to supplement with zinc!

Chromium – the secret of balancing blood sugar

The older you are, the less likely you are to be getting enough chromium[24] – an essential mineral that helps stabilise blood sugar levels and, hence, weight. The average daily intake is below 50mcg, while an optimal intake, certainly for those with a weight and blood sugar problem, is around 200mcg. Chromium is found in wholefoods and is therefore higher in wholewheat flour, bread or pasta than in refined products. (Flour has 98 per cent of its chromium removed in the refining process – another reason to stay away from overprocessed products.) Beans, nuts and seeds are other good sources, and asparagus and mushrooms are especially rich in it.

Since chromium works with insulin to help stabilise your blood sugar level, appetite and weight, the more uneven your blood sugar level, the more chromium you use up. Hence a sugar and stimulant addict, eating refined foods, is most at risk of deficiency.

Two studies carried out at Bemidji State University in Minnesota have shown that chromium supplementation helps to build muscle and burn fat.[25] Because it helps to lower cholesterol as well as stabilise blood sugar levels, it is especially helpful for people at a high risk of developing diabetes.[26] And, in trials where it was taken by people who made no change to their diets, chromium had a small effect on weight loss compared with placebos.[27] The real benefit of chromium supplementation is that it reduces sugar cravings and hence your appetite for the wrong foods. So, all in all, taking chromium, following the Holford Diet and exercise are a winning formula.

Whether or not you can achieve an optimal intake of chromium from diet alone is debatable. It is therefore wise to take supplements of this fatburning mineral as well as eat wholefoods. The best form of chromium is chromium polynicotinate, which means it's bound with vitamin B3 (also called *nicotinic acid*). Most good multivitamins will contain 30mcg of chromium, but you can help balance your blood sugar and reduce sugar cravings more quickly by taking 200–400mcg a day for the first three months of the Holford Diet. Chromium supplements, usually in 200mcg amounts, are readily available in any health-food store.

Slimming pills – the next generation

I'm hardly a fan of slimming pills. Few actually work, and those that do often act like stimulants, speeding up your metabolism and giving you short-term weight loss – and potential *long*-term problems. Over time, some may end up slowing down your metabolism, and may even promote weight gain. This category includes ephedra (now banned), guarana and other sources of caffeine. Others, such as conjugated linolenic acid (CLA for short), promised great results on animal studies, but failed to deliver significant weight loss in human trials.[28]

There are two, however, that I like and recommend: hydroxycitric acid (HCA for short) and 5-hydroxytryptophan, or 5-HTP.

HCA curbs your appetite

HCA is extracted from the dried rind of the tamarind fruit (*Garcinia cambogia*), which you may know from Indian and other Eastern cuisine. HCA is not a vitamin, but it will help you lose weight. Originally developed by the pharmaceutical giant Hoffmann-LaRoche, it has been proved to slow down the production of fat and reduce appetite. It has been extensively tested and found to have no toxicity or safety concerns.

HCA works by inhibiting the enzyme that converts sugar into fat. The carbohydrate in a meal is first used to provide fuel and short-term energy stores as glycogen. Any excess is then converted to fat by the enzyme ATP-citrate lyase. HCA dampens down the activity of this enzyme. Evidence of HCA's fat-burning properties has been accumulating since 1965.[29] For example, participants in one eight-week, double-blind trial reported an average weight loss of 11lb 2oz per person, compared with 4lb 3oz on a dummy pill.

HCA also reduces the synthesis of fat and cholesterol. Animal studies have confirmed this, and it may be that HCA has a role to play in helping those with high triglyceride (fat) or blood cholesterol levels. There is also evidence that HCA may enhance the burning of calories and increase energy levels. According to John Sterling, whose company BioCare was among the first to introduce HCA in the UK, 'People are reporting very positive results. HCA doesn't help everybody, but it is helping about 50 per cent of those who've tried it.'

A recent trial conducted by the University of Maastricht in the Netherlands confirms that HCA acts as a powerful appetite suppressant, reducing weight with no harmful effects. In the study – which was the best kind, a so-called double-blind, placebo-controlled, randomised, crossover trial – 12 men and women were given a tomato juice drink three times a day for two weeks. They then had a two-week break. Following this, the group were divided up, unbeknown to them. Some participants drank tomato juice with a placebo, others one containing 300mg of HCA, three times a day for the next two weeks.

Only those taking the HCA-loaded drink ate less – a total of 15 to 30 per cent fewer calories. However, they didn't report that they tried to eat less, tried to restrict their diet or experienced any loss of enjoyment regarding their food. They just happened to eat less. They also lost more weight, averaging 1lb extra weight loss a week.[30]

I recommend taking HCA, especially during the first three months of the Holford Diet. You need 750mg a day. Most supplements provide 250mg per capsule, so take one capsule three times a day, ideally anywhere from immediately before, to 30 minutes before, a main meal. It is widely available as a supplement.

5-HTP helps you 'think thin'

Have you ever thought about why you get hungry? You might think the obvious answer is because you haven't eaten. But that isn't always true, is it? And don't you often find yourself craving something sweet even though you've just eaten more than enough food?

The two most powerful controllers of your appetite are your blood sugar level and your brain's level of serotonin, the 'happy' neurotransmitter. Serotonin is made from an amino acid, or building block of protein, called *tryptophan*. Many people have low levels of this vital brain chemical and feel depressed as a result. This is especially true of people on weight-loss diets, most of which are notoriously low in tryptophan.

But that isn't all. Serotonin controls appetite. The more you have, the less you eat – and the less you have, the more you eat (most people eat more when they are depressed, and low in serotonin).

If you are low in serotonin, one of the quickest way to restore normal levels, and normal mood, is to supplement your diet with a special form of tryptophan called 5-hydroxytryptophan, or 5-HTP for short. It's found in meat, fish and beans, although in rather small amounts. But one, the African *Griffonia* bean, contains significant amounts, and extracts of this are sold as 5-HTP supplements.

It's not just speculation that 5-HTP works: it's been proven to make you feel happier and want to eat less. While it's been known for some time that giving 5-HTP to animals causes a reduction in appetite, followed by a loss in weight,[31] two recent studies, conducted Dr C. Cangiano and colleagues at the Department of Clinical Medicine, University of Rome (La Sapienza), in Italy, show that 5-HTP does the same thing in overweight people.

In the first study, 20 obese volunteers took either 5-HTP (900mg) or a placebo for 12 weeks. During the first six weeks, volunteers could eat what they liked. During the second six weeks the volunteers were recommended a low-calorie diet. In both phases those taking 5-HTP consistently ate less, felt more satisfied and consequently lost weight.[32] What was particularly interesting was that they ate less carbohydrate.

The second study gave 25 overweight non-insulin-dependent diabetic volunteers either 5-HTP or a placebo for two weeks, with no dietary restriction. They could eat what they liked. In the words of the researchers, 'Patients receiving 5-HTP significantly decreased their daily energy intake, by reducing carbohydrate and fat intake, and reduced their body weight.'[33]

Why the reduced craving for carbohydrates? Imagine two breakfasts. One is an Atkins-style bacon and eggs, high in protein. The other is cornflakes with chopped banana and a muffin. Which will give your serotonin a boost, thereby satisfying you the more? If you think about it logically, you'd say the protein-rich, hence tryptophan-rich, breakfast. But you'd be wrong. It's the cornflakes, banana and muffin breakfast.

Why? Even though the bacon and eggs do contain tryptophan, it has a hard time getting from your blood into your brain – it just doesn't compete well with all the other amino acids in these high-protein foods. However, it does get into the bloodstream. So what drives it into your brain? The answer is insulin. Insulin, which is released by a high-carbohydrate breakfast, carries tryptophan into the brain, and gives you a mood boost. What this means is that when you are feeling tired, hungry and a little blue you crave something sweet, not a sausage. Sound familiar?

> **TOP TIP**
>
> Have one low-**GL** carbohydrate-only snack a day. This raises the brain's level of serotonin, which makes you happier and reduces sugar and carbohydrate cravings.

One big secret of successful weight loss is to (a) ensure you have enough serotonin so you have less desire to eat in excess and (b) keep your blood sugar level, and insulin release, even, so you don't have increased appetite due to blood sugar dips. Remember, too much insulin drives blood sugar into body fat, while too little means low serotonin levels and increased carbohydrate cravings. It's a careful balancing act and one that the Holford Diet takes into account. Here's what I recommend to maximise weight loss.

Fatburning supplements – the basics

I recommend that you supplement your well-balanced diet with fatburning vitamins and minerals, to ensure your metabolism is working at peak efficiency. The ideal intake is different for every individual and can be worked out individually for you by a nutritional therapist (see page 475). However, the chart below gives a good approximation of the optimal supplement levels for an average person, given they're eating a healthful, balanced diet.

Vitamins	Optimum daily intake
Vitamin A	1,500mcg
Vitamin B1 (thiamine)	25mg
Vitamin B2 (riboflavin)	25mg
Vitamin B3 (niacin)	50mg
Vitamin B5 (pantothenate)	50mg
Vitamin B6 (pyridoxine)	50mg
Vitamin B12 (cobalamine)	10mcg
Folic acid	200mcg
Biotin	50mcg
Vitamin C	1,000mg
Vitamin D	5mcg
Vitamin E (d-alpha tocopherol)	100mg

Minerals	Optimum daily intake
Calcium	200mg
Magnesium	150mg
Iron	10mg
Zinc	10mg
Manganese	3mg
Chromium	30mcg

In summary, what this means is taking, on a daily basis:

Daily supplements
2 × multivitamin/mineral
1 × vitamin C 1,000mg

Most health-food shops can help you find supplements to meet these levels in the simplest and least expensive way, choosing from a variety of good brands. Decent, high-strength multi-vitamin/mineral supplements will tell you to take two a day – you just can't get these optimum levels in one tablet. Supplements should be taken with food, preferably with breakfast, or spread throughout the day, since it is during the day that we make most energy and hence need a good supply of these nutrients.

Fatburning supplements – pulling out the stops

During the first three months, if you want all the help you can get in stabilising your appetite and sugar cravings, I recommend the combination of HCA, 5-HTP and chromium. These are the daily levels you need for maximum effect

	Optimum daily intake
Hydroxycitric acid (HCA)	2,250mg
5-hydroxytryptophan (5-HTP)	100–200mg
Chromium	200–400mcg

Bear in mind that 5-HTP is much more effective at normalising the brain's serotonin levels if taken with some carbohydrate, such as a piece of fruit. This will also help prevent the slight abdominal discomfort that a small minority of people get when they take 5-HTP. My advice, therefore, is to supplement both your morning and afternoon snacks with 50mg of 5-HTP.

A word of caution: don't take 5-HTP if you are on sero-tonin-reuptake inhibitor drugs (SSRIs) such as Prozac, Xeroxat, Paroxetine or Lustral, to name just a few. These drugs block the reuptake of serotonin, while 5-HTP provides the brain with the raw material to make enough in the first place. (Logically, 5-HTP should be a more effective antidepressant with fewer side effects. It is – and if you want the proof, see my book *Optimum Nutrition for the Mind*.) Theoretically, taking both could overload you with serotonin. Although I know of no case as such, I don't recommend taking both antidepressant drugs and 5-HTP.

Also take 200mcg of chromium twice a day, with your mid-morning and afternoon snack. Both these supplements tend to reduce sugar cravings and make you feel less hungry and more satiated.

HCA works best before meals. Most supplements supply 750mg per tablet or capsule. You need three times this amount to make a difference, so take one capsule up to half an hour before each meal.

All these supplements are easy to find in most health-food shops.

- Supplement with a high-strength multivitamin and mineral, plus vitamin C every day.

- Supplement with additional chromium, HCA and 5-HTP, especially if you are prone to sugar cravings and have poor appetite control, for the first three months.

Part Three shows you how you do all this.

11

Step 5 – Do 15 Minutes of Exercise a Day

The body is designed to be active. If you've ever truly enjoyed exercise – be it anything from a brisk walk in the park to trekking in the Himalayas – you'll know that wonderful feeling of being at ease and at one with your body. But, even if you've hated exercise, were 'bad at sports' as a child and wouldn't touch an activity holiday with a barge pole, you'll find that the kind of exercise I advocate is amazingly easy to get into, and enjoy.

Exercise is the final puzzle piece in the fatburning picture. Let's take a look at why, and how, it works.

Why exercise?

If you haven't led a very active life, or did once but have gradually become more sedentary, it's not surprising. Life in the West conspires against it. Cars, remote controls, food processors, home-delivery restaurants, 'home entertainment centres', escalators, lifts . . . every year, there are more gadgets and mod cons that do away with the need to expend energy. Ultimately, all roads here lead straight to the sofa, and, if you give in, couch-potato syndrome awaits.

Once that happens, it's all too easy to pile on the pounds. There is no doubt that part of the reason for the massive increase in the number of overweight people is that we are becoming less active.[34] And not only does less activity means fewer calories burned, but also it interferes with the body's appetite mechanisms, rate of metabolism and ability to keep blood glucose levels stable. In other words, some exercise is essential for the body's chemistry to stay 'in tune'.

Now, according to calorie theory, exercise is a poor method of losing weight. After all, running a mile burns up only 300 calories. That's equivalent to two slices of toast or a piece of apple pie. But this argument misses three key points.

1. The effects of exercise are cumulative. OK, so running a mile a day burns up only 300 calories. But if you do that three days a week for a year, that's 22,000 calories, theoretically equivalent to a weight loss of 11lb! Also, the number of calories you burn up depends on how fat or fit you are to start with. The fatter and less fit you are, the more benefit you'll derive from small bouts of exercise.

2. Moderate exercise decreases your appetite. A degree of physical activity is necessary for appetite mechanisms to work properly. Those who do not exercise have exaggerated appetites and hence the pounds gradually creep on.

3. Exercise boosts your metabolic rate. The most important reason exercise is a key to weight loss is its effect on your metabolic rate. According to Professor William McArdle,[35] exercise physiologist at City University, New York, 'Most people can generate metabolic rates that are eight to 10 times above their resting value during sustained cycling, running or swimming. Complementing this increased metabolic rate is the observation that vigorous exercise will raise metabolic rate for up to 15 hours after exercise.'

Dynamic duo – diet and exercise

Combining diet and exercise is the best way to lose weight. Weight lost through restrictive dieting is often half fat and half lean tissue, such as muscle. Since muscle burns up more energy (calories) than fat, the less muscle you have, the slower your metabolism is. Combining the Holford Diet with a good exercise programme ensures you lose fat, not lean muscle. The best kind of exercises to help to burn fat efficiently are brisk walking, jogging, cycling, swimming, aerobic dance, stepping, cross-country skiing, circuit training or any aerobic exercise that is steady, continuous and of a certain intensity.

Such exercises also tone the body, reduce the risk of osteoporosis, increase muscle tissue and reduce one's body fat percentage (high ratios of body fat to lean tissue have been linked to heart disease, diabetes and some cancers). They will strengthen your heart and lungs, reduce your risk of heart disease, help control stress and improve circulation.

Exercise improves insulin sensitivity

But exercise does more than make you leaner. It also helps regulate body chemistry that's essential for fatburning. According to Vanessa Hebditch of the British Diabetic Association, 'Being overweight reduces insulin sensitivity so the risk of developing diabetes is higher. However, there is proof that exercise increases insulin sensitivity, thereby reducing risk." A 24-year study of nearly 6,000 men found that increased physical activity was linked to a reduction in the risk of diabetes, regardless of the level of obesity.

Exercise is especially important in middle age because we are less likely to be able to maintain an even blood sugar level as we age.[36] Unsurprisingly, our sensitivity to insulin decreases with age, along with our control of blood sugar. But physical activity in middle and old age improves insulin sensitivity, therefore helping to stabilise blood sugar levels and weight.[37] Athletes have vastly improved blood sugar control, enhanced insulin sensitivity and faster metabolic rates.[38]

And there's more. High-intensity exercises such as aerobics reduce insulin levels and raise glucagon levels. This means you improve your production of good prostaglandins, boost circulation (and thus the supply of oxygen and nutrients to cells) and increase your ability to burn fat.

Anaerobic exercise such as using weights doesn't burn fat in the same way, or to the same extent. If it is intense enough, though, it may release human growth hormone (controlled by good prostaglandins), which builds muscle and burns fat.

In short, exercise offers a huge array of benefits. If you haven't really got into it before, it opens up an undiscovered world of vitality, health – and sheer enjoyment.

TOP TIP

Go for a stroll after a meal, especially if you tend to get sleepy after meals. It helps to stabilise your blood sugar and insulin level.

How much exercise?

Exercise shouldn't mean a fanatical struggle for some mythical level of fitness. The important thing is merely to stay within the 'training heart rate zone' for your age. Appendix 5 shows you how to work this out (see page 468).

The most traditional formula for calculating your 'training heart rate zone' is to subtract your age from two hundred and twenty. This allows you to estimate your maximum heart rate. This is not the level at which you need to work, this is the predicted maximum your heart can perform at. Once you have calculated your maximum then it is one small step to calculating your training zone.

An overweight, out-of-condition person may reach their training heart rate zone by walking just a few hundred yards. A fitter, leaner person may have to walk briskly for at least five minutes to push their pulse up to their training zone. This is why you need to monitor your pulse while exercising to make sure you do not over- or underexercise, and achieve the best fatburning benefits. As you get fitter and leaner, you'll find that you will have to push harder – perhaps by walking faster or adding more hill walking to your programme – to reach your training zone.

According to surveys, the best benefits in terms of longevity come from expending more than 2,000 calories a week. Walking uses up 300kcals an hour, so you'd need to walk for six hours a week. Jogging is twice as efficient, so you'd need to do only three hours a week. The more overweight you are, the more calories you burn up, so you may need to do only two hours.

If you are doing the right kind of exercise, all you need to do is 15 minutes a day. And this will be enough both for losing weight and for trimming your figure. If you want to confine your exercising to the working week, you can do 21 minutes Monday to Friday and leave the weekend free. Alternatively, you may choose to 'double up' and exercise three times a week for 35 minutes. It doesn't sound that difficult, does it? And it isn't.

When to exercise

The best time to exercise is two hours after eating. If you exercise first thing in the morning, make sure you have breakfast straight after. Even better, if you aim to eat some fruit, perhaps an apple, with your breakfast, have half before you exercise, then the other half with breakfast.

Don't exercise late at night. Exercise promotes adrenal hormones including cortisol. Cortisol should be lowest at night and too much can make it hard to sleep. Also, if possible, exercise in natural daylight because you'll make vitamin D in your skin, which means stronger bones.

One great way to up your general level of exercise is to simply to get more active generally. Use the stairs instead of the lift. Walk or cycle instead of driving everywhere. Run around with your kids, or take up a sport. There are many ways in a day to develop fitness, and soon, this way of living becomes a habit.

The Fat Way	The Fit Way
Take a lift	Use the stairs
Use a trolley when shopping	Use a hand basket
Drive to work	Walk or cycle some of the way
Drive to the shops	Walk to the shops
Spend the night watching TV	Take up an active hobby
Get other people to make you a cup of tea	Get up and make yourself a cup of tea

continues ▶

The Fat Way	The Fit Way
Use powered tools for gardening or DIY work	Use manual tools when it's just as quick
Go upstairs as little as possible at home	Run upstairs as often as possible
Use automatic car washes	Wash it yourself
Stick children in front of TV	Actively play with them
Have business meetings inside	Go for a walk where possible

The more you exercise, the less you eat

Contrary to popular belief, moderate exercise actually decreases your appetite. According to new evidence on appetite research, both animals and humans consistently show decreased appetite with small increases in physical activity. One study looked at an industrial population in West Bengal, India. Those doing sedentary work ate more and consequently weighed more than those doing light work. As the level of work increased from light to heavy, workers ate more, but not relative to their energy output. The result was that the heavier the work, the lighter the worker.

Job classification	Daily caloric intake (kcal)	Body weight (lb)
Sedentary	3,300	148
Light work	2,600	118
Medium work	2,800	114
Heavy work	3,400	113
Very heavy work	3,600	113

Building muscle, burning fat

Having the right balance of hormones, especially insulin – the fat-storage hormone – helps the body to use protein and, if you're exercising, to turn the protein you eat into muscle. And muscle, in its turn, burns fat. Thus the exercise plan I've outlined above works brilliantly with the Holford Diet to turn you into a lean and healthy Fatburner.

A word of warning for the scale-watchers, though: when you start a committed exercise programme, and lose fat and gain lean muscle, you will lose inches faster than pounds. In the first month you'll look trimmer and feel fitter but may lose less weight than you wished. This is because muscle is denser and hence heavier than fat. In other words, a pound of muscle takes up less space than a pound of fat.

Remember, the enemy is not so much your weight, but having too high a body fat percentage. So check this every month using the chart in Appendix 1 (page 429), rather than only jumping on the scales. The more lean muscle you gain, the more ability you'll have to burn fat – and that's what counts.

How do you fit the food around your exercise? Generally, as I've said above, it's good to eat a balanced meal one to two hours before training. Or you can have a light snack half an hour before. Drink plenty of water while you're exercising and eat either a balanced snack or a light meal within an hour of finishing a hard workout. Don't let yourself get so hungry that you eat the wrong food. Glucose drinks, energy bars and the like abound, but by now you'll realise that they're not the way to go for fatburning.

Now we're ready to look in depth at how you're going to put all the pieces together, in Part Three.

● Exercise at least 15 minutes a day, or 35 minutes three times a week.

● Choose aerobic types of exercise that raise your heart rate into the training zone.

- Choose exercise that helps you to build more muscle, which, in turn, burns fat.

References: Part Two

1 Y. Granfeldt, I. Byorck and B. Hagander, 'On the importance of processing conditions, product thickness and egg addition for the glycaemic and hormonal responses to pasta: a comparison of bread made with "pasta ingredients"', *European Journal of Clinical Nutrition*, Vol 45 (1991), pp. 489–99

2 H. Delargy et al., 'Effects of amount and type of dietary fibre (soluble and insoluble) on short-term control of appetite', *International Journal of Food Sciences and Nutrition*, Vol 48 (1997), pp. 67–77

3 H. Kissilef, *American Journal of Physiology* (1980), 238, pp. 14–22; S. Konnyyaku, *Agricultural Biological Chemistry*, Vol 34 (4) (1970), pp. 641–3; M. Matsuura, *Japanese Diabetic Association*, Vol 23 (3) (1980), pp. 209–17

4 A. Mito, data held in ION library, source unknown

5 D. Walsh, unpublished study at GNC Research Center, Fargo, North Dakota (1982)

6 P. Holford, 'The Effects of Glucomannan on Weight Loss', ION (1983)

7 Jenkins D et al., 'Glycemic index of foods: a physiological basis for carbohydrate exchange', *American Journal of Clinical Nutrition*, Vol 34 (1980), pp. 362–6

8 C. B. Pert, *The Molecules of Emotion*, Pocket Books (1999)

9 J. Cleary et al., 'Naloxone effects of sugar-motivated beaviour', *Psychpharmacology*, Vol 176 (1996), pp. 110–14; S. A. Czirr and Reid, 'Demonstrating Morphine's potentiating effects on sucrose-intake', *Brain Research Bulletin*, Vol 17 (1986), pp. 639–42; E. Blass et al., 'Interactions between sucrose, pain, isolation distress', *Pharmacology, Biochemistry of Behaviour*, Vol 26 (1986), pp. 483–9; L. Leventhal et al., 'Selective actions of central mu and kappa opioid antagonists upon sucrose intake in sham-fed rats', *Brain Research*, Vol 685 (1995), pp. 205–10; A. Moles and S. Cooper, 'Opioid modulation of sucrose intake in CD-1 mice', *Physiology and Behaviour*, Vol 58 (1995), pp. 791–96; E. Cheraskin and W. M. Ringsdorf, 'A biochemical denominator in the primary prevention of alcoholism', *Journal of Orthomolecular Psychiatry*, Vol 9 (3) (1980), pp. 158–63

10 G. B. Keijzers et al., 'Caffeine can decrease insulin sensitivity in humans', *Diabetes Care*, Vol 25 (2) (2002), pp. 364–9

11 N. J. Richardson et al., 'Mood and performance effects of caffeine in relation to acute and chronic caffeine deprivation', *Pharmacology, Biochemistry and Behavior,* Vol 52 (2) (1995), pp. 313–20

12 C. Ebbeling et al., 'A reduced-glycemic load diet in the treatment of obesity', *Archives of Pediatrics and Adolescent Medicine,* Vol 157 (8) (2003), pp. 773—9

13 Garg A., 'High mono-unsaturated fat diets for patients with diabetes mellitus: a meta-analysis', *American Journal of Clinical Nutrition,* Vol 67 (1998) (suppl), pp. 577S–582S

14 T. Hung et al., 'Fat versus carbohydrate in insulin resistance, obesity, diabetes and cardiovascular disease', *Current Opinion in Clininical Nutrition and Metabolic Care,* Vol 6 (2) (2003), pp. 165–76

15 C. Bolton-Smith et al., 'Dietary composition and fat to sugar ratios in relation to obesity', *International Journal of Obesity,* Vol 18 (1994), pp. 820–8

16 C. M. Albert et al., 'Blood levels of long-chain n-3 fatty acids and the risk of sudden death', *New England Journal of Medicine,* Vol 346(15) (2002), pp. 1113–18

17 M. Morris et al., *Archives of Neurology,* Vol 60 (2003), pp. 940–6

18 J. Geleijnse et al., 'Reduction on blood pressure with a low sodium, high potassium, high magnesium salt in older subjects with mild to moderate hypertension', *British Medical Journal,* Vol 309 (1994), pp. 436–40

19 T. Gerarduzzi et al., *Journal of Pediatric Gastroenterology and Nutrition,* Vol 31 (2000) (suppl), S29, Abst. 104

20 R. Williams, *The Wonderful World Within You,* BioCommunications Press (1998)

21 'The Vitamin Controversy', ION (1988)

22 R. Wunderlich, *Sugar and Your Health,* Good Health Publications (1982)

23 S. Davies, 'Zinc, Nutrition & Health', in *1984/5 Yearbook of Nutritional Medicine* (1985)

24 S. Davies et al., 'Age-related decreases in chromium levels in 51,665 hair, sweat and serum samples from 40,872 patients – implications for the prevention of cardiovascular disease and type II diabetes mellitus', *Metabolism,* Vol 46(5) (1997), pp. 1–4

25 G. Evans, 'The effect of chromium picolinate on insulin controlled parameters in humans', *International Journal of Biosocial & Medical Research,* Vol 11 (2) (1989), pp. 163–80

26 R. Riales et al., 'Effects of chromium chloride supplementation on glucose tolerance and serum lipids including high density lipoprotein of adult men', *American Journal of Clinical Nutrition*, Vol 34 (1981), pp. 2670–8; A. Abraham et al., 'The effects of chromium supplementation on serum glucose and lipids in patients with and without non-insulin-dependent diabetes', *Metabolism*, Vol 41 (1992), p. 768; W. Glinsmann et al., 'Effects of trivalent chromium on glucose tolerance', *Metabolism*, Vol 15 (1966), pp. 510–15; R. Levine et al., 'Effects of oral chromium supplementation on the glucose tolerance of elderly human subjects', *Metabolism*, Vol 17 (1968), pp. 114–24; K. Hambidge, 'Chromium: A Review' in *Disorders of Mineral Metabolism Vol 1: Trace Minerals*, Academic Press (1981), pp. 272–94

27 M. H. Pittler, C. Stevinson and E. Ernst, 'Chromium picolinate for reducing body weight: meta-analysis of randomized trials', *International Journal of Obesity and Related Metabolic Disorders*, Vol 27(4) (2003), pp. 522–9

28 T. Larsen, S. Toubro and A. Astrup, 'Efficacy and safety of dietary supplements containing CLA for the treatment of obesity: evidence from animal and human studies', *Journal of Lipid Research*, Vol 44(12) 2003, pp. 2234–41

29 D. Clouatre and M. Rosenbaum, *The Diet and Health Benefits of HCA*, Keats Publishing (1994)

30 M. S. Westerterp-Plantenga and E. M. Kovacs, 'The effect of hydroxycitrate on energy intake and satiety in overweight humans', *International Journal of Obesity and Related Metabolic Disorders*, Vol 26(6) (2002), pp. 870–2

31 A. Amer et al., '5-Hydroxy-L-tryptophan suppresses food intake in food-deprived and stressed rats', *Pharmacological Biochemical Behaviour*, Vol 77(1) 2004, pp. 137–43.

32 C. Cangiano et al., 'Eating behavior and adherence to dietary prescriptions in obese adult subjects treated with 5-hydroxytryptophan', *American Journal of Clinical Nutrition*, Vol 56(5) (1992), pp. 863–7

33 C. Cangiano et al., 'Effects of oral 5-hydroxy-tryptophan on energy intake and macronutrient selection in non-insulin dependent diabetic patients', *International Journal of Obesity and Related Metabolic Disorders*, Vol 22(7) (1998), pp. 648–54

34 A. Prentice and S. Jebb, 'Obesity in Britain: gluttony or sloth?', *British Medical Journal*, Vol 311 (1995), pp. 437–9

35 W. McArdle, chapter in *Medical Aspects of Clinical Nutrition*, Keats Publishing (1983)

36 D. Broughton et al., 'Review: Deterioration of Glucose Tolerance with age: The Role of Insulin Resistance', *Age and Ageing* Vol 20 (1991), pp. 221–5

37 C. Hollenbeck et al., 'Effect of habitual exercise on regulation of insulin stimulated glucose disposal in older males', *Journal of the American Geriatric Society*, Vol 33 (1986), pp. 273–7

38 P. Ebelin et al., 'Mechanism of enhanced insulin sensitivity in athletes', *American Society for Clinical Investigations*, Vol 92 (1993), pp. 1623–31

PART THREE

The Action Plan

12

In a Nutshell

The Holford Diet is not a gimmick. It has been tested over 20 years of clinical experience, and is backed by hundreds of scientific trials. It is the best way of helping you lose weight and gain health, easily and enjoyably, because it works with your body's natural design. All you have to do is get your blood sugar balance back to normal, to kick-start your body's own formidable fatburning ability. And in this section I'll show you how – every step of the way.

The key principles behind the Holford Diet are explained in Part Two. Make sure you understand these before you start.

If you're ready – here are the ground rules:

Food

OUT

- **Avoid sugar** in its many disguises and foods that contain fast-releasing carbohydrates with a high-**GL** score – that is, above 10 **GL** per serving.

- **Avoid foods high in saturated, hydrogenated, processed fats or damaged fats**, such as sausages, fried food and junk food.

- **Eliminate any foods you're allergic to.** You can do an avoidance/reintroduction test, but in the long run it's better to have a proper quantitative IgG ELISA test. (After three months you can reintroduce the foods you tested positive for, ideally not eating them every day.)

IN

- **Eat no more than 40 Ⓖ a day**, choosing foods that contain low-Ⓖ carbohydrates, below 10 per serving.

- **Eat low-Ⓖ carbohydrates with protein-rich foods.**

- **Eat whole, unadulterated food, high in soluble fibre** (beans, lentils, oats).

- **Eat foods high in the essential fats** omega-3 and omega-6, with an emphasis on omega-3 fats from fatty cold-water fish, seeds and their oils.

Drink

OUT

- **Limit or avoid alcohol.** Ideally, drink no more than three small glasses of wine, half-pints of beer or lager, or measures of spirit a week.

- **Limit or avoid caffeinated drinks.** Ideally, drink no more than one regular coffee or two weak teas a day. Avoid all caffeinated fizzy drinks.

IN

- **Drink the equivalent of eight glasses of water a day,** including non-caffeine herbal teas or diluted juices.

Supplements

IN

- **Supplement your diet with a high-strength multivitamin and mineral, plus vitamin C, every day.**

- **Supplement your diet with additional chromium, HCA, 5-HTP or konjac extract (glucomannan fibre)** if you are prone to sugar cravings and have poor appetite control, for the first three months.

Exercise

IN

- **Exercise at least 15 minutes a day,** or 35 minutes three times a week.

Each one of these makes a difference in its own right. Put them all together and amazing things can happen, because the whole is far greater than the sum of its parts. This is the most effective way to reduce body fat percentage, lose excess weight and gain health without a rebound effect. Do all this for 30 days and you will switch your body's metabolism from storing fat to burning fat. You will be a fatburner.

Putting all this into practice is even simpler than it sounds. In essence, all you have to do is:

- **Eat any recommended breakfast, lunch or dinner, plus two of the snacks.**

- **Take the recommended supplement programme every day.**

- **Do fatburning exercise on a regular basis.**

There are two ways to do this. Either follow the four weeks of sample menus, together with recipes, in Part Four. Or, for the more independent fatburner, or any time you're eating out (including working lunches), you can devise your own regime using the chart on pages 434–50. Simply follow the golden rules, and you'll be following the Holford Diet.

Whichever way you choose, it's a good idea to stick to the Week 1 menu. This will give you a good idea about quantities, and how to prepare some of the fatburning foods that may be new to you.

Exercise is important for everybody. Combining the Holford Diet with a regular exercise programme (at least three times a week) will undoubtedly give you top results.

It's as simple as that!

One of the first things you'll feel is the satisfaction – you won't have that starved feeling some diets give you. According to Hilary Evans, the first ever Fatburner, 'I have never felt hungry on this diet.' She lost over 20lb.

Chances are you'll also feel more energised and alert within days of starting the Holford Diet. Beyond that, it just gets better.

Now let's look at what you need to do before you start.

13

Getting Ready

Getting ready for the diet is a bit like a warm-up before you exercise. You need a week to prepare – restock your fridge with fatburning foods, find the best alternative foods and drinks and your nearest suppliers, and get used to some of the new foods.

As I said in Part Two, if you're addicted to coffee, tea, chocolate, alcohol and/or cigarettes, you'll need to cut them all out of your life when you start the diet. I realise that cigarettes might take a bit more time, although you'll be surprised how a combination of resolve, modern techniques for quitting and getting into the Fatburning way of life will help cut the cravings. This is also a great time to try out your exercise options (see Chapter 22) and fit them into your weekly routine.

Remove temptations

You'll also need to remove any edible temptations. Start by using up or throwing away any of the foods you'll need to avoid (see the following chapters) from your fridge or larder. This is a great time to have people round for dinner! Restock your kitchen with the recommended foods and drinks. Do the same at work.

Some of the foods on this diet may be new to you, but all of them are readily available in your local health-food shop, supermarket or good greengrocer's. There's a shopping list for you, as well as guidance on how to prepare foods that may be new to you, in Chapter 18.

Setting your targets

Most people start diets hoping to lose in a month what they gained in a year. They vow never to eat chocolate again and to exercise every day. This approach usually ends in failure.

Remember, the purpose of the Holford Diet is to reprogramme your body to burn fat. While it is specifically designed for you to lose weight, equally important is changing your body's chemistry so that you become more inclined to burn unwanted fat than to store it. This takes about 30 days. Once this is achieved, losing weight becomes much easier.

In the meantime, you don't want to start out like a rookie in diet boot camp. So here's my advice on easing into this new way of eating and exercising.

Be realistic

Be realistic, and take it one step at a time. Set yourself targets for changing your diet and taking exercise that you know you will reach. The weight will look after itself. It is far better to take one step towards permanently changing your lifestyle than to take four steps forward and four steps back because you were overambitious to start with.

After all, we often eat because we are under pressure or stressed. Boredom, frustration, anger or a lack of direction all lead to feelings that can be temporarily suppressed with food. Even making small dietary changes is, to begin with, stressful. It takes time to adjust. So don't add to your stress by expecting too much from yourself and then failing to meet your targets.

Be patient

It took years to get that fat. Does it really matter if you take months, rather than weeks, to lose it? Our impatience drives us towards the countless 'get-slim-quick' diets that have been shown, time and time again, not to produce long-term results.

It is very hard for the body to lose more than 2lb of actual fat in a week, although you can also lose a lot of excess fluid when you stop eating something you're allergic to. Anything more rapid is likely to be mainly the short-term loss of fluid caused when you eat too little carbohydrate for energy production, leaving the body to break down stores of glycogen. Glycogen is stored with water – hence the apparent loss of fat that's really loss of water.

Obviously, this won't be happening with the Holford Diet: good-quality, low-Ⓖ carbs are an important part of it, as is sure and steady weight loss.

What results can I expect?

According to studies on the Holford Diet, the average weight loss achieved is 1–2lb a week over a 12-week period. That's 1–2 stone (14–28lb) in less than three months. It is better not to lose weight faster than this. Weight loss of over 2lb a week will not be all fat loss.

Generally speaking, a good target during the first 30 days is to lose 6lb. This is easily achievable on the Holford Diet. But don't forget that your body fat percentage is far more important than your weight, so don't rely on your scales as the only means for checking your progress. As you begin to make more lean muscle you won't lose so much weight, because lean muscle is heavier than the fat your burn off. But you will lose inches, since muscle is more compact than fat.

Making muscle is good news not only because you'll look leaner. Muscle cells are more metabolically active and therefore have the capacity to burn off fat, while fat cells don't. So, as you make more lean muscle, your ability to burn fat increases. Therefore, with the Fatburner System, you'll be able to lose weight and inches consistently, month after month, as well as gain health and vitality.

How do you measure your body fat percentage? You can do this roughly on a week-by-week basis using the equation in Appendix 1. If you do have access to the equipment for measuring it, perhaps at your gym, aim to reduce it by 10 per cent each month until you reach the optimal level of not more than 15 per cent for a man and 22 per cent for a woman.

The chart in Appendix 1 shows your ideal weight range for your height. These figures are calculated from life insurance figures. If you're within your ideal range, I recommend that you don't aim to lose more than 4lb a month until you reach your target. If you are above the ideal range your target should be no more than 8lb a month.

Week-by-week planning

When you're setting your target, it is good to have long-term and short-term objectives. Let's call your long-term objective your goal. What weight would you like to be, ideally? The following questions help to give you a realistic yardstick to go by. What do you weigh now? What, in your opinion, is your ideal weight? How does that compare with the chart in Appendix 1?

When were you last that weight? What is the most you've ever lost on a diet?

When you've answered these questions, you'll have a good idea of your ultimate goal. Once you've set it, you can work out your target, week by week, and fill it in on the chart on page 461. For example, if you want to lose 15lb, your target after one week would be to weigh 1½lb less and so on for 10 weeks, after which you'll have achieved your goal.

Now you are ready to get fatburning! The next three chapters tell you what to eat for breakfast, lunch, dinner and snacks.

14

What to Eat for Breakfast

First of all, don't skip on breakfast. It's the most important meal of your day. You may feel that the old adage 'Breakfast like a king ...' is being taken down and dusted off, but it's absolutely true, and here's why.

When you wake up your blood sugar is low because you haven't eaten. So you need to eat. But many people in the grip of a firm resolve to lose weight make the fatal mistake of trying not to eat anything for as long as possible. Unless propped up with liquid stimulants (coffee or tea), nicotine, or instant sugar in the form of a piece of toast or a croissant, that resolve becomes weaker and weaker as your blood sugar level dips lower and lower, until the chances of making the right food choices become smaller and smaller. So you buckle under the strain and end up bingeing out on high-ⓖⓛ foods. Sound familiar?

That's why you must eat breakfast. The only question is what and how much. Nutritionists at Oxford Brookes University set out to test this by giving children either a low-ⓖⓛ breakfast or a high-ⓖⓛ breakfast, then measuring who ate the most as children helped themselves to a buffet lunch. While both breakfasts were rated as equally satisfying by the children immediately after eating, by lunchtime those who'd had the high-ⓖⓛ breakfast were more hungry and ate more food.[1] Exactly the same thing has been shown in adults, too.[2]

The message is clear. Eat a low-ⓖⓛ breakfast. It will satisfy you for longer so you'll eat less later.

There are two ways to do this. The simplest is to choose from any of the Fatburner breakfasts listed on page 307. These are already calculated to give you no more 10 ⓖⓛ, plus the right amount of protein and essential fats.

Or you can 'do it yourself'. The DIY Fatburner breakfast is also very straightforward. The fundamental rules are shown in the diagram overleaf.

There are five fundamental breakfasts that give you the right balance of both carbohydrate and protein. These are:

Carbohydrates		Protein
Cereal/fruit	+	seeds/yoghurt/milk
Fruit	+	yoghurt/seeds
Fruit	+	Get Up & Go/milk
Bread/toast	+	egg
Bread/toast	+	fish (e.g. kippers)

The question is which and how much cereal, fruit, toast and so on. Let's kick off with the cereal-based breakfast, sweetened with fruit rather than sugar.

The best cereal-based breakfasts

A good cereal-based breakfast needs to include a low-ⓖⓛ cereal, a low-ⓖⓛ fruit as a sweetener and a source of protein and essential fats. The goal, remember, is no more than 10 ⓖⓛ.

Breakfast

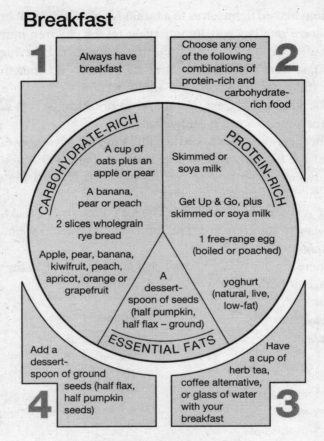

1 Always have breakfast

2 Choose any one of the following combinations of protein-rich and carbohydrate-rich food

CARBOHYDRATE-RICH

A cup of oats plus an apple or pear

A banana, pear or peach

2 slices wholegrain rye bread

Apple, pear, banana, kiwifruit, peach, apricot, orange or grapefruit

PROTEIN-RICH

Skimmed or soya milk

Get Up & Go, plus skimmed or soya milk

1 free-range egg (boiled or poached)

yoghurt (natural, live, low-fat)

ESSENTIAL FATS

A dessert-spoon of seeds (half pumpkin, half flax – ground)

4 Add a dessert-spoon of ground seeds (half flax, half pumpkin seeds)

3 Have a cup of herb tea, coffee alternative, or glass of water with your breakfast

The Holford Diet: breakfast

In the chart opposite you'll see how much of the following six cereals you can have to total 5 ⓖ. As you can see, the best 'value' in terms of your appetite are oat flakes, either cooked as in porridge or eaten raw, just as you would cornflakes. Basically, you could eat as many as you like, given that two servings will fill anybody up.

CEREAL 5 🄖🄻

Oat flakes	2 servings
All-Bran	1 serving
Unsweetened muesli	1 small serving
Alpen	half a serving
Raisin Bran	half a serving
Weetabix	1 biscuit

Below, on the right-hand side you can see how much of these six fruits you could eat to equal 5 🄖🄻.

FRUIT 5 🄖🄻

Strawberries	1 large punnet
Pear	1
Grapefruit	1
Apple	1 small
Peach	1 small
Banana	less than half

So your best bet out of these would be to have porridge or raw oat flakes with as many strawberries as you could eat. Alternatively, you could have a bowl of All-Bran and a grapefruit, or a bowl of unsweetened muesli with a small grated apple. Or you can build your own breakfast using the full 🄖🄻 chart in Appendix 2 on pages 434–50.

As far as protein is concerned, there's some in milk (or in soya milk, if you're allergic to dairy). Rice milk is high-🄖🄻 and best avoided. Yoghurt (unsweetened) is also high in protein. So, have a spoonful of yoghurt, some milk or some soya milk on your cereal if you'd like to.

Another source of protein, as well as countless vitamins, minerals, essential fats and fibre, is seeds. I recommend you have a tablespoon of ground seeds on your cereal as well. This really adds flavour and, by giving yourself the essential fats you need, you won't crave less desirable food sources of fat.

TOP TIP

Smart animals – from parrots to people – eat seeds. Seeds are incredibly rich in essential fats, minerals, vitamin E, protein and fibre. You need a tablespoon a day for 100% health. Here's the magic formula:

1. Fill a glass jar that has a sealing lid half with flax seeds (rich in omega-3), half with sesame, sunflower or pumpkin seeds (rich in omega-6).
2. Keep the jar sealed and in the fridge to minimise damage from light, heat and oxygen.
3. Put a handful in a coffee/seed grinder, grind up and put a tablespoon on your cereal. Store the remainder in the fridge and use over the next few days.

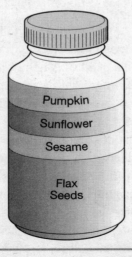

The best cereal-based breakfast is Fatburner Muesli, made by mixing porridge oat flakes, oat bran and ground seeds, fresh berries and yoghurt. See the recipe on page 310. A serving has a 🄶🄻 of 8 and is completely satisfying.

The best yoghurt-based breakfasts

If you are fond of yoghurt, you could dispense with the cereal altogether and have yoghurt, fruit and seeds. Let's take a look at how this adds up. In the chart below you'll see how much yoghurt you can eat for 5 🄶🄻. (A small pot of yoghurt is 150g.)

YOGHURT	5 🄶🄻
Plain yoghurt	2 small pots (330mg)
Non-fat yoghurt	2 small pots
Low-fat yoghurt with fruit and sugar	less than 1 small pot (100g)

So provided you choose a yoghurt that doesn't have added sugar, you can eat two small pots, sweetened with any of the fruits you like from the fruit chart above, plus a tablespoon of ground seeds.

Get Up & Go-based breakfasts

Get Up & Go is a powder that you blend with a piece of fruit, choosing from any of the 5-🄶🄻 servings of fruit shown above and half a pint of skimmed milk (or sugar-free soya milk if you are allergic).

Get Up & Go is made from a special blend of quinoa, brown rice and soya flour, giving an excellent quality of protein balanced with carbohydrate, mainly from whole apple powder, together with oat bran, rice bran and psyllium husks for added soluble fibre, plus sesame, sunflower and pumpkin seeds and some almond meal, cinnamon and natural vanilla for flavour. In addition, it has added vitamins and minerals, including 50mcg of chromium and 1,000mg of vitamin C, plus all the B vitamins.

When it's made up, it's guaranteed to fill you up till lunchtime, and yet is only 283 calories. The best fruits to use in Get Up & Go are strawberries, raspberries, a soft pear, black-currants (which you can buy in cans in apple juice) or banana. If you use banana, use only half a fruit. Get Up & Go provides about 5 Ⓖ, so you're looking for no more than another 5 from the fruit you blend in with it. (See page 480 for Get Up & Go stockists.)

The best egg-based breakfasts

While it is true that more than half the calories in an egg come from fat, the kind of fat depends on what you feed the chicken. Most eggs come from battery chickens. If you know how unhealthy they are, you don't eat their eggs, which are high in saturated fat.

However, there are two egg producers in the UK (and many more abroad) that give their chickens feed rich in fatty acids, for example flax seeds. These egg brands are Columbus and Intelligent. These are both free-range and rich in omega-3 fats, and much better for you than ordinary eggs. I recommend you have no more than four eggs a week on the Holford Diet – and only these kinds of egg. Have either two small eggs, or one large egg, at one meal. Poach, boil or scramble them, but don't fry them, since the high heat damages the essential fats.

As eggs are pure protein and fat, what carbohydrate can you have with them? If this is your entire breakfast you can use up your entire 10-🔵 quota by having any of the following bread servings.

BREAD	10🔵
Oatcakes	4
Rye 'pumpernickel' style	2 thin slices
Sourdough rye bread	2 thin slices
Rye wholemeal bread (yeasted)	1 slice
Wheat wholemeal bread (yeasted)	1 slice
White, high-fibre bread (yeasted)	less than 1 slice

As you can see, your best-'value' breads are oatcakes, which are a Scottish favourite, or Scandinavian-style pumpernickel, son-nenbrot- or volkenbrot-type breads, or sourdough rye bread, made without yeast. Unlike the light, white, fluffy 'fake' breads we've been conditioned to eat, which are full of air, super-refined and nutritionally inferior, sourdough and the like are real breads, substantial, fibre-rich and delicious. You may find the change a bit of a shock at first, but you'll find that they are very satisfying.

Real breads are better for two reasons. One is the way they're processed, which I discussed in Part Two. They have far fewer additives, use coarsely ground flours and, in the case of sour-dough, have no added yeast. All this keeps the 🔵 score lower.

Also, some grains are better than others because of the type of carbohydrate, or sugar, they contain. Wheat and corn are high in a fast-releasing sugar called *amylopectin*, while barley, rye and quinoa are higher in one called *amylose*, which is slower-releasing. Most rice, by the way, has a high 🔵 score because it contains a large proportion of amylopectin. Basmati rice, however, has more amylose and is therefore slower-releasing. Brown basmati is best.

· Of the grains, oats are among the best. While the Ⓖⓛ of wheat varies depending on what's done to it, oats are the same in any shape or form. Whole oat flakes, rolled oats or oatmeal, as used in oatcakes, all have a low glycemic effect.[3]

Kippers, anyone?

Kippers (smoked herring) have gone out of fashion, but they make a fabulous fatburning breakfast – tasty and highly nutritious. Rich in protein and omega-3 fats, one kipper and any of the bread portions shown above will meet your needs for a fatburning breakfast.

Now let's move on to snacks, since that's the next thing you are going to eat.

15

What to Eat for Snacks

The Holford Diet is all about enjoying your food while losing weight and boosting health, and snacks give you even more scope for enjoyment. But what to eat? Those with sugar sensitivity are likely to reach for snacks that compensate for changes in blood sugar levels and hormonal responses. Most commercial snacks are incredibly high in sugar or fat. It won't surprise you that a Mars Bar is almost two-thirds sugar with the rest mainly fat; but even some so-called 'muesli' bars are deceptively unhealthy, made with refined sugar and masses of hydrogenated fat.

However, research shows clearly that 'grazing' (eating little and often) is healthier for you than 'gorging' (having one or two big meals in the day).[4] Grazing helps keep your blood sugar level even and this makes overeating far less likely, as you'll never experience any between-meal hunger pangs. For this reason I recommend you have a mid-morning and a mid-afternoon snack. The ideal snack is one that provides no more than 5 ⒼⓁs and also some protein, and the simplest snack food is fruit. Let's see what you could eat to stay within 5 ⒼⓁ for your snack.

FRUIT	**5 ⑮**
Strawberries	1 large punnet
Plums	4
Cherries	1 small punnet
Pear	1
Grapefruit	1
Orange	1
Apple	1 small (can fit in the palm of your hand)
Peach	1 small
Melon/watermelon	1 slice

Berries, plums and cherries are your best-'value' fruit snacks. Berries include raspberries, blueberries, blackberries and any others that you can get your hands on in season. You can further slow down the ⑮ score of these fruits by eating them with five almonds or a dessertspoon of pumpkin seeds. Other than chestnuts, almonds are the best nut because they have the most protein compared with calories. Pumpkin seeds are also high in protein and in omega-3 fats. Flax seeds are the highest for omega-3 but are too small to make good snacks, and need to be ground up because they have a hard outer coating.

Another snack option would be some kind of bread with a protein-based spread. Cottage cheese, hummus and peanut butter are good examples. Hummus, if you haven't encountered it before, is a Middle Eastern chickpea spread or dip, deliciously rich-tasting although low in ⑮. It tastes great with oatcakes, on rye bread or with a raw carrot (see recipe on page 328). (A large carrot is still less than 5 ⑮). If you like peanut butter, buy the kind with no added sugar. A slice of any of the bread servings below with either hummus or peanut butter gives you the right kind of low-⑮ carbohydrate with some protein to keep your blood sugar level even.

Oatcakes, and oats in general, are excellent as far as weight and blood sugar are concerned. Oats contain beta-glucans, a type of fibre that helps to slow down the release of glucose into the blood, lessen insulin response and also lower cholesterol and heart disease risk. Of all the grains, it's the best for losing weight, and for controlling your blood sugar.[5]

Watch out when buying oatcakes, though. Many contain sugar. The best are Nairns, since not only do they have sugar-free, organic types, but also they use palm fruit oil, which contains unsaturated fat, as opposed to palm oil, which is higher in saturated fat.

BREAD	**5 ⒼⓁ**
Oatcakes	2 biscuits
Rye 'pumpernickel' style	1 thin slice
Sourdough rye bread	1 thin slice
Rye wholemeal bread (yeasted)	half a slice
Wheat wholemeal bread (yeasted)	half a slice
White, high fibre bread (yeasted)	less than half a slice

So here are a selection of 5-ⒼⓁ snacks to choose from:

- a piece of fruit, plus five almonds or a dessertspoon of pumpkin seeds;

- a thin slice of rye bread or two oatcakes and half a small tub of cottage cheese (150g);

- a thin slice of rye bread/two oatcakes and half a small tub of hummus (150g);

- a thin slice of rye bread/two oatcakes and peanut butter;

- crudités (a carrot, pepper, cucumber or celery) and hummus;

- crudités and cottage cheese;

- a small yoghurt (150g), no sugar, plus berries; or

- cottage cheese plus berries.

As you can see, you won't be bored between meals, as there's masses of scope for mixing and matching. But these are only to give you an idea of what to expect. You'll find an array of snack recipes in Chapter 28, including Flageolet Bean Dip, Smoked Salmon Pâté with oatcakes and crudités, and Quinoa Tabbouleh.

16

What to Eat for Lunch and Dinner

Main meals are really something to look forward to on the Holford Diet, as you'll see from the recipes and menus in Part Four. But how do you put it all together? The easiest way to get the right nutritional balance is to imagine all the different foods a plate. I showed you this method in Part Two, and you'll find it described again below.

Half the plate will consist of very low-ⓖⓛ vegetables. This includes peas, broccoli, carrots, runner beans, courgettes and kale, among many others. These vegetables, listed on page 221, will account for no more than 4 ⓖⓛ, and I'm going to show you how to prepare them in minutes. If you haven't been all that interested in veg up to now, you'll be amazed by how fresh and zingy they can taste when they're cooked in these ways.

The other half of your plate is divided into two, one for protein-based food such as meat, fish or tofu, and the other for more 'starchy' vegetables, which account for 6 to 7 ⓖⓛ. There's a chart showing this on page 217. So, a quarter of what's on your plate is protein-rich, a quarter is carbohydrate-rich and half is made up of very low-Ⓖ vegetables. You'll soon get the hang of it. It's dead simple.

More fish, less meat

Let's kick off with the protein serving on your plate. Remember from Part Two that the overall amount of protein – by which I mean the protein contained in the various foods, not protein-rich foods – at each meal will be 20g. The protein-rich food on your plate will provide 15g of this, and the table below tells you how much you need to eat of each of these to get that 15g. (The one serving of carbohydrate-rich starchy vegetables and two servings of very low-Ⓖ vegetables will provide the remaining 5g.)

In the table I've listed a lot of fish options and fewer meat options. In fact, red meat is missing entirely. White meat tends to be much lower in fat and fish is much higher in the essential omega-3 fats, so, becoming a 'fishichicketarian' is a great way to lose weight and gain health.

Does this mean you can never eat red meat again? Certainly not. Once you've attained your target weight you can have lean red meat once a week.

How big is a protein serving?

Food	Weight	Serving
Tofu and tempeh	160g	¾ packet
Soya mince	100g	3 tbsp
Chicken (no skin)	50g	1 very small breast
Turkey (no skin)	50g	½ small breast
Quorn	120g	⅓ pack
Salmon and trout	55g	1 very small fillet
Tuna (canned in brine)	50g	¼ tin
Sardines (canned in brine)	75g	⅔ tin

Cod	65g	1 very small fillet
Clams	60g	¼ can
Prawns	85g	6 large prawns
Mackerel	85g	1 medium fillet
Oysters	–	15
Yoghurt (natural, low fat)	285g	½ large tub
Cottage cheese	120g	½ medium tub
Hummus	200g	1 small tub
Skimmed milk	440ml	c. ¾ pint
Soya milk	415ml	c. ¾ pint
Eggs (boiled)	–	2
Quinoa	125g	large serving bowl
Baked beans	310g	¾ tin
Kidney beans	175g	⅓ tin
Black-eyed beans	175g	⅓ tin
Lentils	165g	⅓ tin

Starchy vegetables

As we see on the plate on page 228, carbohydrate-rich 'starchy vegetable' servings should be roughly the same size or weight as protein servings. But this depends on how each food weighs up. For example, if you are eating chicken with rice, the serving size of rice is somewhat larger than the piece of chicken for each to be roughly the same weight, because chicken is dense and heavy and rice is relatively light.

Remember, starchy vegetables will account for a maximum 7 🄶🄻 of your meal (out of a total of 10 🄶🄻). Let's take a look at what quantity of different starchy vegetables you can eat to keep within that limit, leaving 3 🄶🄻 for the very low-🄶🄻 veg that occupy half the plate.

STARCHY VEGETABLES	7 🔵
Pumpkin/squash	big serving (186g)
Carrot	one large (158g)
Swede	big serving (150g)
Quinoa	big serving (131g)
Beetroot	big serving (112g)
Cornmeal	a serving (116g)
Pearl barley	a small serving (95g)
Wholemeal pasta	half a serving (85g)
White pasta	third of a serving (66g)
Brown rice	a small serving (70g)
White rice	a third of a serving (46g)
Couscous	a third of a serving (46g)
Broad beans	a serving (31g)
Corn on the cob	half a cob (60g)
Boiled potato	three small potatoes (74g)
Baked potato	half (59g)
French fries	tiny portion (47g)
Sweet potato	half (61g)

As you can see, there are some obvious winners. Wholemeal pasta – for example spaghetti – and brown rice are much better than white pasta and white rice. (As we saw earlier, brown basmati rice has the lowest 🔵 score of all the different types of rice.) Swede, carrot and squash are much better than potato. Boiled potato is better than baked potato, which is in turn better than French fries.

Some of these foods may be new to you. If so, you'll be bowled over by, say, the nutty flavour of quinoa and the smooth, rich savour of the squashes. If you love pasta, switching to the wholemeal variety is painless. It cooks the same way, but you can eat more of the unrefined variety and stay slim.

TOP TIP

Try a new food every week. For example, have you ever eaten barley or quinoa? Barley can be cooked like rice and is very tasty in soups and casseroles. So is quinoa – actually a seed rather than a grain – which takes only 13 minutes to cook and is packed with extra protein, iron and vitamins.

Beans and lentils

It's telling that beans and lentils are no longer widely eaten in many of the world's fattest nations. These are the best foods for both balancing your blood sugar and giving the right mix of protein and carbohydrate. It's this rare double whammy that keeps their ⒼⓁ score low. (Another reason why lentils and soya are so low is that they contain a substance that prevents the digestion of amylose, therefore slowing down its release further.) Soya also keeps your arteries healthy by lowering the 'bad' LDL cholesterol. A serving a day, either as soya milk or tofu, can lower your LDL cholesterol by over 10 per cent.

Any meal containing beans and lentils can be quite generous with the portion size because you are getting both the protein and the carbohydrate from the same food. However, when you are eating these foods as your source of protein, combine with only *half* the serving size of a carbohydrate-rich food, instead of an equal serving. For example, if you were making Dhal (Lentil Curry) (see page 352), you'd have a cup of lentils and half a cup of rice. This is, of course, because you're already getting a significant amount of carbohydrate in the lentils.

This is how much you can eat, assuming you are not eating another starchy vegetable, to stay within 7 ⒼⓁ. (Most regular cans of beans provide around 225 to 245g of beans.)

BEANS AND LENTILS	7 ⓖⓛ
Soya beans	2 cans
Pinto/borlotti beans	¾ can
Lentils	¾ can
Baked beans	½ can
Butter beans	½ can
Split peas	½ can
Kidney beans	½ can
Chickpeas	⅓ can

If you're not vegetarian, you may be relatively unfamiliar with beans and lentils. You may have encountered dhal, baked beans, hummus or cassoulet, but never actually thrown a packet or tin of lentils or beans into your shopping basket. These are great foods, immensely satisfying in flavour and texture, and they feature in all of the world's great cuisines – as well as kitchen classics such as beans on toast. You'll be making mouthwatering dishes with them, from hummus and Flageolet Bean Dip to Lentil and Lemon Soup, Dhal and a fiery chilli, to name just a few.

Unlimited vegetables

Now it's time to move on to the other half of your plate. This is made up of what I call the 'unlimited vegetables'. Of course, there are limits, but these are vegetables for which a serving is less than 2 ⓖⓛ. A serving of peas, for instance, is a cup.

> ### TOP TIP
>
> Eat your food slowly. Chew each mouthful twenty times, as this will further 'slow-release' the carbohydrate in your food.

UNLIMITED VEGETABLES

Asparagus	Endive	Radish
Aubergine	Fennel	Rocket
Beansprouts	Garlic	Runner beans
Broccoli	Kale	Spinach
Brussels sprouts	Lettuce	Spring onions
Cabbage	Mangetout	Tenderstem
Cauliflower	Mushrooms	Tomato
Celery	Onions	Watercress
Courgette	Peas	
Cucumber	Peppers	

If the word 'cabbage' makes you think of watery soup, and runner beans have always been something you pushed around on your plate, be prepared: I have some seriously delicious recipes for these. You'll end up eager to find new ways of eating them – and looking amazing, thanks to the vitamins, minerals and other phytonutrients they're brimming with.

So, to recap: I want you to eat two servings of unlimited vegetables, one serving of 'starchy' vegetables and once serving of protein-based food. Together, they'll help you feel full at the end of every meal.

Vegetarians

If you're a strict vegetarian, you'll need to eat more tofu, beans, lentils, soya produce and Quorn than usual to achieve the target for protein intake. A serving size of tofu for a main meal is 160g, which is roughly three-quarters of a packet. Part Four contains a number of recipes and ways to use tofu – the vegetarian Fatburner's best friend – along with recipes using a variety of beans and lentils. And many of the recipes containing chicken or fish can be adapted by replacing them with tofu or a tofu steak, and I make a point of mentioning this. (For more detailed general advice for vegetarians, see Chapter 20.)

Fats and oils

This diet is not low-fat; you'll be able to eat enough to keep you satisfied. As far as fats and oils go, what's important is which fats you use, and how you use them.

Creams: If you want to make a savoury dish creamier, try adding a teaspoon of tahini (sesame spread) or a tablespoon of coconut milk or coconut cream.

Salad dressings: When using seed oils for salad dressings, pick either flax seed oil or a blend of oils that gives at least one part of omega-3 fats to one part of omega-6 fats. These seed oils need to be cold-pressed and stored in a lightproof container.

Two good seed-oil blends are Essential Balance and Udo's Choice, available in health-food shops. Also good is walnut oil. You can lightly drizzle these oils onto vegetables instead of butter.

Cooking oils: For steam-frying (see below) and sautéing, use a small amount of butter, coconut butter or olive oil. Coconut butter adds a great flavour to steam-fries.

Cooking methods

All carbohydrate foods release their carbohydrate somewhat faster once cooked. The longer you cook something and the higher the temperature, the faster-releasing the food becomes. It's therefore best to eat food as close to raw as possible.

This doesn't mean endless salads. You can steam, steam-fry,

boil and poach food without cooking it to death. Next best is baking, grilling, sautéing and stir-frying. Worst is frying and deep-frying.

Steaming is the best way of cooking green, leafy, less starchy vegetables, since it preserves a lot of their vitamins and minimises any raising of ⓖⓛ. This method can be used with any food and is very successful with fish – but perhaps not ideal with starchy vegetables, which require longer cooking, or with red meat. Many different kinds of steamers are available, or you can improvise with a colander, pot and lid.

Boiling raises the ⓖⓛ of foods more than steaming, but less than baking. Changes can be kept to a minimum by using as little water as possible, keeping the lid on, and cooking the food as whole as possible. Also, eat all vegetables *al dente* – a little crisp, not soft.

Steam-frying figures large in the Holford Diet because it adds loads of taste without compromising on health. The great advantage of this style of cooking is that the lower temperature of steaming doesn't destroy nutrients to anything like the extent that frying does, and you use only a small amount of oil, if any. As with boiling and ordinary steaming, aim to keep veg *al dente*.

To steam-fry, use a shallow pan or a deep frying pan with a thick base and lid that seals well. You can steam-fry without oil by first adding two tablespoons of liquid to the pan – water, vegetable stock, soy sauce or a watered-down bit of the sauce you'll use for the dish. Once it boils, immediately add some vegetables, 'sauté' rapidly for a minute or two, turn the heat up, add a tablespoon or two more of the liquid and clamp the lid on tightly. After a minute add the rest of the ingredients. Turn the heat down after a couple of minutes and steam in this way until cooked.

Or you can add a teaspoon to a tablespoon of olive oil, butter or coconut oil to the pan, warm it, add the ingredients and sauté. After a couple of minutes, add two tablespoons of liquid as above and clamp the lid on. Steam ingredients till done.

Poaching is like steam-frying without the sautéing. You can make delicious water-based sauces. For example, you could cook fish in vegetable broth flavoured with ginger, garlic, lemongrass, spices and wine (the alcohol boils off).

Waterless cooking requires specially designed pans in which you can 'boil' foods by steaming them in their own juice and 'fry' foods with no oil. Both methods are excellent, for preserving both nutrients and flavour.

Baking is useful, especially if the food is large and has a thick skin (such as a whole or half pumpkin). Avoid coating food with oil, because the oil will oxidise with cooking, which creates free radicals (highly reactive, harmful molecules). You can roast a potato without adding oil. The higher the temperature and the longer you cook something, the higher the ⓖⓛ becomes.

Frying should be kept to a minimum, and deep-frying avoided altogether. When you do fry use butter, coconut oil (saturated fat) or olive oil (mono-unsaturated) rather than other vegetable oils (polyunsaturated oils), since these are much more prone to oxidation.

Grilling foods that contain fat is less damaging than frying, but browning or burning a food does create free radicals. Try to avoid barbecued food, or at least ensure what you eat is not charred.

Microwaving is a problematic cooking method, although admittedly fast. As food cooks in its own water, it seems better than most cooking methods for preserving the water-soluble vitamins B and C. A Spanish study, however, found that microwaved broccoli lost vast amounts of major antioxidants (nutrients working to rid the body of free radicals) compared with steaming.

Moreover, the temperatures reached in fat particles are very high, so avoid microwaving oily fish: it will destroy the essential fats it contains. And remember that microwave ovens do give off electromagnetic radiation, even six feet away.

If you must microwave, it is better to use lower-voltage/heat settings for longer. Cover dishes to encourage steaming, although you do need to leave some room for steam to escape.

TOP TIP

- Buy foods as fresh and unprocessed as possible and eat them soon afterwards.
- Eat more raw food. Be adventurous. Try raw beetroot and carrot tops in salad.
- Cook foods as whole as possible, slicing or blending before serving.
- Use as little water as possible, preferably steaming, poaching or steam-frying.
- Fry foods as infrequently as possible.
- Favour slow-cook methods that introduce less heat.
- Don't overcook, burn or brown food.

What to limit and avoid

The trick with any diet is to fill yourself up with the good stuff so there's little room left for less desirable foods. Some of the goodies, however, such as oily fish, still need to be limited because, although they contain valuable fats, too much of any fat is bad for you.

Foods to limit

The chart below shows you which foods to limit and how much to limit them to. Some of these are included in the recipes in specific amounts because they contain important nutrients. Some are high in fat, while others are high in sugar, so do not have more than the recommended amounts.

Dried fruit	choose fresh fruit or soak dried fruit
Coconut	can be used in small amounts to flavour dishes
Seeds	limit to two dessertspoons a day maximum, or one heaped tablespoon
Nuts	same as seeds (don't have both, and seeds are better)
Salad dressings	stick to the measures given in Part Four
Avocados	twice a week, maximum
Vegetable oil and butter	use sparingly, as in the recipes
Tahini (sesame spread)	use a small amount of instead of butter
Fatty fish such as herring, mackerel, tuna, kippers	three times a week, maximum
Chicken (no skin), game	twice a week, maximum
Milk and yoghurts	stick to skimmed milk and low-fat yoghurt
Eggs	three a week, maximum

Foods to avoid

These foods are high in fat and/or fast-releasing sugar, or are devoid of nutrients, so they're best strictly avoided. Once you have attained your target weight they may be eaten on rare occasions.

High-fat meats including beef, pork, lamb, sausages and processed meats

Lard, dripping, suet and gravy

Deep-fried foods

Cream and shop-bought ice cream

High-fat spreads and mayonnaises

All cheeses except cottage cheese, low-fat quark or fromage frais, and half-fat Cheddar cheese such as Shape

Rich sauces made with cream, cheese or eggs

Sugar, sugar-laden sweets and foods with added sugar

Pastries, cakes and biscuits

White bread

Snack foods such as crisps

Main Meals

1 Choose one serving of a protein-rich and one serving of a carbohydrate-rich food, plus two servings of any of the vegetables.

2 The serving size of the carbohydrate food (such as rice or pasta) should be more or less the *same size or weight* as the serving size of the protein food.

3 Vary your diet. If you eat meat and fish, have meat no more than twice a week, fish three times a week and vegetarian meals the rest.

4 Have a glass of water with your meal.

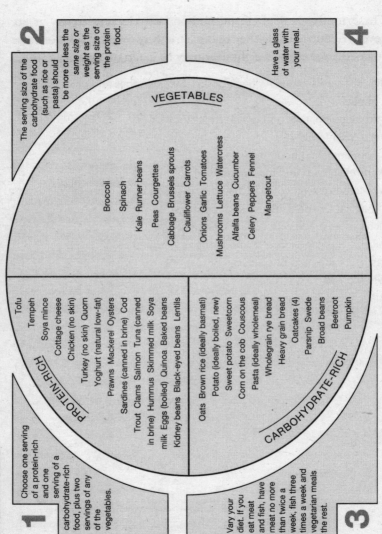

VEGETABLES

Broccoli
Spinach
Kale Runner beans
Peas Courgettes
Cabbage Brussels sprouts
Cauliflower Carrots
Onions Garlic Tomatoes
Mushrooms Lettuce Watercress
Alfalfa beans Cucumber
Celery Peppers Fennel
Mangetout

PROTEIN-RICH

Tofu
Tempeh
Soya mince
Cottage cheese
Chicken (no skin)
Turkey (no skin) Quorn
Yoghurt (natural low-fat)
Prawns Mackerel Oysters
Sardines (canned in brine) Cod
Trout Clams Salmon Tuna (canned in brine) Hummus Skimmed milk Soya milk Eggs (boiled) Quinoa Baked beans
Kidney beans Black-eyed beans Lentils

CARBOHYDRATE-RICH

Oats Brown rice (ideally basmati)
Potato (ideally boiled, new)
Sweet potato Sweetcorn
Corn on the cob Couscous
Pasta (ideally wholemeal)
Wholegrain rye bread
Heavy grain bread
Oatcakes (4)
Parsnip Swede
Broad beans
Beetroot
Pumpkin

The Holford Diet: main meals

17

Drinks, Desserts and Sweets

So far, we've looked only at food. But what about drinks – including alcohol? You'll have a broad choice of hot drinks and juices, and will be able to have a few convivial glasses of wine a week. And there are plenty of mouthwatering desserts in Part Four to choose from, as well as sweets that won't overshoot your ⒼⓁ allowance by a mile, available at your local health-food shop.

As you now know by heart, the food you eat will have 40 ⒼⓁ a day. On top of this, the ⒼⓁ allowance for drinks, desserts and sweets is 5 ⒼⓁ. Your 5 daily ⒼⓁ could be a glass of juice or wine, a Fatburner dessert or even some chocolate – just not all four in the same day.

As before, if you're drinking a lot of coffee or tea, getting through a fair bit of chocolate, drinking alcohol fairly frequently – or doing all three – you will need to stop all of them for at least two weeks to a month when you start the Holford Diet. Thus any withdrawal symptoms will be short-lived: the nutrients and supplements you're taking in will be getting to grips with the bottoming out of your blood sugar. You could feel a bit rough for several days, but this will dissipate fast.

Gradually, you should see any cravings for super-sweetness or alcohol begin to disappear. By the time you're ready to reintroduce the odd piece of chocolate, cup of tea or glass of Sancerre, the switchover to fatburning will have begun and you'll be able to handle the occasional treat without encouraging any imbalance in blood sugar.

Cold drinks

The best drink for fatburning is water – and you need to drink the equivalent of 2 litres, or 8 glasses, a day. If that seems an enormous amount, be aware that you can factor in any herbal teas, coffee substitutes and juices you drink. Leaving a bottle on your desk at work makes it easier to remember to keep it topped up. When you're thoroughly hydrated, you'll feel much better in every way. This is a habit that will – like the rest of the Holford Diet – become second nature.

Fruit juices, whether concentrated or fresh, have a relatively high ⑮ because the fibres have been removed. The best is apple juice, although even this should be drunk diluted – half juice, half water, or, even better, two-thirds water, one-third juice.

Here's how much you can drink for 5 ⑮ points.

DRINK	5 ⑮
Tomato juice	1 pint
Carrot juice	small glass
Grapefruit juice, unsweetened	small glass
Apple juice, unsweetened	small glass, diluted 50:50 with water

Orange juice, unsweetened	small glass, diluted 50:50 with water; or juice of one orange
Pineapple juice	half a small glass, diluted 50:50 with water
Cranberry juice drink	half a small glass, diluted 50:50 with water
Grape juice	an inch's worth of liquid!

Stay away from all fizzy, sweetened, caffeinated drinks and sugar-sweetened cordials. You can use cordials sweetened with apple juice concentrate, which contains more slow-releasing fructose, rather than grape juice concentrate, which has a much higher score.

A good rule of thumb is to have no more than one glass of juice a day, diluting it as you need to in order to have no more than 5 ⑬ a day. So have, say, either a glass of carrot juice, or a diluted apple juice.

TOP TIP

Drink slowly. Sip rather than gulp your drinks. This helps to slow-release the sugars in fruit juice, as does diluting them.

Alcohol

The effect of alcohol is similar to that of sugar, and if you want to burn fat fast it is best avoided during the first two weeks to a month of the Holford Diet. Aqua Libra, Amé and other soft drinks made of natural ingredients with no added sugar are good alternatives if you remember to keep within the 5 ⑬ rule.

After the initial 'cold turkey' period of two weeks to a month, you can start drinking again, in moderation. That means three drinks a week, either a small glass of good-quality wine, half a pint of beer or lager or a small shot of spirits. Of these, the best is neat spirits, then white wine, red wine and finally beer. Beer has the highest carbohydrate content, double that of red wine and eight times that of white wine.

Hot drinks

Refer to pages 112–19 for a full discussion of coffee, tea and all their permutations. By now you'll know that, whether you're addicted to endless cuppas or are a real espresso fiend, you'll need to abstain completely for two weeks to a month on the diet. Luckily, there are many wonderful, non-addictive alternatives around – really delicious and inventive herbal teas, excellent coffee substitutes – so it should be positively enjoyable to do so. After all, when you're positively fizzing with energy from diet alone, stimulants lose their sparkle pretty fast.

That said, when the time comes, you can reintroduce weak tea. Drinking it from time to time shouldn't be a problem. Coffee has several addictive substances in it, however, and should be reserved as an occasional treat.

> ### TOP TIP
>
> If you're addicted to coffee try a Teeccino with some frothed milk and a touch of cinnamon. If you're addicted to tea try Rooibosch (red bush) tea with milk.

Sugar and sweets

Sugar is perhaps a greater addiction than many people realise, and kicking the habit could prove a little tough (see page 110). But your taste buds will become acclimatised. Fruit will help when you crave something sweet (see the list on page 212 for the low-🅖🅛 fruits). Also, get used to diluting fruit juices with water, as outlined above. Once you're sugar-free, the odd sweet food is no big deal.

Many 'sugar-free' foods use grape juice concentrate as a sweetener. They might as well use glucose. Some use apple juice concentrate and, as it's high in fructose, it is much better for you. Some health-conscious drinks use blue agave cactus nectar, which is better still.

The best sugar-free alternative is xylitol (see page 476 in Resources). It is a natural sweetener found in many fruits and vegetables, but has a much lower 🅖🅛 score – a seventh that of sugar and half that of fructose. Plums, for example, are naturally high in xylitol and hence taste sweet but have a very low 🅖🅛 score. So, if you are addicted to having three teaspoons of sugar in your tea, cutting to one teaspoon of xylitol will have cut your 🅖🅛 load by 14.

SUGAR	5 🅖🅛
Xylitol	10 teaspoons (50g)
Blue agave cactus nectar	10 teaspoons (50g)
Fructose	5 teaspoons (25g)
Lactose	2 teaspoons (10g)
Sucrose	1 heaped teaspoon (7g)
Honey	1 teaspoon (6g)
Glucose	1 teaspoon (5g)
Malt	1 teaspoon (5g)

Chocolate

As we've seen, chocolate is full of sugar and cocoa, which contains stimulating substances including caffeine, theobromine and theophylline. Higher-quality dark chocolate tends to have less sugar, but obviously more of the stimulants. Some chocolates even use some of the 'healthier' sugars described above. But the fact is that, whichever way you cut it, chocolate is addictive and contributes to blood sugar problems and hence weight. When you're two weeks to a month into the diet, you may well find you've lost any cravings for it. But, if you still fancy some here and there, limit it, like desserts, to once a week.

So, how much equals 5 ⓖⓛ?

SWEETS	**5 ⓖⓛ**
GoodCarb Real Belgian Chocolate Brownie (all varieties)	one and a half bars
Fruitus oat and fruit bar	a bar (24g)
Rebar fruit and vegetable bar	half a bar
Muesli bar	less than half a bar
Regular chocolate bar, milk or plain	less than a quarter of a bar
Mars Bar	a fifth of a bar

One way of quitting the chocolate or sweets habit is to stop, and find good alternatives, which luckily abound in good health-food shops. My favourites are Shepherdboy's Sunflower Bars and Panda Liquorice bars, which are sweetened with molasses.

But you can't munch on these all the time, either: they'll simply keep your sweet tooth going. And be aware, too, that many so-called healthy bars are packed with sugar, hydrogenated fat and other not-so-healthy ingredients – so always check labels.

Desserts

It's the same story with desserts. If you eat a lot of desserts, or if you are insulin-resistant, you will probably crave something sweet at the end of each meal. It is very important to break this habit because, if you don't, it will keep your blood sugar level seesawing. It takes only three days in most cases to stop the craving. So, after your initial stimulant- and sugar-free period, limit desserts to one a week, perhaps at the weekend.

You'll find wonderful recipes for Fatburner desserts in Chapter 28, including Chocolate Ice Cream and Kiwi and Coconut Pudding. These don't exceed 5 🅖🅛 and aren't loaded with saturated fats. Don't have desserts when you are eating out (see Chapter 19), because almost all restaurant desserts are heavily loaded with sugar and saturated fat.

You can have a 5-🅖🅛 dessert with your meal and leave out one of your snacks, but having the snack is better because you are grazing more than gorging. This helps to keep your blood sugar level even, which as we've seen prevents weight gain.

So, in summary, once you've started the diet, you can be drinking unlimited hot drinks such as Teeccino, Rooibosch tea or herbal teas, and one glass of diluted juice a day. After you've gone through two weeks to a month with no coffee, tea, sweets or alcohol, you can have, taking the place of juice on that day, a small glass of wine, a half-pint of beer or a shot of spirits up to a maximum of three times a week; or six pieces of chocolate, or a Fatburner dessert, once a week. And don't forget your 2 litres of water a day.

But, whichever option you choose, the goal for your drinks, sweets and desserts is to keep within 5 🅖🅛 a day. Enjoy!

18

Shopping

Everything you need for the Holford Diet is easily available in the supermarket, greengrocer's and, for a few speciality items, your local health-food shop.

Some of the ingredients may be new to you, so this chapter will tell you where to get them and give you some guidance on what to do with them. Below you'll find a shopping list containing all you need to get stocked up and ready for fatburning.

This list includes anything that lasts for a week or more. Fresh fruits and vegetables form a large part of what you eat and need to be stocked up on a regular basis, but you may want to check the recipes and menus in Part Four first to see what you'll need. The same holds true for fresh fish – just buy what you need for that week. As for supplies from the health-food shop, these are becoming far cheaper than they once were as demand is growing. And some items once available exclusively from such stores, such as wholemeal pasta, are now widely available from supermarkets. So scout around for products, and prices, that suit you.

Your shopping list

From the supermarket

Foods for the fridge

Apples, pears, oranges, raspberries (fresh or frozen), gooseberries or
cooking apples, rhubarb, blackcurrants

Mushrooms, celery, spring onions, avocado, parsley, carrots,
beansprouts, peppers, courgettes, aubergine, cucumber, lettuce,
frozen peas

Fresh root ginger

Flat leaf parsley and basil plants

Skimmed milk

Very low-fat, live natural yoghurt (with no additives)

Cottage cheese, low-fat quark or fromage frais, half-fat Cheddar
cheese, such as Shape

Very low-fat mayonnaise

Free-range eggs

Tofu – plain, smoked and marinated pieces

Tahini

Cod, haddock, mackerel, herring, salmon (go for wild salmon if
possible)

Store-cupboard staples

Bananas, lemons

Potatoes and sweet potatoes, onions, garlic

Rolled oats and oat flakes

Wheat germ

100 per cent rye bread, pumpernickel bread

Oatcakes (the best are Nairns sugar-free variety)

Brown rice

Soba noodles

Bulgur (cracked wheat)

Couscous

Millet

Wholemeal spaghetti and other wholemeal pasta

Wholemeal flour

Chickpeas, various dried beans, lentils

Cooked chestnuts

Raw (unroasted/unsalted) mixed nuts, cashews, almonds, walnuts

Sunflower, sesame, pumpkin and flax seeds

Raisins, dried apricots

Tinned pineapple chunks (unsweetened, in juice)

Tinned tomatoes, tomato purée

Tuna fish in brine

Anchovies in olive oil (drain on kitchen towel before use)

Sardines in tomato sauce

Olive oil (cold-pressed, extra-virgin)

Cider vinegar

Balsamic vinegar

Dried herbs (turmeric, cumin, paprika, cayenne pepper, coriander)

Honey

Vanilla essence

Herbal teas

Aqua Libra, Amé

From the health-food shop

Foods for the fridge

Alfalfa seeds or sprouts

Seed oil blends such as Udo's Choice

Store-cupboard staples

Vecon, Hugli, Morga, Marigold and the like (instant vegetable stocks)

Tamari (an alternative to soy sauce)

Yeast extract – low-salt (Natex)

Wholemeal lasagne and macaroni, and wholemeal or buckwheat spaghetti

Millet
Quinoa
Pear and apple spread (a sugar-free alternative to jam)
Whole Earth sugar-free jam
Higher Nature's Get Up & Go
Dandelion coffee (Symingtons)
Barleycup, Caro or Teeccino

How to use the new foods

In Part Four, you'll be discovering how to cook with all these foods. For now, here's a bit of background on some that may be new to you.

Quinoa is actually a seed rather than a grain, and looks much like millet. It was once eaten by the Inca and was reputed to be the source of their empire's strength – and it is still eaten widely in the Andes. The flavour is slightly nutty and something like that of rice, and it's an excellent source of protein, as well as slow-releasing carbohydrate.

You cook quinoa like rice, adding up to three times as much water as quinoa and cooking it for about 13 minutes. It's best eaten as an accompaniment to, for example, a steam-fry or casserole. You could also add it to a soup to thicken it up or eat it cold as part of a salad, much like couscous, and it makes a tasty pilaf cooked with onions, brown rice and peas.

Tofu is, in terms of protein quality, second only to quinoa – and is also an excellent source of both protein and slow-releasing carbohydrate. Both tofu and quinoa, when eaten with carbo-hydrate-rich foods, slow down the release of their sugars.

Tofu is made from the soya bean and is something like a bland cheese. It comes in different textures: soft (good for desserts or making things 'creamy') or hard (better for steam-fries and main meals). While rather flavourless itself, it rapidly absorbs the flavour of any sauce. So if you are cooking a Chinese steam-fry flavoured with soy sauce, garlic and ginger, the tofu will readily soak up these flavours and taste delicious. With plain tofu, you need to drain the liquid off first.

You can also buy tofu ready-flavoured – smoked, marinated or braised (but avoid fried tofu). These varieties, which are firmer than plain tofu and already delectable-tasting, make an excellent substitute for meat or chicken in steam-fries, stews and casseroles. You can also add flavour to tofu by marinating it for 20 minutes before you cook with it. You can even make a tofu steak, or include it in sandwiches. I recommend suppliers who guarantee soya that has not been genetically modified, such as Cauldron Foods.

Lentils and beans are excellent and inexpensive foods that are very much underused in traditional British cooking. Both lentils and beans need to be boiled in plenty of water. Lentils, depending on the type, take between 15 and 25 minutes. Beans need to be soaked overnight, then boiled usually for up to two hours. You can buy pre-soaked, cooked beans and lentils in tins which you can simply drain and add to recipes.

If you've never cooked with beans, you'll soon become an enthusiast. Their taste and texture are very satisfying, and, as they're such a big part of cuisine round the world – from India, Mexico and South America to the Far East – the range of dishes you can make from them is huge. Hummus and other dips, chilli, casseroles, lentil roast and soups are only part of the story, as you'll see in Part Four.

Salad ingredients can be used much more imaginatively than most people think. With a few exceptions, most vegetables can be eaten raw. Raw, uncooked and grated beetroot, cabbage, broccoli, courgettes and carrot tops can all be used along with peppers, tomatoes, grated carrots, baby sweetcorn and a variety of green leafy vegetables such as watercress, rocket, lettuce, chicory, red cabbage and spinach. You can also add marinated tofu pieces, almonds and, less frequently, avocados, to increase the protein content. There are plenty of salad and salad-dressing recipes to choose from in Part Four.

Tahini is a spread made from sesame seeds and their oil. As it's high in essential fats, it's a lot better for you and more flavourful than butter. I use tahini on bread and toast instead of butter, and often add some to savoury dishes at the end for a creamier texture and added flavour. Use in moderation, as instructed in the recipes, and keep in the fridge.

Seeds contain vitamins, minerals, protein, fibre and essential fats. They are therefore a superfood, yet many people shy away from them because of fat phobia or simply ignorance about how to use them. Flax seeds (linseeds) and pumpkin seeds are the best for the essential omega-3 fats, while sesame and sunflower are the best for the omega-6 fats. A combination of all four, stored in a glass jar in the fridge to minimise oxidation, then ground in a coffee grinder, makes a great addition to any cereal. Two dessertspoons give you a good daily intake of essential fats plus lots of other key nutrients, including bone-building calcium, magnesium and zinc. They're best uncooked or thrown in at the last moment of cooking, such as in a steam-fry, since heating them lowers the quality of their essential fats.

Seed-oil blends need to be cold-pressed and preferably organic, stored in a lightproof container and kept refrigerated. The best blends of oils are those that provide roughly equal proportion of omega-3 and omega-6 fats, usually by combining flax seed oil, pumpkin seed oil, sesame oils, sunflower oil or borage oil. Two such oils are Essential Balance, available from Higher Nature (see page 480 in Resources) and Udo's Choice, available from health-food shops. These can't be cooked, so they're for adding to soups at the end of cooking, or to cereals, vegetables and salad dressings.

19

Eating Out

You don't need to stay in every night, slaving over a hot stove (or a salad bowl) on the Holford Diet. But when it comes to eating out you will need to be choosy. As I've said, I travel the world on lecture tours and I always find excellent restaurants as I go, simply by choosing Chinese, Japanese, Malaysian or Thai establishments.

The reason? These countries have the leanest, healthiest people, and much of that is down to the way they eat. And, because the Chinese, for instance, have emigrated to so many countries round the world, it's usually possible to find a Chinese restaurant at least, whether in the US, Canada, Australia, continental Europe, South America – or the Far East! But this doesn't mean you can't eat French, Italian, Mexican, Indian or other foods. You just need to know what to order.

The trick, as ever, is to fill yourself up with the good stuff. That means having a starter and a main course, or just a main course, but not a dessert. It also means avoiding any breads, prawn crackers or the like. In fact, it's best to ask the waiter to take it away, thus removing the temptation. Instead, ask them to bring some olives, or a dish of hot pickles. Order water and say you won't be drinking anything else.

When you are choosing items from the menu, watch out for the hidden sugar and high-⑬ carbohydrates in sauces, pickles and dips. For example, all Thai restaurants do very tasty fish-cakes and spring rolls. The fishcakes are better than the spring rolls because they have more protein. Both come with a sweet sauce, and you'll need to leave this on the side.

Where possible, choose food that hasn't been deep-fried. So go for boiled noodles rather than fried, or boiled rice rather than fried rice. Share a portion between two or even three people. Remember, you want about as much weight of the carbohydrate food as the protein-rich food, such as a steamed or poached fish.

Japanese restaurants are great, especially if you like fish. All offer wonderful fish dishes, from teriyaki salmon to sashimi. (Sushi isn't as good because it includes a lot of sweet white rice.) This can be very satisfying without filling you up with fast-releasing carbohydrates or saturated fat.

Always order some vegetable dishes, whether it's a salad or a side order of green beans or broccoli. Make sure you eat your greens and, if you haven't had enough, order some more.

By the time you get to the end of your main course you should be full. This is the time to make your exit, asking for the bill and letting your perhaps dejected waiter know that the food was so good and so filling that you don't want coffee or dessert!

Most of all, remember who is in charge of what goes in your mouth. Think of the menu as only a small selection of what's on offer, opening up the possibility of ordering 'off menu'. For instance, if you like the sound of the fish, but not the cream sauce, ask for it without, or swap it for another method of cooking. Ask what's in various dishes and have a look around at what other people are eating.

Indian food uses a lot of vegetables, beans and lentils, but there's also a lot of hidden sugar and fat in some of the sauces. You have to choose very carefully indeed in an Indian restaurant, so I'd recommend going to them only as an occasional treat. The same applies to cheaper Italian restaurants that specialise in pizza and pasta. These dishes are based on high-GL carbohydrates and the pasta can come with fatty, cheesy or creamy sauces, so they're best avoided. But authentic Italian and French restaurants will have plenty of excellent main dishes, such as grilled chicken, plus good salads and vegetables, so be on the lookout for these.

Here are some typical items from Chinese, Thai, Japanese, Malaysian and Indian restaurant menus to choose, or avoid.

Choose

Sashimi (Japanese raw fish dish)

Fish/chicken teriyaki

Tom yum soup

Thai fish/chicken/prawn tikkas, curries (but avoid the creamier ones listed under 'Avoid' below)

Fish/chicken satay (peanut-based sauce)

Indian bhunas or baltis – ask for less oil

Steamed fish and other non-fried fish dishes

Tofu-based dish

Omelettes

Noodles with vegetables, such as chop suey (share a portion)

Vegetable dishes such as chana masal or dhal (Indian) or stir-fried beansprouts, bamboo shoots, water chestnuts or mushrooms (Chinese)

Avoid [B]

Fried fish/meat

Sweet-and-sour dishes

Creamy curries such as
kormas and masalas

Rice (unless brown, then
share a portion)

Potato dishes

Bread such as naans and
chapattis

Prawn crackers

The fallback in any restaurant is to choose something simple, without sauces with unknown ingredients. So you can't go wrong with grilled fish or chicken and vegetables or salad.

Restaurants are a good proving ground for your new relationship with food. Now that you understand so much more about why you feel the way you do and what food has to do with it, make good food your friend. Become the master of your own weight and health by becoming the master of your diet.

The best way to do this is to get your hands dirty preparing your own meals. Experiment. Make mistakes. Try new foods. Get involved with creating a way of eating that really works for you.

Choose to follow this diet because it makes sense and you want to change. I guarantee the results will be worth it. I want you to make this *your* diet, and simply use what's in this book as a springboard. That means finding the balance between eating out and eating in, breaking your addictions and having the odd treat. Be moderate in everything, including moderation.

20

Fatburning for Vegetarians

Being vegetarian is generally healthier than being a carnivore, but you have to know what you are doing. The key is making sure you get enough protein, vitamin B12 and iron (see Chapter 21), and don't live off dairy and wheat, which are the most common allergy-provoking foods.

The Holford Diet's emphasis on vegetables and plant-based protein makes it very easy for vegetarians and vegans to follow. There are a number of delicious dishes listed in Chapter 28 that are suitable for anyone avoiding meat and fish, from Chestnut and Mushroom Pilaf and Quinoa Tabbouleh to Thai-Style Vegetable Broth and Pasta with Pumpkin Seed Pesto. The diet has also been designed to be as versatile as possible, so you can simply substitute tofu or pulses such as chickpeas or kidney beans for the meat or fish in most of the recipes.

To make this easier for you, in Part Four I have given recommendations for suitable replacements alongside recipes in the meat and fish sections, where appropriate. This is also a good opportunity to try some of the more unusual vegetarian and vegan-friendly ingredients that are on offer. We've already had a look at some of these in Chapter 18, but let's delve a little deeper here and see how they can be used as dietary staples.

Soya stars

Plain, marinated and smoked tofu (see page 239) are the protein stars of the vegetarian Holford Diet. You can now buy imaginative flavours of marinated tofu, such as sesame and ginger, or almond and hazelnut. Tempeh is made of fermented soya beans, and has a much nuttier taste and firmer texture than tofu. Rather like Marmite, it is not for everyone, but I love it. Silken tofu is a very soft type that is useful for blending to thicken sauces, dips or smoothies. There is a recipe in the vegetarian section of the main meals in Chapter 28 that makes use of smoked tofu, Japanese Noodles (page 360), and many in the meat sections that are easy to adapt.

Finger on the pulse

I've already discussed beans and lentils in Chapter 18, and as a vegetarian you're very likely highly familiar with legumes and pulses such as chickpeas and kidney beans. But we'll be cooking with many others, such as the delicious green-hued flageolet (Flageolet Bean Dip has a very delicate flavour and is a delicious and unusual alternative to hummus), while black-eyed beans add a great texture to salsas and in Gazpacho soup. If you have previously dismissed lentils as mushy and bland, try Puy lentils cooked with a little vegetable stock. These green, shiny lentils hold their shape and texture when cooked, and are rightly considered a delicacy in France.

With the grain

You've seen how amazing quinoa is already. Containing all the essential amino acids for our protein requirements, it is a nutritionally perfect food as well as being very versatile, working as both carbohydrate and protein in a meal. You can use quinoa in all kinds of dishes, such as salads (Quinoa Tabbouleh), main dishes (Roasted Vegetables with Mediterranean Quinoa), and even desserts (Coconut Quinoa Pudding).

But good grains and seeds don't stop there. You can experiment with couscous, bulgur and millet, which are excellent served with all sorts of casseroles. And the range of available yeast-free pumpernickel and other low-Ⓖ breads, as well as delicious flaked grains, increases yearly.

Not from the cow

If you are vegan, you can substitute soya milk or rice milk for dairy milk. Rice milk has a much higher Ⓖ and is therefore not so good. There are other milks now available in health-food stores, from oat milk to quinoa milk. These have a lower Ⓖ.

21

Supplements

Good nutrition is achieved by eating the right foods, *and* by supplementing. There is no question that the levels of many nutrients required to help your body function at its best are above those easily achieved by diet alone. Such optimal levels of nutrients can also help you to reprogramme your body to burn fat. If you want to know more about the vitamins and minerals that help you to burn fat, refer back to Chapter 10.

If you have never taken supplements before, you may find they have many beneficial side effects. In a survey at ION, 79 per cent of people, after six months on a supplement programme, reported improved energy, while 61 per cent felt physically fitter, and had fewer colds.

The basics

The starting point for any supplement programme is a good, all-round multivitamin and mineral supplement plus 1,000mg of vitamin C. Do check that the multivitamin/mineral that you've chosen meets the amounts shown on page 175. You'll also probably need to supplement your diet with chromium (200mcg) separately – check the label on your multi.

So an ideal supplement programme looks like this:

	Breakfast	Lunch	Dinner
High-strength multivitamin and mineral	1	1	
Vitamin C 1,000mg	1		
Chromium 200mcg	1		

A good quality multi will direct you to take two per day. This is simply because you can't fit adequate quantities of vitamins and minerals into a single tablet or capsule. To get the most value out of your multi, I recommend taking one with breakfast and the second with either lunch or dinner. If you're having Get Up & Go for breakfast, you won't need to supplement it with vitamin C that day, as it already includes 1,000mg.

If you are struggling with your appetite or sugar cravings, I recommend you add hydroxycitric acid (HCA) and 5-HTP:

HCA (250mg)	1	1	1
5-HTP (50mg)	1	1	1

HCA helps encourage fatburning and is good for everyone. Take before each meal.

5-HTP is especially good for those with sugar cravings and a tendency to mild depression. If you crave something sweet when your mood is low, try 5-HTP. It is best absorbed either on an empty stomach or with a piece of fruit. Try with your mid-morning and mid-afternoon snack.

For details on suppliers and brands of supplements I recommend, see page 479 in Resources.

Fibre supplements

Generally speaking, fibre is not something you add to food. It's in food anyway unless a food manufacturer has processed it out. The Holford Diet is a high-fibre diet. However, there is one special kind of fibre that can help you to lose weight by slowing down the release of carbohydrates. It is called glucomannan and comes from the Japanese konjac plant (see page 104 in Chapter 17 for more details).

Three grams of glucomannan a day has been proved to assist weight loss. Konjac extract, which is 60 per cent glucomannan, comes in 500mg capsules. It's recommended that you take nine of these capsules a day. Take three, with a large glass of water, three times a day just before meals. As it swells to a hundred times its volume by absorbing water, it is very important to drink a large glass of water whenever you take konjac extract or glucomannan. Suppliers are given on page 480.

The when and how of supplements

Vitamin and mineral supplements are best taken with food and, if they are involved in energy regulation, during the day. They should also be taken *every* day. While most people notice the effects of taking them after 30 days, it is best to stick to a supplement programme for three months to see a real difference.

There are no dangers with taking any of these supplements on a long-term basis. However, once you've achieved your desired weight, you may wish to stop taking HCA, 5-HTP and additional chromium. These are included specifically to help stabilise your blood sugar levels. Most decent multivitamin and mineral supplements will provide around 30mcg of chromium, which is enough when you're on the maintenance phase of the Holford Diet.

22

Exercise

While the main thrust of the Holford Diet is food, we've also seen how exercise helps you to keep your blood sugar level even and to burn fat. But it's important to do the right kind, and this is a combination of aerobic exercise and resistance or toning exercise.

To be a Fatburner, the minimum you need to exercise is 15 minutes a day, or 35 minutes three times a week. The exercise programme you choose needs to include both aerobics, which burns fat directly, and toning exercises, which build muscle which burns fat. If you are significantly underlean (see page 64), you may need to do more to build up enough lean muscle to keep you thin.

Earlier I suggested that you start to experiment with some of the exercises in this chapter right before you start the diet, to get used to including it in your week. Take that time to find an exercise routine that suits you. You may wish to join a gym, get a workout video and find a friend to do it with so you can keep each other motivated. Set yourself a specific time to exercise during the day. You may wish to double the time you exercise, and do it every other day, which will let you have more days off.

If you've never really exercised, or are very overweight or unfit, it's best to go to your local gym and get advice from a fitness instructor before you start. It's important, too, to let your doctor know what you're doing so that he or she can advise, if necessary.

Aerobic exercise

Aerobics has to be intense enough to raise your pulse rate into the training zone (see the chart below), but not so intense that you exceed your capacity to produce muscular energy using the oxygen you breathe. Sprinting, for example, is too intense – it demands more oxygen than is available, so the muscles switch to making energy anaerobically. This results in a build-up of toxic by-products.

Training heart rate zone (while exercising)

Age	65–80% of maximum heart rate (beats in 1 minute)	(beats in 10 sec.)
20	130–160	22–27
22	129–158	22–26
24	127–157	21–26
26	126–155	21–26
28	125–154	21–26
30	124–152	21–25
32	122–150	20–25
34	121–149	20–25
36	120–147	20–25
38	118–146	20–24
40	117–144	20–24

45	114–140	19–23
50	111–136	19–23
55	107–132	18–22
60	104–128	17–21
65	101–124	17–21
70	98–120	16–20

The centre column shows how many beats you should have in one minute; beginners should aim for the lower figure on the left-hand side (that is, 65% of their maximum heart rate for their age), then slowly increase to 80%. Do not exceed this higher level. The column on the far right gives you how many beats you should have in a 10-second pulse count. Beginners should stay at the lower end of their exercise range.

You may never have done aerobics, but don't view it as a hard slog before you've begun. It can be hugely fun. Think of swimming, a volleyball game with friends or colleagues, or a long ramble through stunning countryside.

Here are just some of your choices:

Walking	Aerobics
Rambling	Dance classes
Jogging	Cycling
Swimming	Team sports
Circuit training	Video workouts

But whichever you choose, you need to follow the same golden rules with each:

1. **Warm up first.** This is especially important if you are unfit and overweight. Warming up is necessary to prepare the body for an increased level of activity. The body needs

time to transport the oxygen you breathe into your muscles. Gradually increasing a walk from a slow to a medium pace gives the body the time that is needed. Or starting with breaststroke before you move on to front crawl when swimming may be a good way to slowly increase the intensity.

If you start too quickly then inevitably you will start to feel uncomfortable and will need to slow down in order to continue. This can be discouraging if you are new to exercise. Take 2–3 minutes to warm up. Think of it as a gradual increase rather than stop–start. It's like driving a car – you need to pull away in first gear and work your way up through the gears, slowly building up to a level you can maintain. If you tried to pull away in top gear when driving a car, it would struggle and stall. In the same way, you will feel very uncomfortable very quickly if you do not warm up.

Remember: you warm up to work out, you don't work out to warm up.

2. **Exercise at a level that keeps you in your training zone for at least 15 minutes.** If you are swimming, for example, don't stop every couple of lengths. It is better to swim more slowly and keep going than to stop frequently and catch your breath. If you are attracted to team sports such as tennis, badminton, squash or football, the trick is to keep moving. Short bursts of activity won't do you much good for developing aerobic fitness, which is what burns fat.

The purpose of training in your training zone is to develop your aerobic fitness. This will in turn increase your body's ability to use fat as a fuel. As you get fitter the body increases the cells where it produces energy. These cells (mitochondria) increase in size and number with activity that is continuous in nature and of a moderate intensity. They can turn you into an incredibly efficient fatburning machine. It is no surprise that distance runners and cyclists have the highest levels of these cells. Your goal is to build up to a level that allows you to keep exercising continuously for up to 35 minutes.

How will you know if you are exercising within your training zone? Well, it will be a faster pace than your normal walking speed but not so fast that you can't continue to talk to someone else at the same time.

It is recommended that if you are new to exercise then start by increasing how many times you exercise first and how long you exercise for, before increasing the intensity. Think 'more active, more often'.

3. Set yourself a realistic goal and gradually increase it.
Here's an example. If you like jogging round your local park, you might find that one circuit takes you 10 minutes. In your second week, can you get that time down to 9 minutes? Or you could increase the distance and/or how often you do it. In the beginning, make it easy to reach your goal. Then week by week, reach for higher goals. When you achieve them you'll know you're really Fatburning – you'll be seeing, and feeling, the results.

Find some time in your schedule when you can do some exercise and make a date with yourself. As a benchmark, see how long you can exercise in your training zone. Let's say 5 minutes. Now that you know what you can manage, make sure you do 5 minutes of exercise more frequently. Your goal is to build up to 3–5 times a week. Alternatively, you may want to increase the time. Again, with 5 minutes as your starting point, try to add just 1 minute each time you exercise. Too often people try to add too much at the beginning, become uncomfortable, do not achieve their goal and become discouraged.

Here's an example. If you plan to do more exercise, you may want to start with 10 minutes, three times a week. You could aim to add 1 minute each time you exercise, thereby gradually increasing the total duration. This would mean that in the first week you would complete three sessions: one of 10 minutes, one of 11 minutes and one of 12 minutes. Within four weeks you will have doubled the time you initially exercised for, but the increase will have been so gradual that you'll hardly have noticed it.

	Monday	Wednesday	Friday	Weeks total minutes
Week 1	10	11	12	33
Week 2	13	14	15	42
Week 3	16	17	18	51
Week 4	19	20	21	60

Within two weeks you will have reached the recommended 15 minute minimum and you can then focus on increasing the frequency.

Alternatively, you may want to increase the frequency first. This would require you to plan 15 minutes of exercise into your day. In the first week you might manage to fit in two 15-minute sessions. The following week you should aim to find time to add another session. This should continue gradually and soon you'll find that you are exercising for 15 minutes every day.

Once you have achieved this, you should try to find time elsewhere in your schedule so that you could carry out two 15-minute sessions in a single day. Perhaps you could look at alternatives to driving or taking public transport to work: if you cycle, or get off your bus a few stops earlier, you could gain 15 minutes of exercise when travelling in and another when travelling home.

Your goals need to be achievable and manageable. You are better off planning and attaining small goals that build your success rather than aiming too high initially. Remember that just becoming more active is an achievement. Finding time to be more active and planning exercise maybe your initial goal.

4. **Vary the exercise so that you don't get bored.** Variety can add a dimension to your exercise routine. In the same way that you don't plan to eat the same meals every day, you can vary the types of exercise that you do. This will also allow you to work different muscles and develop your general fitness.

Try to find activities that you enjoy. If you don't enjoy one form of exercise, try something else. Finding the right environment can be very important.

Exercise won't always be fun. At times you may find it uncomfortable, time-consuming or solitary. However, ask anyone who exercises on a regular basis and they will tell you that while they don't always enjoy the sessions, they do enjoy the results.

5. **Exercise with a friend, at a gym, or in classes for extra motivation.** When you start to plan your exercise programme consider several options.

Who do you want to exercise with? Some people prefer to exercise in groups or with other like-minded people. However, others prefer to exercise alone and use the time to think. You may want both. Time passes more quickly when you are with someone else.

Where do you want to exercise? The gym can be a really good place to get support. The fitness instructors want to help. They enjoy developing new exercise programmes for people. You may prefer to do exercise classes. If you're not sure which would be most effective, ask for advice. Remember that you want something that is aerobic in nature rather than a 'Legs, bums and tums' class which is better for toning.

Plan to reward to yourself with something other than food for completing certain targets. These rewards can be symbolic or practical. A new piece of training gear, a massage or a new book. Anything that will motivate you to achieve your goal.

6. **Drink plenty of water before, during and after exercising.** The body is two-thirds water and you lose significant amounts of it through sweating and breathing. Drink a glass of water for every half-hour of exercise.

7. **Cool down when you finish and stretch the muscles you've been exercising.** If you have been exercising for 15 minutes, take 2–3 minutes to cool-down before starting your stretches. The cool-wdown is the opposite to the warm-up. Again, think of your body as a car you would not change from fifth gear to first in one go. So make sure you slow down gradually.

Stretching will promote recovery as well as relaxing your muscles. It is often neglected; however, it is essential that you stretch the muscles you have worked to reduce the risk of injury. Depending on which muscles you've been working, stretch them out immediately after exercising. It is best to hold a stretch and count to twenty, rather than stretching, then releasing, then stretching again.

8. Keep it up. The real benefits of exercise are seen after weeks or months, not days. Make exercise a part of your daily routine.

It can be quite an achievement to plan and complete exercise on a daily basis. Remember that every exercise session that you complete takes you closer to your goal; every session missed keeps you further away. Try not to focus only on the physical changes to your body, as this does not recognise your accomplishment in being a regular exerciser (with all the planning and organisation this entails).

Don't think of it as taking up exercise, but as giving up being inactive.

The psychological benefits of exercise are just as well established as the physical benefits. You won't just enjoy a healthier, more efficient body, but you will sleep more soundly, have more energy for other tasks and think more clearly.

Toning exercises

By toning specific muscle groups you can lose inches as well as pounds. As we've seen, the more muscle you build, the greater your ability to burn fat: muscle uses up more calories. Some workouts include both aerobic and toning exercises. Alternatively, you could do a mainly aerobic exercise one day and a mainly toning exercise another.

The trick for toning exercises is to get some good advice. Your local gym is probably the best place for that. If you prefer to exercise as part of a group, ask your local gym for an exercise programme. Classes focusing on toning exercises (such as 'Legs, bums and tums') are very popular and you will often have a variety to choose from. Many celebrities swear by yoga

– if you can't attend a class you could try one of the yoga videos on sale. There are different types of yoga and you need to find a style and level of class to suit you.

Ask your gym instructor to include compound exercises in your workout. These exercises use the large muscle groups and help keep the total number of exercises to a minimum.

Typical exercises used in circuit classes can be completed at home. Traditional press-ups and their modifications can be performed in the living room, as can many of the other bodyweight movements. Here is an example of a set of exercises that could be performed one after another in a circuit fashion, to give you the toning effects you want. (For detailed descriptions of the exercises please visit www.theholforddiet.com).

Example circuit workout

Exercise	Circuit 1	Circuit 2	Circuit 3
Squats	10	12	15
Press-ups	10	12	15
Sit-ups	10	12	15
Upright rows	10	12	15
Back extensions	10	12	15
Triceps dips	10	12	15
Lunges	10	12	15
Side leg lifts	10	12	15
Lateral raises	10	12	15
Biceps curls	10	12	15

You do not have to start by doing all of the exercises at once or all three circuits the first time; you can build up to completing this over a period of time.

Psychocalisthenics®

One of my favourite exercise routines is Psychocalisthenics. You can learn it in five hours, by watching a video or, ideally, doing a course, and do it in about 15 minutes wherever you are.

Psychocalisthenics is a precise sequence of 23 exercises that leave you feeling fantastic. I've been doing it for 20 years and I've yet to find anything that keeps me trimmer and makes me feel better – which isn't bad for 15 minutes a day! Each exercise is driven by the breath and, somehow, my body feels lighter, freer and thoroughly oxygenated after this simple routine, which anyone can do.

Psychocalisthenics is the brainchild of Oscar Ichazo. Ichazo founded the Arica School in the 1960s as a school of knowledge for the understanding of the complete person. A practitioner of martial arts and yoga since 1939, he developed Psychocalisthenics to be a daily routine that can be done in less than 20 minutes. At first glance it looks like a powerful kind of aerobic yoga. 'In the same way that we have an everyday need for food and nourishment we have to promote the circulation of our vital energy as an everyday business,' says Ichazo.

While most exercise routines simply treat the body as a physical machine that needs to be worked to stay fit, Psychocalisthenics is designed to generate both physical fitness and vital energy by bringing mind and body into balance. The key lies in the precise breathing pattern that accompanies each physical exercise. Energy generation happens when you have stable blood sugar, plus a good supply of oxygen. According to Jane Alexander of the *Daily Mail*, 'Psychocalisthenics is exercise, pared to perfection. I wasn't sweating buckets as I would after an aerobics class. But I had exercised far more muscles. I was clear-headed and bright rather than wiped out.'

The best way to learn Psychocalisthenics is to do a short course. For details see www.patrickholford.com/psychocalisthenics. You can also teach yourself from a DVD, but it is best to learn it 'live'.

My ideal weekly Fatburning exercise regime is to do Psychocalisthenics every other day, three or four times a week; walk, run, swim or cycle three times a week; and do one Ashtanga yoga class a week that involves 'resistance' training, building muscle more than stamina. Enjoy experimenting and finding your favourite routine – once you've done this, it'll be easier to stick to it.

23

Monitoring Your Results

Once you've got going on the Holford Diet, you will feel and see the results. You may not be able to measure your new energy levels – but you can certainly monitor the pounds you're dropping and the inches you're losing. And here's how.

Weigh and measure yourself at the start of this diet and at the end of every week. Always weigh yourself in the morning, before breakfast, without clothes. Keep monitoring your progress week after week. If you have a bad week, notice what effect that is having on your progress, and get back on course. If you reach a 'plateau', don't worry. This can happen. You can encourage weight loss by following the diet more precisely. Soon, you'll find what you need to do to lose weight and, once you've reached your ultimate goal, what you need to do to stay there.

There's a Fatburner progress report for each of the first four weeks in Appendix 4. Fill out the report for Week 1, setting your long-term goal weight and your weekly target weight (see page 198 for how to figure these out). You'll need an accurate pair of scales and a tape measure. Since scales do vary, it's best to weigh yourself on the same ones each week. For the measurements, always take the widest part of, for example, your waist, your thighs or your hips. For your thigh measurement, take the average of your left and right thighs.

Waist–hip ratio and total inch loss

I recommend that you also work out your waist–hip ratio. This is your waist measurement divided by your hip measurement. The reason is that it's one of the most important measures in relation to your health. Abdominal weight gain is associated with insulin resistance and hence the risk for diabetes much more than hip and thigh weight gain. The average ratio in Britain is 0.90 for men and 0.79 for women. Once you're above 0.95 for men or 0.85 for women, you do have an increased risk of obesity-related diseases. Broadly speaking, if your waist is greater than 102cm (men) or 88cm (women), you need to lose weight. (Obviously, this does depend a bit on your height.)

Your total inch loss is the sum of all the inches you have lost from measurements of your bust or chest, waist, hips and thighs. (If you've lost an inch from each, your total loss is 4 inches.)

Progress, week by week

At the end of each week, ask yourself honestly how well you've stuck to the diet and exercise programme. There's a space on the progress report to rate yourself out of 100 per cent. This will help you to stay on course. If, at the end of the week, you feel your targets are too hard or too easy, you can adjust the rate of progress you're aiming for.

You'll also find a spare Fatburner progress report that you can copy for subsequent weeks. Keep all these weekly progress sheets and then, when you've reached your ideal weight, I'd greatly appreciate it if you'd fill out the Fatburner questionnaire on page 466. This is how I can get your feedback to keep making this diet even more effective.

With a little help from your friends ...

Let your friends and your family know what you are doing. Show them this book. Maybe they'll want to join in too! Doing the diet with a friend is great, because you can then give each other support. Encourage your family to support you by being tolerant with the new foods you'll be preparing, and not tempting you with forbidden foods. When you're invited out to dinner, let your hosts know about the diet. And when you throw your own dinner party, use the recipes in Part Four. There are plenty that are elegant enough for a formal meal, and they're all delicious.

You may also find it extremely helpful to carry out this diet with the help of a nutrition consultant, who can help you to get started and will work out a personalised vitamin programme for you. He or she can also keep you on track and provide you with moral support and tips on how to deal with any problems you may have. (See the section on nutrition consultations on page 475 in Resources.)

Breaking the rules

Very few people stick to diets 100 per cent, 100 per cent of the time. No doubt there will be the odd occasion when you break the rules. This is not a disaster. In fact, it can be a good idea to give yourself two meals a month when you can eat what you like. This will help you to deal with special occasions and celebrations. So enjoy yourself.

Remember, though, that the more you break the rules, the slower your progress will be. And if you are really addicted, say to double espressos or binge drinking after work, be careful. You can't consume any of these substances in excess and keep your weight down or health up. They have a nasty habit of creeping back into your life and are best avoided if you really feel you can't control your consumption of them.

If you do indulge at a friend's wedding, or find yourself unable to resist pizza and *gelato* on your Italian holiday, the most important thing to do is to get back on track the next day. In one experiment, two groups of slimmers were given an identical milkshake to drink. One group was told it was high in calories, the other that it was low. Each group was then given an unlimited amount of ice cream. Which group, do you think, ate more?

The answer is the group that had been told the milkshake was high in calories. This shows a very common pitfall among dieters – the 'If I've broken my diet I might as well go the whole hog' syndrome. Don't do it. If you blow it one day, get back on track the next.

The first 30 days

If you have more weight to lose and feel good on this diet, keep going for up to 90 days. An excellent target weight loss for an obese person is to decrease body fat percentage by 10 per cent each month or to lose 18 pounds in 90 days. The balance of protein, carbohydrate and fat in the Holford Diet (25 per cent protein, 50 per cent carbohydrate, 25 per cent fat) helps to reprogramme your body to burn fat. This reprogramming is especially important for those of you with a degree of insulin resistance who show signs of sugar sensitivity (see the questionnaire on Page 56), and sometimes it takes longer than 30 days.

If you've achieved your goal you can ease up by eating 50 Ⓖ a day. Chapter 25 is all about how to maintain your weight and health. But first let's look at what to do if this diet simply isn't working for you.

24

What If It's Not Working?

Say you're on Week 4 of the diet, and you've really stuck with it. Congratulations! You've sorted out your coffee addiction, you're feeling much more energetic, and you can definitely see the gloss back in your hair with all the omega-3s you're getting. You love the recipes and your new running regime. There's just one problem: you haven't shed a pound.

I can understand how frustrating this must feel. It's at this point that I have to say no single diet works for everyone, for the simple reason that there are many different causes of overweight or obesity.

But I also have to say that, in truth, I haven't yet had a case of a person failing to lose weight after they looked at all the possible reasons below, and discovered the one that's holding them back.

So let's look at them.

You're not losing weight, but you are losing inches. This is OK for now. What it means is that you are making lean muscle, which is heavier, but has the capacity to burn more fat. Keep going. The weight loss will follow.

You are still insulin-resistant. Have you quit alcohol, sugar and/or caffeine? If not, and you're not losing weight, you'll have to bite the bullet and give them up.

You're not exercising. Exercise really does help kick-start your metabolism. If your weight isn't shifting, then up your levels of activity.

You're not taking the supplements. Supplements do make a difference and, in addition to the basic multivitamin and vitamin C, the combination of chromium, HCA and 5-HTP definitely gives you the edge in appetite control. They are well worth taking.

You have a hidden allergy. Don't underestimate this factor. Many people fail to lose weight until they have their food allergies checked. Your weight can really get stuck until you remove an offending food. Have a food-intolerance test (see page 477 in Resources) and avoid your food allergies.

You are oestrogen-dominant. Hormonal imbalances, especially of the thyroid, can stop you losing weight. You need to get this checked by your doctor. You should also be tested for an underactive thyroid (see page 274.)

Hormone imbalances and weight gain

It is not at all uncommon for weight gain to be precipitated by hormonal changes. In fact, according to the MyNutrition survey ION conducted on almost 30,000 people, those with hormonal issues were twice as likely to have problems losing weight. For some women, the pounds pile on during pregnancy, only to stay on after the birth. For others, going on or coming off the pill or HRT can trigger weight gain.

A common time for weight gain for many women is in the pre-menopausal years (usually from 40 onwards) and even more so at the menopause, when menstruation ceases. Even more common than weight gain is a change in weight redistribution, which we'll look at now.

Apples and pears

Are you an apple, or a pear? Excess weight on the hips and thighs, resulting in a pear-shaped body, is associated with excess oestrogen, the feminising hormone. Too much upper-body and waist gain is associated with excess androgens, the masculinising hormone.

These hormonal differences are partly genetic and partly a consequence of how we live. Some people have more active adrenal glands, a factor encouraged by a stressful and competitive lifestyle. This leads to the release of more adrenal hormones, such as cortisol and adrenalin, as well as androgens, which all help to build protein and muscle.

Hence these 'adrenal types' tend to be more muscular and have more weight in the top half of their bodies. For such people it is very important not to live off adrenal stimulants (see Chapter 7) and to keep fat intake down. Too much fat, coupled with prolonged stress and a lack of exercise, leads to obesity. In fact, too much of the adrenal hormone cortisol can also lead to too much oestrogen (produced in the both adrenal glands and fatty tissue, as well as the ovaries) which can lead to lower-body weight gain, too.

The two key female hormones are *oestrogen* and *progesterone*. They're produced mainly in the ovaries and need to be in balance with each other. An increasingly common problem is that a woman produces too much oestrogen in relation to progesterone. The problem usually stems from a progesterone deficiency, rather than actual excess oestrogen.

Progesterone is produced by the ovaries only once the egg has been released, at ovulation. If a woman doesn't ovulate (which is increasingly common as a woman approaches the menopause), then no progesterone is produced. After the menopause progesterone output falls to almost nothing, while oestrogen levels sink very gradually. Oestrogen is the 'feminising' hormone: it helps to lay down fat as storage, especially on the hips and thighs, creating a more curvaceous shape. Many women gain weight in these places after the age of 35.

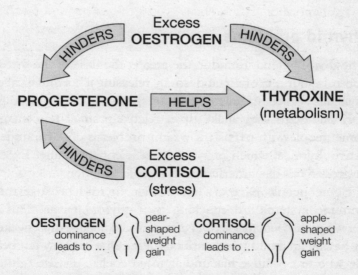

Hormones and their effects on weight distribution. Too much oestrogen (or not enough progesterone) competes with the thyroid hormone thyroxine, resulting in a slow metabolism and weight gain, especially on the hips and thighs. Too much cortisol, the stress hormone, also affects thyroid function, slowing down the body's metabolism which leads to weight gain, especially around the middle.

Full details on this subject are given in my book *Balancing Hormones Naturally*, co-authored with Kate Neil.

Men, too, can suffer from oestrogen dominance. This is most likely to occur when their levels of the male hormone, testosterone, is low, as this counteracts the feminising effects of oestrogen. A diet high in meat, dairy and pesticide-sprayed foods can make a contribution to developing oestrogen dominance.

If you suspect you have a hormonal imbalance and that this is contributing to your excess weight, the best thing to do is to see a nutritional therapist who can work with your doctor to have the necessary tests done and organise appropriate treatment if necessary.

Thyroid problems

The thyroid gland, found in the area at the base of the throat, controls your rate of metabolism by releasing a hormone called *thyroxine*, which stimulates cells to speed up energy production. Although they make up a relatively small percentage, some people with persistent weight problems do have underactive thyroids, which produce insufficient thyroxine. Excess oestrogen can also interfere with thyroid function.

Some people have an underactive thyroid because their immune systems are attacking their thyroid tissue. This is known as *autoimmune thyroid disease*. You can have this checked by having an 'antithyroid antibody test'. One in every ten people who test positive has undiagnosed coeliac disease (gluten sensitivity). It seems that you can become allergic to a food, and your immune system can then attack a part of you, thinking it's the food, perhaps because the food and you share similar proteins. So the next thing to do is get yourself tested for hidden food allergies.

If you've done everything I've mentioned in this chapter and it still isn't working, I recommend that you get professional advice from a qualified nutritional therapist. They can investigate your particular problem or perhaps give the necessary support and guidance you need. There are details on how to find one near you on page 475.

25

Controlling Emotional and Obsessive Eating

Eating is very nearly the first thing most of us do in life. Within minutes of being born, a baby receives sustenance from its mother. But suckling provides far more than food, as Harry Harlow's monkeys showed us.

In this famous experiment in the 1950s, infant monkeys were presented with the choice of two surrogate mothers – constructed dummies complete with teats. One provided nourishment, the other no milk but the tactile experience of fur. The baby monkeys chose the tactile sensation rather than food – comfort, over nourishment.

Eating is emotive

For baby humans, the tactile sense and security of the breast is soon associated with food. Eating is an emotive business. And, later in life, eating can become associated with pleasing, rebelling, imitating, rewarding – even punishment. For example, the girl who eats sparingly, like her mum, because she also wants to be thin; the boy who eats certain foods because they 'make him big and strong' and develops aversions to other foods; the rebellion against 'eat it up or you won't get any pudding'; the reward of sweets if you do something good, or the comfort of sweets when you're hurt. By adolescence, a multitude of psychological factors govern when, how, what and how much we eat.

Does any of this ring bells? Do you reach for chocolate when you're upset? Do you gain or lose weight when you are in love? Do you reward yourself with food? Do you always finish what's in front of you? Are you a fussier eater when you feel unhappy? Do you eat more when you are out with the lads?

'Five hundred people were asked what they fear most in the world and 190 answered that their greatest fear is "getting fat",' wrote Kim Chernin in *The Obsession*, a book about hunger. The fear of fat, and the love and hate of food, is a real social problem of epidemic proportions. With this fear, there has been a rapid rise in maladaptive eating behaviour, compulsive eating, crash dieting, bulimia (weight control by vomiting) and anorexia nervosa.

Conflicting images

At least 95 per cent of the sufferers are women, and there is little doubt that social pressures play a significant role. Torn between the advertising images of the sexual 'perfect' woman and the perpetual sensory bombardment with tantalising foods; between the image of the thin and sensuous woman, designed to attract her man, and the caring, providing 'earth mother' image associated with fat, twenty-first-century women feel they must be all things to all people. And twenty-first-century men are also meant to bring home the bacon, yet look like Brad Pitt. But who has the time, the money or the inclination to live in gyms with today's work pressures?

There's a simple set of exercises to get a handle on emotional eating so you have more choice about how to eat, rather than being a victim of your immediate desires or emotions. The exercises are divided into three steps called 'the three As':

> Awareness
> Acceptance
> Action

Step 1: Awareness

Awareness is the first: awareness of when, how, what you eat, your beliefs, facts and fantasies about eating, being fat, being thin. To get the most benefit from these exercises, answer each question accurately and write down your answer on a separate sheet of paper.

1. What do you weigh?

2. What is the heaviest you have ever been?

3. What is the lightest?

4. What is your ideal weight?

5. How long have you been overweight?

6. What personality characteristics do you associate with being fat?

7. What personality characteristics do you associate with being thin?

8. What do you fear most about being overweight (think about this in relation to health, sex, relationships, work and so on)?

9. What do you like most about being overweight?

10. Imagine you're at a party and you are your ideal weight. What feelings would you experience? How would this change the way you relate to the people around you?

11. Now imagine you become very overweight. How do you feel now, and how does this change the way you relate to others?

12. If you were your ideal weight, how do you think your life would change (think of your feelings, relationships, sex, career, clothes, sports)?

When

At this stage do not reason 'why', just observe your own behaviour in relation to eating – the hows, whens, whats. Now make a comprehensive list of all the circumstances that precipitate eating for you, other than hunger:

I eat when I'm bored

I eat when I get home from work

I eat when ...

I eat when ...

What

The next exercise will take a little longer.

Keep a food diary for one week, listing the circumstances, feelings before and feelings after each meal or snack, as well as detailed listings of what, and how much, you ate.

This can be done as follows:

Day 1 (time)	Food/drink	Circumstances	Feelings before	Feelings after
E.g. Monday 9 a.m.	Cup of coffee	Need to wake up	Tired	Bit more energy

Be precise in your answers. This will help you become aware of the situations in which you eat, as well as showing you what you eat. You may find there are some foods or snacks you feel guilty about, that you would rather not commit to paper. You may make excuses to yourself – 'I don't usually eat …' or 'It would have been rude to refuse.' Again, observe your own reactions as if you were watching your behaviour and thoughts, without judgement, on a TV screen.

How

The next series of questions will help you examine how you eat. Answer these as precisely as possible.

1. What eating and mealtime rules did your parents teach you (such as, 'Always eat everything on your plate')?

2. Do you:
   a) eat your food very fast?
   b) eat your food at a normal rate?
   c) savour each mouthful and chew it well?

3. How fussy are you? What foods will you not eat and for what reasons?

4. When you shop for food do you:
  a) go for the best quality even if it's a little expensive?
  b) go for the best value in terms of money?

5. Do you enjoy cooking and preparing food?

6. Do you usually work, read or watch TV when you eat?

7. Do you have set mealtimes?

8. How much of what you eat is snacks and nibbles?

9. Do you usually eat beyond the point of feeling full?

10. Do you prefer to eat with other people or by yourself?

Now go back over all the questions and make any additions or changes until you are sure that you have a comprehensive picture of all aspects of your eating behaviour (if there are aspects of your eating behaviour that are not covered by the questions, write these down too). Review your eating behaviour by reading your answers back to yourself as if you were hearing an impartial commentary on someone else.

Step 2: Acceptance

All eating behaviour, however destructive or counterproductive, has a purpose. We may overeat to help us deal with anger or boredom, or as a rest after a hard day. Sometimes we overeat because we *want* to be fat. For some being fat is a mark of authority. Suzie Orbach, in *Fat Is a Feminist Issue*, cites a number of clients for whom fat was a rebellion against the sexy, dependent, ineffective model imposed on women. By being fat one could be stating, 'I'm a real person with ambitions and independence.' Fat means many different things to many different people. For all, overeating has a purpose, is a means for compensation. The first step to acceptance is to understand this.

Only by seeing your eating behaviour as it is – and understanding that, in the past and the present, this behaviour has been an attempt to compensate, find pleasure or security – is it possible to eat (and on occasions overeat) without guilt or remorse. However, to accept our habits is not to give in, to surrender to food. It's a step nearer to being in control of your eating behaviour.

Acceptance is the opposite of resistance. To resist any desire or want means that desire will persist. Nothing is really solved. If you continually crave chocolate you can resist for only so long. You may overeat 'good' food with the hope that your craving for chocolate will go away. You may believe that eating chocolate is bad, that you're bad, and as you give in to this irresistible urge you may have feelings of guilt and self-disgust at your unhealthy tastes and lack of willpower. With these feelings can come more desire to eat, to compensate for these feelings. It is better to accept your initial desires and to understand them.

As an exercise in acceptance, go to your favourite food shops and buy all the foods you like most, whether 'good' or 'bad'. Stock up your fridge and larder with all the foods you could possibly want. For one week eat what you want, how you want it. If what you really want is the dessert, start with this.

Step 3: Action

We are all programmed to survive. We have a built-in mechanism that makes us hungry when we are deprived of nutrition. Any baby will cry if it wants food. If the food doesn't satisfy the baby's nutritional needs it will still feel hungry. We are no different.

For many of us hunger is rarely the motive for eating. We have learned that eating suppresses feelings that certain foods are addictive, that it is sociable to eat and encourage others to eat. We have learned how to eat against our instincts. Only by unlearning these habits is it possible to discover or uncover our inbuilt desire to eat nutritious food in the right quantities.

From the questions on previous pages you will have a list of when you eat and what you eat, as well as the feelings you associate with eating. These are some of the commonest 'when's' from clients at my clinics:

- I eat when I'm bored.
- I eat when I'm happy.
- I eat when I'm frustrated/angry/upset.
- I eat when I'm sexually frustrated.
- I eat when I'm tired.
- I continually nibble after work from 6 p.m. onwards.
- I eat when I'm under pressure at work.

According to the psychologist Oscar Ichazo, these are examples of using eating to compensate for feelings we cannot handle. For instance, boredom may result from our having more energy than we know how to deal with. Drinking or overeating is one way to dissipate that energy, leaving us psychologically in balance. It's as if we had a steam boiler full of energy, and when the pressure builds up we experience negative feelings like frustration or boredom. To compensate, we must let off steam by opening safety valves, one of which is gluttony, which includes overeating. Others include panic, phobia, overexertion, cruelty and toximania (such as getting drunk).

Ichazo calls these 'doors of compensation' because we develop the habit of losing energy through one 'door' or another. (I've discussed these more fully in my book *Beat Stress and Fatigue*). If, for example, gluttony is one of your favourite doors (using food to excess), or toximania, then the goal is to find a better way to deal with the situation you are compensating for.

Breaking the habits

The object of the next exercise is to break each part of your overeating habits, initially for a period of one week. Only then are you in a position to decide whether curbing overeating is the most effective way to deal with the particular situation. With objective awareness and acceptance of our eating behaviour and the following exercise, habitual eating becomes easier to stop.

Pick a 'when' such as, 'I eat when I'm frustrated.'

QUESTION 1. Is there any way you can deal with the situation directly? For example, how can you most effectively express the anger/frustration to achieve the results you want? Depression is often anger without enthusiasm!

QUESTION 2. Is there any way you can deal with the situation indirectly? For example, go for a run, call a friend, energetically do some housework, beat the hell out of a carpet, or rip the weeds out of your garden instead.

SET YOUR TARGET. Now set yourself this target for the next week:

'I eat as much as I want, when I want, and I do not eat when … [I'm frustrated].'

Write this down on a card and keep it in a prominent place. When you have completed your first target, reward yourself by doing something you really enjoy. You are now in a position to choose whether eating is the best way of dealing with this 'when' situation. You are in control.

Now move on to your next 'when'. Ask yourself Questions 1 and 2 each time this situation arises. Set your target for the next week, write this down on a card and keep it in a prominent place. Do this for each 'when' until you've completed your list.

Remember: *you* are not your eating behaviour. Your eating behaviour consists of habits you have consciously or unconsciously learned as a result of experiences in the past. Some of these habits are still useful and some of them are not. By stopping each eating habit for a week you are in a position to choose how, when and what you eat. You are in control.

These simple exercises will help you get a handle on emotional and obsessive eating, helping you to follow my diet to its successful conclusion.

26

Maintenance

As I said at the start, the Holford Diet is all about optimum health, and weight loss is just one facet of this. It's a diet for life, and that's why 90 per cent of the principles covered in this book are consistent with ongoing good health and weight maintenance. However, there are some aspects of the diet that you don't need to keep up for ever.

Once you have lost most of the weight you wanted to lose, are feeling full of energy and vitality, and have lost any cravings for stimulants and sugary foods (check your score on the 'Are you insulin-resistant?' questionnaire on page 56), you don't need to keep eating quite so much protein every day. You can reduce the amount from 25 per cent of your daily calories to between 15 and 20 per cent. The chart below shows you what this means in practice.

Protein servings on the maintenance diet

Food	Weight/Vol	Serving
Tofu	85g	½ packet
Soya mince	72g	2 tbsp
Chicken (no skin)	35g	¾ very small breast
Turkey (no skin)	35g	¼ small breast
Quorn	85g	¼ pack
Salmon	40g	¾ very small fillet
Tuna (canned in brine)	35g	⅕ tin
Sardines (canned in brine)	55g	½ tin
Cod	45g	¾ very small fillet
Clams	45g	⅕ can
Prawns	60g	4 large prawns
Mackerel	60g	¾ medium fillet
Oysters	–	11
Yoghurt (natural, low-fat)	205g	¼ large tub
Cottage cheese	85g	¼ medium tub
Hummus	145g	¾ small tub
Skimmed milk	315ml	*c.* ½ pint
Soya milk	300ml	*c.* ½ pint
Eggs (boiled)	–	1½
Quinoa	90g	5 heaped tbsp
Baked beans	225g	½ tin
Kidney beans	125g	1 tbsp
Black-eyed beans	125g	1 tbsp
Lentils	120g	1 tbsp

But, while you eat less protein-rich food, you'll eat more carbohydrate-rich food. Go by the chart on page 228, but this time aim to eat between half to two-thirds of the protein portions given, and one and a half to twice the carbohydrate portion. This means upping your daily GL score for what you *eat* from 40 to 55 points, which will include unchanged GL of 10 for two snacks, and 5 for drinks, sweets and desserts. So each meal will have 15 ⓖ.

As a result, you'll have to alter some of the recipes a bit to up the proportion of carbohydrate-rich foods. The chart below gives you some guidelines on common combinations.

Protein-rich food	Carbohydrate-rich food
¾ small breast/3 slices chicken	1 medium serving brown rice (150g)
¾ small fillet salmon	1 serving wholewheat pasta (175g)
¼ medium pot cottage cheese	6 small (new) boiled potatoes (150g)
1 tbsp beans	6 oatcakes

Everyone is different, so you'll have to experiment with ratios of carbohydrate and protein till you find what suits you best. Your best guide is your body and your instincts. Eat what works for you.

Supplements for life

While it's a great idea to keep supplementing your diet with a good high-strength multivitamin and mineral, plus 1,000mg of vitamin C, you don't need to keep taking additional chromium (provided there's 40mcg or more in your multi), HCA or fibre supplements for ever. So you can safely stop these, too, when you've achieved your final weight. Chromium is particularly helpful at keeping your blood sugar level stable, so if you ever find yourself craving stimulants or sweet things – perhaps when you're under a lot of stress – you may find it helpful to take additional chromium for a few weeks.

Stimulants – don't drift back

One of the most important, yet most difficult, times to stay on track is when you're stressed. This is when the old familiar stimulants (tea, coffee, chocolate, cigarettes, sugar) remind you of their existence. If you've really been addicted to one or more of these, don't let them creep back, even when you've achieved your final goal. The daily use of any stimulant is a bad sign. The odd cup of weak tea or coffee when you eat out or on holiday, or the odd chocolate dessert, is no big deal, though.

100 per cent health

Losing weight and gaining all that energy is just the beginning. Why not go all the way, and start to incorporate into your diet and lifestyle all the advice given in my books *The Optimum Nutrition Bible* and *Optimum Nutrition for the Mind*? Each encourages you to go deeper in both your understanding and your application of optimum nutrition, to help you achieve higher and higher levels of health in all aspects of mind and body. And you can produce even more delectable gourmet dishes with my *Optimum Nutrition Cookbook*, co-authored with Judy Ridgway.

(TOP TIP)

Fatburner research
You can help with ongoing Fatburner research. If you've completed the diet for four or more weeks, let us know your results by filling the simple questionnaire at the end of Appendix 4, on page 466. Answer as many questions as you can and send or fax the questionnaire to Fatburner Research, Holford & Associates, Carters Yard, London SW18 4JR; fax: 020 8874 5003. Alternatively, you can fill in this information online at www.theholforddiet.com.

References: Part Three

1 J. Warren, C. Henry and V. Simonite, 'Low glycemic index breakfasts and reduced food intake in preadolescent children', *Pediatrics*, Vol 112(5) (2003) p. 414

2 D. Ludwig D., 'Dietary Glycemic Index and Regulation of Body Weight', *Lipids*, Vol 38(2) (2003), pp. 117–21

3 K. Heaton et al., 'Particle size of wheat, maize and oat test meals: effects on plasma glucose and insulin responses and on the rate of starch digestion in vitro', *American Journal of Clinical Nutrition*, Vol 47 (1988), pp. 675–82

4 E. Cheraskin, 'The Breakfast/Lunch/Dinner Ritual', *Journal of Orthomolecular Medicine*, Vol 8(1) (1993), pp. 6–10

5 J. T. Braaten et al., 'High beta-glucan oat bran and oat gum reduce postprandial blood glucose and insulin in subjects with and without type 2 diabetes', *Diabetic Medicine*, Vol 11(3) (1994), pp. 312–18

PART FOUR

Food: Menu Plans and Recipes

27

Menus

You may have followed diets with insipid low-fat recipes, or, in the case of high-protein regimes, super-rich and filling ones. The Holford Diet is all about freshness, flavour, zing – and satisfaction. And there's no end to the variety of meals you can make that fit within the Fatburner principles.

So now is the time to get to grips with all the new ingredients in your fridge and larder. I'll start with a menu plan for the first four weeks, which I recommend you follow for at least the first week so you get a clear idea of the quantity and balance of foods on this diet. Once you're familiar with them and with the basic rules, you can use these recipes and your imagination to create a feast of Fatburning gastronomic delights.

Should you wish to do it your own way and work out your menus yourself, that's fine too. You can swap meals around from one day to another. However, do bear in mind that each day of the menus in this book is well balanced. The menus are also balanced for fat, giving you two measures of the essential fats (explained in Chapter 8) each day.

If you make up your own daily menus, make sure you are not getting too much or too little essential fat. Don't pick, for example, the highest-fat recipe and have that every day. Oily fish, for example, occurs in the menus no more than three times a week. So, as you work out each day's menu, ensure you have enough variation. Also, be sure to ring the changes with your snacks. Try a ripe pear with pumpkin seeds; a couple of oat-cakes with a dollop of hummus; cottage cheese with berries; or a handful of delicious Spiced Chickpea Chews (page 390).

Bear in mind that puddings are a treat I recommend having just once a week, starting in Week 3.

If you're a vegan or vegetarian, you've got both recipes that you can go with right away and recipes in which you can sub-stitute tofu, tempeh or other protein sources for fish or chicken. Chapter 20 also has useful information and suggestions for the rich array of options this diet offers you.

Please note the portion sizes you should consume for the following, as either snacks or components of a meal:

- Nuts/seeds – 50g

- Berries – ½ cup

- Steamed vegetables (taken from the 'unlimited' table on page 221) – half a dinner-plateful, unless stated otherwise

Week One

Day 1

Breakfast: Scots Porridge with berries or one chopped apple or pear and milk

Lunch: Apple and Tuna Salad with three oatcakes

Dinner: Steam-Fried Vegetables with tofu with 70g brown basmati rice

Snacks: Pear with pumpkin seeds/two oatcakes with hummus

Drinks: Unlimited water, herbal teas and coffee alternatives, plus one glass of diluted juice

Day 2

Breakfast: Fatburner Muesli

Lunch: Fatburner Sandwich with Green Salad

Dinner: Chicken Tandoori with 70g brown basmati rice and steamed vegetables

Snacks: Apple with sunflower seeds/cottage cheese with berries

Drinks: Unlimited water, herbal teas and coffee alternatives, plus one glass of diluted juice

Day 3

Breakfast: Fruit Yoghurt/Yoghurt Shake

Lunch: Beany Vegetable Soup with two oatcakes

Dinner: Pasta with Pumpkin Seed Pesto

Snacks: A punnet of strawberries/one thin slice of rye bread with peanut butter

Drinks: Unlimited water, herbal teas and coffee alternatives, plus one glass of diluted juice

Day 4

Breakfast: Scots Porridge with ½ cup berries or one chopped apple or pear and milk and yoghurt

Lunch: Quinoa Tabbouleh

Dinner:	Tuna Steak with Black-Eyed Bean Salsa and Rocket and Watercress Salad
Snacks:	An apple and five almonds/two oatcakes and peanut butter
Drinks:	Unlimited water, herbal teas and coffee alternatives, plus one glass of diluted juice

Day 5

Breakfast:	Fatburner Muesli
Lunch:	Fatburner Baked Potato with Coleslaw
Dinner:	Chicken Chermoula with Oriental Green Beans
Snacks:	A small yoghurt with blueberries/crudités (one carrot, two sticks of celery and five broccoli florets) and hummus
Drinks:	Unlimited water, herbal teas and coffee alternatives, plus one glass of diluted juice

Day 6

Breakfast:	Fruit Yoghurt/Yoghurt Shake
Lunch:	Walnut and Three-Bean Salad with Green Salad
Dinner:	Chestnut and Mushroom Pilaf with steamed spinach and broccoli
Snacks:	Pear with pumpkin seeds/two oatcakes with hummus
Drinks:	Unlimited water, herbal teas and coffee alternatives, plus one glass of diluted juice

Day 7

Breakfast:	Scrambled Egg with one thin slice of rye toast
Lunch:	Stuffed Peppers with Green Salad

Dinner:	Thai Baked Cod with 70g brown basmati rice and Crunchy Thai Salad
Snacks:	Apple with sunflower seeds/cottage cheese with berries
Drinks:	Unlimited water, herbal teas and coffee alternatives, plus one glass of diluted juice

Week Two

By now you'll be getting a taste for the Fatburner recipes. Note the ones you like, and remember that you can exchange lunches or dinner from one day with another day. However, keep your choices varied, since some meals are less balanced than others. By Weeks 3 and 4 you can add in one dessert per week, and continue to introduce new and delicious recipes.

Day 1

Breakfast:	Scots Porridge
Lunch:	Fatburner Sandwich with Green Salad
Dinner:	Ratatouille Sausage Bake with three steamed baby new potatoes and a quarter of a plateful of broccoli
Snacks:	Two pieces of fruit with nuts/seeds
Drinks:	Unlimited water, herbal teas and coffee alternatives, plus one glass of diluted juice

Day 2

Breakfast:	Fatburner Muesli
Lunch:	Thai-Style Vegetable Broth, Crunchy Thai Salad
Dinner:	Trout with Puy Lentils and Roasted Tomatoes on the Vine

Snacks:	Two pieces of fruit with nuts/seeds
Drinks:	Unlimited water, herbal teas and coffee alternatives, plus one glass of diluted juice

Day **3**

Breakfast:	Fruit Yoghurt/Yoghurt Shake
Lunch:	Smoked Salmon Pâté on two thin slices of toasted rye bread
Dinner:	Thai Green Curry with a quarter plateful of steamed mangetout
Snacks:	Two pieces of fruit with nuts/seeds
Drinks:	Unlimited water, herbal teas and coffee alternatives, plus one glass of diluted juice

Day **4**

Breakfast:	Scots Porridge
Lunch:	Flageolet Bean Dip with crudités (one carrot, two sticks of celery and five broccoli florets) and three oatcakes
Dinner:	Roasted Vegetables with Mediterranean Quinoa
Snacks:	Two pieces of fruit with nuts/seeds
Drinks:	Unlimited water, herbal teas and coffee alternatives, plus one glass of diluted juice

Day **5**

Breakfast:	Fatburner Muesli
Lunch:	Fatburner Baked Potato with Green Salad
Dinner:	Dhal (Lentil Curry) with 70g brown basmati rice and steamed broccoli
Snacks:	Two pieces of fruit with nuts/seeds

Drinks: Unlimited water, herbal teas and coffee
alternatives, plus one glass of diluted juice

Day **6**

Breakfast: Fruit Yoghurt/Yoghurt Shake
Lunch: Chestnut and Butterbean Soup with two oatcakes
Dinner: Spiced Turkey Meatballs with 85g of wholegrain
spaghetti and one courgette (sliced lengthways
and grilled)
Snacks: Two pieces of fruit with nuts/seeds
Drinks: Unlimited water, herbal teas and coffee
alternatives, plus one glass of diluted juice

Day **7**

Breakfast: Boiled Egg with one thin slice of rye toast
Lunch: Gazpacho, Baba Ganoush and one thin slice of
rye bread
Dinner: Chicken Dumplings with Chilli Dipping Sauce,
with 85g soba (buckwheat) noodles and steam-
fried pak choi
Snacks: Two pieces of fruit with nuts/seeds
Drinks: Unlimited water, herbal teas and coffee
alternatives, plus one glass of diluted juice

Week Three

Day **1**

Breakfast: Scots Porridge
Lunch: Green Bean, Olive and Roasted Pepper Salad in
one wholemeal pitta bread

Dinner: Borlotti Bean Bolognese with two steamed courgettes

Snacks: Two pieces of fruit with nuts/seeds

Drinks: Unlimited water, herbal teas and coffee alternatives, plus one glass of diluted juice

Day 2

Breakfast: Fatburner Muesli

Lunch: Hummus with crudités (one carrot, two sticks of celery and five broccoli florets) and four oatcakes

Dinner: Fajitas with Mediterranean Tomato and Courgette Salad

Snacks: Two pieces of fruit with nuts/seeds

Drinks: Unlimited water, herbal teas and coffee alternatives, plus one glass of diluted juice

Day 3

Breakfast: Fruit Yoghurt/Yoghurt Shake

Lunch: Beany Vegetable Soup with two oatcakes or one toasted pitta bread

Dinner: Garlic and Lemon Roast Chicken with two small boiled new potatoes and steamed broccoli
Chocolate Coconut Cookies

Snacks: Two pieces of fruit with nuts/seeds

Drinks: Unlimited water, herbal teas and coffee alternatives, plus one glass of diluted juice

Day 4

Breakfast: Scots Porridge

Lunch: Blueberry and Cottage Cheese Salad with three oatcakes

Dinner: Chickpea Curry with 70g brown basmati rice or 50g couscous and steamed runner beans
Snacks: Two pieces of fruit with nuts/seeds
Drinks: Unlimited water, herbal teas and coffee alternatives, plus one glass of diluted juice

Day 5

Breakfast: Fatburner Muesli
Lunch: Fatburner Baked Potato with Mediterranean Tomato and Courgette Salad
Dinner: Stuffed Peppers with Tomato and Red Onion Salad
Snacks: Two pieces of fruit with nuts/seeds
Drinks: Unlimited water, herbal teas and coffee alternatives, plus one glass of diluted juice

Day 6

Breakfast: Fruit Yoghurt/Yoghurt Shake
Lunch: Walnut and Three-Bean Salad with Coleslaw
Dinner: Sticky Mustard Salmon Fillets with 100g quinoa and steam-fried leeks and peppers
Snacks: Two pieces of fruit with nuts/seeds
Drinks: Unlimited water, herbal teas and coffee alternatives, plus one glass of diluted juice

Day 7

Breakfast: Scrambled Egg with one thin slice of rye toast
Lunch: Lentil and Lemon Soup with three oatcakes
Dinner: Indian Spiced Chicken with 70g brown basmati rice and steam-fried vegetables

Snacks: Two pieces of fruit with nuts/seeds
Drinks: Unlimited water, herbal teas and coffee alternatives, plus one glass of diluted juice

Week Four

Day 1

Breakfast: Scots Porridge
Lunch: Fatburner Sandwich with Tomato and Red Onion Salad
Dinner: Grilled Goat's Cheese on Portabella Mushrooms with mixed salad leaves (such as spinach, rocket and watercress) and either dressing
Snacks: Two pieces of fruit with nuts/seeds
Drinks: Unlimited water, herbal teas and coffee alternatives, plus one glass of diluted juice

Day 2

Breakfast: Fatburner Muesli
Lunch: Spicy Pumpkin and Tofu Soup
Dinner: Chicken with Roasted Courgettes and Red Onion
Snacks: Two pieces of fruit with nuts/seeds
Drinks: Unlimited water, herbal teas and coffee alternatives, plus one glass of diluted juice

Day 3

Breakfast: Fruit Yoghurt/Yoghurt Shake
Lunch: Sardines on Toast with Celeriac Rémoulade

Dinner: Nick's Beef Burgers with Mexican Bean Dip and as much lettuce as you can squeeze into a toasted wholemeal pitta bread
Individual Berry Cheesecake
Snacks: Two pieces of fruit with nuts/seeds
Drinks: Unlimited water, herbal teas and coffee alternatives, plus one glass of diluted juice

Day **4**

Breakfast: Scots Porridge
Lunch: Chestnut and Butterbean Soup with a Green Salad on the side
Dinner: Tarragon and Lemon Roast Chicken Breast with 70g brown basmati rice and Mediterranean Tomato and Courgette Salad (or steamed vegetables)
Snacks: Two pieces of fruit with nuts/seeds
Drinks: Unlimited water, herbal teas and coffee alternatives, plus one glass of diluted juice

Day **5**

Breakfast: Fatburner Muesli
Lunch: Fatburner Baked Sweet Potato with Rocket and Watercress Salad
Dinner: Grilled Burgers with one wholemeal pitta bread and mixed salad leaves (such as spinach, rocket and watercress) with either dressing
Snacks: Two pieces of fruit with nuts/seeds
Drinks: Unlimited water, herbal teas and coffee alternatives, plus one glass of diluted juice

Day 6

Breakfast: Fruit Yoghurt/Yoghurt Shake
Lunch: Mexican Bean Dip and crudités (one carrot, two sticks of celery and five broccoli florets)
Dinner: Trout with Puy Lentils and Roasted Tomatoes on the Vine with steamed courgettes
Snacks: Two pieces of fruit with nuts/seeds
Drinks: Unlimited water, herbal teas and coffee alternatives, plus one glass of diluted juice

Day 7

Breakfast: Boiled Egg with one thin slice of rye toast
Lunch: Quinoa Tabbouleh with Tomato and Red Onion Salad
Dinner: Chestnut and Mushroom Pilaf with mixed salad leaves (such as spinach, rocket and watercress) and either dressing
Snacks: Two pieces of fruit with nuts/seeds
Drinks: Unlimited water, herbal teas and coffee alternatives, plus one glass of diluted juice

28

Recipes

In the end, all diets stand or fall by their recipes. Huge amounts of research, care and thought may have gone into the principles behind them, but, if the food itself is tasteless or monotonous, the diet will fail.

The Holford Diet passes this test with flying colours. I promise you wonderful flavours, intriguing textures, fantastic freshness and great variety. I've borrowed from the best in world cuisine to create dishes bursting with health and flavour. Hundreds of thousands of people have found these recipes seriously delicious, so, if you're ready, let's get going on them.

Almost all the recipes are sugar-free, using the natural sweetness present in food, or they use a proprietary product called xylitol, a natural plant sugar that has all the taste of sugar but a third of the calories, and does not disrupt your blood sugar, giving it a very low ⓖⓛ. Another added bonus is the fact that it protects your teeth from cavities. It is available from Health Products for Life (you'll find their address on page 479 of Resources).

The recipes are also high in fibre, so you don't need to add any. The foods used are naturally high in key vitamins and minerals. I recommend you buy the freshest ingredients, organic if possible, since these tend to contain more nutrients as well as being chemical-free.

As this diet is mainly based on fresh vegetables, fruits, beans, lentils and wholegrains, with some fish and chicken, you will find it very economical, too. You may, however, need to vary the fruits and vegetables depending on what's in season.

To follow the diet, all you need to do is select a breakfast, lunch and dinner for each day, based on the menus in the previous chapter. Not all the recipes have exactly the same balance of nutrients, so it's best to vary your choices.

Note that, unless otherwise stated, all lunches and main meals, except for things like sandwiches, give quantities for two people. If there's only one of you, halve the portion sizes or make enough for two meals and pop one in the fridge. (Note also that I often suggest you season a dish with Solo, a special kind of salt; for more on this product, see Resources, page 476.)

Bon appétit!

Breakfasts

Yes, it's true: breakfast *is* the most important meal of the day. It's all down, literally, to your body's sugar level, which is at its lowest ebb first thing in the morning. If you go to work very early, take your breakfast to work and have it during the first break you take. All recipes are for one person. (For the size of a serving of various kinds of fruits, see page 205.) Remember, breakfast can have a maximum 10 Ⓖ.

ⒼⓁ scores:

Get Up & Go

Get Up & Go is a powdered breakfast drink, which is blended with skimmed milk or soya milk and banana or berries. Nutritionally speaking, it is the ultimate breakfast: each serving gives you more fibre than a bowl of porridge, more protein than an egg, more iron than a cooked breakfast and more vitamins and minerals than a whole packet of cornflakes. In fact, every serving of Get Up & Go gives you at least 100 per cent of every vitamin and mineral and a lot more of some key nutrients. For example, you get 1,000mg of vitamin C – the equivalent of more than 20 oranges.

Get Up & Go is made from the best-quality wholefoods, ground into a powder. The carbohydrate comes principally from apple powder, the protein comes from quinoa, soya and rice flour, the essential fats from ground sesame, sunflower and pumpkin seeds, the fibre from oat bran, rice bran and psyllium husks, and additional flavour from almond meal, cinnamon and natural vanilla.

It contains no sucrose, no additives, no animal products, no yeast, wheat or milk, and it tastes delicious. Each serving, with half a pint of skimmed milk or soya milk and some fruit, provides fewer than 300 calories and, when mixed up, only 10 ⓖ, making it ideal as part of the Holford Diet. It is nutritionally superior to any other breakfast choice and is totally suitable for adults and children alike. It is fine to have this for breakfast every day, if you choose.

Make it up with berries such as strawberries, raspberries or blueberries, or a soft pear. If you use a banana have a small, less ripe banana or use half a larger banana. It is widely available in health-food shops. (See Resources, page 479, for stockists.)

Get Up & Go

> 1 serving Get Up & Go powder
> ½pt (300ml) skimmed milk or low-fat soya milk
> 1 small banana, or ½ larger banana, or 1 pear or 2 heaped tbsp
>   berries

Blend milk, fruit and Get Up & Go powder.

Fatburner Muesli

You can make this delicious muesli yourself. Experiment with fruit combinations. It tastes best when the oats/rye are soaked overnight in enough water to cover ingredients.

> ½ cup soft porridge oat flakes
> ½ cup oat bran
> 1 tbsp ground seeds (see page 206 for the seed mix recipe)
> as many berries as you want (strawberries, raspberries,
>   blueberries)
> 2 tbsp plain, natural yoghurt

Scots Porridge

On a cold winter day nothing can be more warming than porridge. Oats have special properties, making them known to promote a healthy heart and arteries, and are full of fibre and complex carbohydrates.

½pt (300ml) water
½pt (300ml) skimmed or soya milk
2oz (57g) porridge oats
1 tsp honey
1 dessertspoon ground flax and pumpkin seeds

1 Put the water and half the milk in a saucepan and sprinkle in the oats.
2 Bring to the boil and simmer for 3–5 minutes, stirring all the time.
3 Serve with milk, seeds and a little honey.

Fruit Yoghurt/Yoghurt Shake

Low-fat, live, natural yoghurt is a first-class food, unlike its commercial counterpart, in which most bacteria have been destroyed for a longer shelf life. Live yoghurt is packed with friendly bacteria that have a spring-cleaning effect on your digestive system, as well as being a good source of protein.

10oz (283g) very low-fat live yoghurt
1 tsp honey
1 serving fruit – banana, apple, pear, berries, kiwi
1 dessertspoon ground flax and pumpkin seeds

1 Combine all the ingredients. Use any fruit in season.
2 If you prefer, make a shake by processing the mix in a blender.

Scrambled Egg

While eggs are rather high in fat, as part of a balanced diet they are a good source of protein and add variety. Limit to five a week, and seven a week in the maintenance phase.

> 1 large free-range egg
> dash of skimmed or soya milk
> 1 tbsp parsley
> small knob of butter

1 Beat eggs with milk and parsley.
2 Melt butter in a small saucepan.
3 Pour in egg mixture. Cook slowly, stirring constantly.
4 Serve with one thin slice of rye toast.

Boiled Egg

This simple breakfast makes a wholesome start to the day.

> 1 large free-range egg

1 Boil the egg to taste (3–4 minutes for soft-boiled).
2 Serve with very lightly buttered wholegrain rye toast.

Salads, soups, dips and light meals

As you saw in the menus, you can include salads on the side with many of the main dishes. They add vitamins, crunch and flavour to mealtimes and are all fast and easy to prepare.

A number of the soups in this section can take the place of main dishes. There's a wide and delicious selection. To save time you may want to make enough for two or three days and store some in the fridge, or make in even larger batches and freeze some. If you're in a tearing hurry, you could choose a serving of one of the better-quality soups now available commercially, such as Baxter's tinned soup or Covent Garden fresh soups. Remember to include a serving of protein if you choose a vegetable soup, and to avoid the creamy ones.

Most of these recipes would make great packed lunches for work, too (just invest in an insulated flask for the soups), and I have included some dips and dressings to liven up salads and vegetable accompaniments. Quantities given are for two servings unless otherwise stated.

Remember, salads and soups will make up a variable number of ⑬ within your ultimate meal allowance of 10 ⑬.

⑬ scores:

continues ▶

Salads

French Dressing

This standard French dressing can be jazzed up by adding fresh and dried herbs. Also, experiment with other oils such as cold-pressed sesame oil or flax oil, which contains essential fatty acids. Use as little dressing as possible on salads.

3 tbsp olive oil

2 tbsp Essential Balance Oil (from Health Products for Life, whose address you'll find in Resources), or olive oil

2 tbsp cider or balsamic vinegar

1 tsp French mustard

1 clove garlic, crushed

Put all the ingredients in a screw-top jar and shake vigorously. Any extra dressing can be stored in the fridge.

Tahini Dressing

Tahini is made of crushed sesame seeds and their oil – it makes a dressing thicker and creamier.

Either

2 tbsp homemade French Dressing (see above)

1 tbsp tahini

or

½ tsp honey

1 tsp mustard

2 tbsp Essential Balance Oil (from Health Products for Life – see Resources), or olive oil

1 tbsp tahini

juice of ½ lemon

Put all the ingredients in a screw-top jar and shake vigorously. Any extra dressing can be stored in the fridge.

Rocket and Watercress Salad

Watercress is rich in iron and vitamin A and is delicious in salad.

> 2 good handfuls of rocket
> good handful of watercress, torn
> 1 gem lettuce, torn into pieces
> 1 tbsp cress

Combine all the ingredients and toss with 1 tbsp French or Tahini Dressing.

Green Salad

This simple green salad is a good accompaniment to any meal. It's subtly different because of the aniseed flavour from the fennel, and has plenty of crunch.

> ⅓ cos or other lettuce, torn into bite-sized pieces
> ¼ bulb fennel, finely sliced, or 2 tbsp fresh peas, uncooked or
>   just blanched (if you don't like fennel)
> ¼ cucumber, finely sliced
> 1 stick celery, finely sliced

Combine all the ingredients and toss with dressing.

Mediterranean Tomato and Courgette Salad

Raw courgette has a subtle flavour that makes an interesting change from cucumber.

> 3 tomatoes, thinly sliced
> 1 small courgette, very thinly sliced widthways (using a
>   mandolin grater is easiest)

6 large, fresh basil leaves, roughly torn
1 dessertspoon olive oil
2 tsp balsamic vinegar
1 dessertspoon pine nuts (lightly toasted in a dry pan if time)
black pepper

Toss all ingredients together and season.

Crunchy Thai Salad

This is a variation on one of the most popular street food dishes in Thailand, where it is freshly made to order with a pestle and mortar. It originally comes from the north-east of the country. Now you can save the airfare and make it in your own kitchen!

¼ medium white cabbage, finely shredded
4oz (113g) mangetout, parboiled (for 2 minutes) and shredded
   sugar snap peas, sliced
½ medium tomato, finely chopped
1 small, mild, red chilli, deseeded and very finely chopped
juice of 1 lime
½ tsp mirin (Japanese rice wine, available from supermarkets)
2 tbsp tamari or soy sauce
1 ½ tsp sesame oil
½ inch chunk ginger root, finely chopped
2 tbsp sesame seeds (toast in a dry pan until they go brown,
   shaking from time to time)

Combine all ingredients in a large bowl and toss well. If you are not keen on hot food, leave out the chilli, although if you are careful to remove the inner pith and seeds you will find it provides flavour without excessive heat.

Tomato and Red Onion Salad

A classic salad with a strong taste, full of flavour and goodness.

> 1 beefsteak tomato, diced
> ½ red onion, finely sliced into rings
> 1 dessertspoon extra-virgin olive oil
> juice of ½ lemon
> 2 tsp balsamic vinegar
> black pepper
> small handful fresh basil leaves, torn

Toss all ingredients together.

Coleslaw

Cabbage is packed with vitamins and minerals. So are carrots, high in vitamin A, and onions, high in sulphur-rich amino acids, which help to remove toxins from the body. This coleslaw is nothing like the limp supermarket variety: it really packs in the power and crunch.

> 7 oz (198g) red or white cabbage, finely shredded
> 3oz (85g) carrots, grated
> ½ small onion, finely chopped
> 1 tbsp low-fat mayonnaise
> 1 tbsp very low-fat live yoghurt

Mix all ingredients well in a large bowl.

Celeriac Rémoulade

If you haven't eaten celeriac before, you'll find it's a revelation. This is a great addition to a Fatburner picnic, and the perfect alternative to shop-bought coleslaw.

½ a celeriac, peeled and thinly grated
½ tsp smooth mustard
2 tsp chopped fresh parsley
2 tbsp live natural yoghurt
Solo sea salt

Stir all the ingredients until the celeriac is well coated and serve.

Oriental Green Beans

Tender green beans go well with this dressing. This recipe works brilliantly with tofu steam fries.

9oz (255g) young green beans, cut in half crossways
1 clove garlic, crushed
1 tbsp tamari
1 tsp sesame oil
1 tsp sesame seeds, dry-roasted in a pan until golden (shake them occasionally)

1 Steam the beans gently for around 3 minutes, or until tender.
2 Place the dressing ingredients in a bowl and stir together, then toss over the beans and serve warm.

Walnut and Three-Bean Salad

No foods are better than beans for satisfying your appetite and giving stamina. It helps if they're served in a delicious, crunchy salad such as this one.

14oz (397g) canned mixed beans (such as chickpeas, haricot and flageolet beans)
handful of walnuts, roughly chopped
½ apple, cubed
1 dessertspoon fresh flat-leaf parsley or chives, chopped
1 tbsp olive oil
1 tbsp walnut oil (or olive oil)
juice of ½ lemon
1 stick celery, finely chopped
black pepper

Combine all ingredients and serve with mixed salad leaves (such as spinach, rocket and watercress).

Apple and Tuna Salad

Tuna is a fairly good source of essential fatty acids – which keep our hormones and brain in shape – as well as other vital nutrients and protein. Combining it with apple is a bit unusual, but highly successful in the flavour stakes.

6oz (170g) tuna in brine, drained
1 apple, chopped
1 stick celery, sliced
1 little gem lettuce, ripped into bite-sized pieces
1 tbsp low-fat mayonnaise
3oz (85g) natural live yoghurt

2 tsp lemon juice
Solo sea salt
black pepper

Drain the tuna and mix well with the apple, celery, lettuce, yoghurt, mayonnaise, lemon juice and seasoning.

Green Bean, Olive and Roasted Pepper Salad

A Spanish-style salad that goes well stuffed in a pitta pocket. Or optionally add some black-eyed beans (5 ⓖⓛ per half-cup).

7oz (198g) French beans, topped and tailed
2 medium eggs
1 small red onion, finely chopped
2 roasted red peppers, finely chopped
handful of black olives, stoned and halved
1 tbsp olive oil
1 tsp red wine vinegar
black pepper

1 Hard-boil the eggs (8 minutes), then cool rapidly under cold water until they are stone-cold. Shell and slice.
2 Steam the beans until *al dente*, then refresh under cold running water in order to keep the deep green colour. Dry well on kitchen towel and put in a bowl.
3 Whisk the vinegar into the oil and season, then toss over the beans.
4 Place the beans in a serving dish, stir through the onion, red pepper and olives, then gently scatter the egg over the top.

Quinoa Tabbouleh

Using quinoa instead of bulgur wheat in this Middle Eastern dish provides first-class protein. You could double up the quantities and keep some in the fridge to take to work.

> 5oz (142g) quinoa
> vegetable stock or bouillon made up into liquid (2 parts liquid
>   to 1 part quinoa)
> ¼ medium-sized cucumber, sliced lengthways into quarters,
>   then finely sliced horizontally (making tiny triangles)
> 2 good handfuls of cherry tomatoes, chopped to the same size
>   as the cucumber
> 4 spring onions, finely sliced
> good handful of fresh mint, finely chopped
> good handful of fresh flat-leaf parsley, finely chopped
> 1–2 tbsp olive oil
> 1 tbsp lemon juice
> 1 dessertspoon balsamic vinegar or to taste
> Solo sea salt
> black pepper

1 Bring the quinoa to the boil in a saucepan with the bouillon, then cover, reduce the heat and simmer for approximately 10–15 minutes until the liquid is absorbed and the grains are fluffy. Place the quinoa in a bowl and leave to cool.
2 When at room temperature, mix in the chopped vegetables and herbs with a fork, then add the oil, juice and vinegar and season. Taste to check the flavour and adjust accordingly.
3 Place in the fridge for at least an hour to allow the flavours to develop.

Blueberry and Cottage Cheese Salad

Blueberries are one of the best sources of bioflavonoids, which are powerful antioxidants. Here they contrast beautifully in colour and taste with apple and kiwi.

1 apple, thinly sliced
1 kiwi fruit, peeled and thinly sliced
2 tsp lemon juice
9oz (255g) cottage cheese
2 handfuls of blueberries
4 fresh mint leaves, finely chopped

1 Arrange the apple and kiwi on individual dishes.
2 Sprinkle with lemon juice and top with cottage cheese, blueberries and mint.

Rice, Tuna and Petits Pois Salad

This is unbelievably tasty – much more interesting than bog-standard tuna mayo. Peas are delicious raw, and of course retain more vitamins this way.

4oz (113g) brown basmati rice, cooked
4oz (113g) tuna in brine, drained
1 tsp sesame oil
2 tsp tamari or soy sauce
2 tsp lemon juice
1 tbsp fresh, uncooked petits pois (or blanched, according to taste)
1 carrot, julienned (finely sliced lengthways)
1 spring onion, finely sliced
black pepper

1 Cook rice and allow it to cool.
2 Combine with all other ingredients, tossing thoroughly to mix all the flavours.

Cottage Cheese, Radish and Watermelon Salad

A refreshing, summertime salad. Don't remove the watermelon seeds, because they are packed full of nutrients and are barely noticeable anyway.

9oz (255g) cottage cheese
¼ watermelon, sliced into thin triangles
⅓ cucumber, thinly sliced
6 radishes, trimmed and thinly sliced lengthways
2 tsp lemon juice
4 fresh mint leaves, finely chopped
black pepper

1 Lay the cucumber, watermelon and radish slices out on a large platter and spoon the cottage cheese over the top.
2 Drizzle with the lemon juice and season with black pepper and mint.

Soups

Beany Vegetable Soup

This one-pot winter warmer is crammed full of fibre and is just the thing to take in a thermos flask to work.

Serves 6
1lb (454g) mixed root vegetables (such as carrot, swede and parsnip), peeled and chopped into bite-sized chunks
3 sticks celery, finely chopped
3 leeks, sliced
2 onions, chopped
2 x 14oz (397g) cans mixed pulses (or your choice of beans, such as kidney, chickpea, borlotti, butter or flageolet)
1½pt (850ml) vegetable stock
fresh flat-leaf parsley, roughly chopped
Solo sea salt
black pepper

1 Put the onion, celery, leeks, root vegetables, stock and seasoning in a large saucepan and stir.
2 Cover and bring to the boil, then reduce the heat and let the soup simmer for 20 minutes.
3 Stir in the mixed pulses, then cover and simmer for 5–10 minutes until the vegetables and beans are both tender.
4 Add the parsley, then check the seasoning before serving.

*Spicy Pumpkin and Tofu Soup**

A wonderfully warming soup that is a completely balanced meal, with hidden protein power from the tofu.

Serves 4
1 tbsp olive oil
1 large onion, finely chopped
2 cloves garlic, crushed
2 large butternut squash, deseeded, peeled and diced
1 ½ tsp cumin
1 tsp dried coriander
½ tsp ground nutmeg
¼ tsp chilli powder
1 tsp fresh thyme, chopped
3 vegetable stock cubes dissolved in 1¾pt (1l) hot water
1 packet Cauldron Organic Tofu, drained
Solo sea salt and pepper to taste
parsley and chives, freshly chopped

1 Heat the olive oil in a large saucepan. Add the chopped onion and garlic and gently cook over a low heat until the onion has softened.
2 Add the diced squash, cumin, coriander, chilli, nutmeg, thyme and stock. Bring to the boil, turn down the heat and simmer for 15 minutes.
3 Blend the tofu in a food processor and set aside.
4 Once the soup has simmered for 15 minutes, allow to cool slightly, then liquidise and return to the pan.
5 Whisk in the tofu using a balloon whisk, a tablespoonful at a time, and gently reheat. Season to taste, then add the fresh herbs and serve.

* Courtesy of Cauldron Foods.

Gazpacho

For a taste of Andalusia, serve this raw cold soup at al fresco meals such as barbecues, or keep for a perfect instant snack. It keeps well in the fridge for up to a week. Add black-eyed beans to make it a main meal – and an ice cube or two on really sultry days.

Serves 6
3 peppers (red, yellow and orange are the sweetest)
1 cucumber
1 red onion
3 sticks celery
1 x 14oz (397g) can chopped tomatoes
¾ pint (about 430ml) tomato juice
2 cloves garlic, crushed
½ jar Peppadew sweet baby peppers, drained and chopped
    (from supermarkets and delis)
black pepper
Solo sea salt

1 Chop the fresh vegetables and put half in the food processor with the tomatoes, tomato juice and garlic and process till smooth.
2 Add the remaining vegetables and the Peppadew peppers, and season.

Chestnut and Butterbean Soup

Chestnuts have the lowest fat content of all nuts and a pleasantly sweet flavour which goes well with the smooth texture of the butterbeans.

> **Serves 4**
> 7oz (198g) cooked and peeled chestnuts (get the vacuum-packed or tinned ones to save time)
> 1 x 14oz (397g) can butterbeans, drained and rinsed
> 1 onion, chopped
> 1 carrot, peeled and chopped
> couple of sprigs of thyme
> 2pt (1.1l) vegetable bouillon or stock
> black pepper

1 Place all the ingredients in a large saucepan, put a lid on it and simmer very gently for 35 minutes.
2 Purée the soup until smooth and add black pepper.

Lentil and Lemon Soup

The spices and lemony sharpness make this lentil soup anything but boring. A satisfying winter warmer.

> **Serves 4**
> 1 tbsp olive oil
> 9oz (255g) onions, chopped
> 4 cloves garlic, coarsely chopped
> 9oz (255g) red lentils, rinsed
> 2pt (1.1l) chicken or vegetable stock
> 1 tsp ground cumin
> 1 tsp ground coriander
> juice of ½ lemon
> Solo sea salt and black pepper

1 Heat the oil in a saucepan and add the onion and garlic, cooking them gently for 10 minutes until soft. Stir frequently to prevent sticking.

2 Add the lentils and cook for a further 2 minutes. Add the stock and bring to the boil before reducing the heat to a simmer for 30–45 minutes, until the lentils are almost soft.

3 In a non-stick frying pan, dry-fry the herbs over a high heat for 1–2 minutes until they release their aroma, then add to the soup. Bring soup back to the boil and add the lemon juice, then let it simmer for 5 minutes before seasoning lightly.

Thai-Style Vegetable Broth

This soup is packed with flavour and phytonutrients, and, even better, tastes brilliant. Experiment with different vegetables such as beansprouts.

Serves 4

4 thin slices ginger, cut into thin matchsticks

2 cloves garlic, cut into thin matchsticks

1pt (570ml) vegetable bouillon (Marigold Reduced Salt bouillon powder provides the best flavour for the soup base)

1 head pak choi, finely shredded

2 shiitake mushrooms, sliced

1 carrot, cut in half lengthways, then thinly sliced at a horizontal angle into half-moons

5 spring onions, sliced thinly at an angle

2oz (57g) firm tofu, cut into ½in (1cm) cubes

1 tbsp tamari or soy sauce

1 Place the ginger and garlic in a saucepan with the stock. Bring to the boil, cover and simmer for 3 minutes.

2 Bring the pan back to the boil and add the prepared vegetables and tofu. Season with the tamari, then reduce the heat and simmer for 2/3 minutes.

Dips

Mexican Bean Dip

This spicy red-bean dip is a tasty accompaniment to raw
vegetables, but goes best of all with Nick's Beef Burgers (see
page 368) with lettuce in a pitta bread.

> ¼ onion, finely chopped
> 2 cloves garlic, crushed
> ¼ tsp chilli powder
> 1 tsp lemon juice
> 5oz (142g) kidney beans, cooked and drained
> 3oz (85g) cottage cheese
> ½ tbsp olive oil
> 1 tbsp yoghurt
> Solo sea salt
> black pepper

1 Sauté the onion and garlic gently in the oil for around 2 minutes, then add the chilli powder and cook for a further 3 minutes. Cool.
2 Blend all the ingredients for a fairly smooth creamy dip.

Hummus

Chickpeas, also known as garbanzos, have a unique taste,
which combines well with tahini, a paste of ground sesame
seeds. You may prefer to buy ready-made hummus, which is
widely available in supermarkets.

> 1 x 14oz (397g) can chickpeas, drained
> 2 cloves garlic, crushed
> 2 tbsp olive oil

juice of ½ lemon
Solo
2 tsp tahini
cayenne pepper

1 Place all the ingredients, including a pinch of cayenne, in a food processor and blend until smooth and creamy, adding a bit of water if necessary. Check the flavour and adjust according to preference.
2 Garnish with a little cayenne pepper.

Flageolet Bean Dip

This is an unusual, decorative and tasty alternative to hummus that is delicious on oatcakes or with crudités.

Serves 4 (keeps well in the fridge)
1 x 14oz (397g) can of flageolet beans, rinsed and drained
5 spring onions
1 clove garlic, crushed
handful of flat-leaf parsley, finely chopped
1–2 tbsp lemon juice (according to taste)
1 tbsp olive oil
around 1 tbsp water (if the dip is too thick)
Solo sea salt
black pepper

Place the beans, onions, garlic, parsley, lemon juice and oil into a blender, and blend until smooth. Add the water if necessary, then add the seasoning slowly, according to taste.

Baba Ganoush

I love this Lebanese aubergine dip on oatcakes or pumpernickel bread. Again, it's a great addition to a party, or can form part of a meze platter for an informal dinner, with Hummus and Quinoa Tabbouleh. Just add green and tomato salads.

2 cloves garlic, crushed
1 tbsp olive oil
½ aubergine, cubed
juice of ½ lemon
1oz (28g) sesame seeds
1oz (28g) fresh coriander
4oz (113g) live natural yoghurt (a healthier alternative to the traditional Greek yoghurt)
Solo sea salt and freshly ground black pepper

1 Lightly sauté the garlic in the oil for a couple of minutes, then add the aubergine. Add a tablespoon or so of water to the pan, put on the lid and steam-fry the mixture for 8 minutes or so, until soft.
2 Put into a food processor and add the rest of the ingredients, then blitz till relatively smooth.

Light meals

Pumpkin Seed Pesto

This keeps in the fridge for 2–3 days and can be stirred through soup or pasta, or added to bean salads. It makes a pleasant change from the basil-and-pine-nut variety.

Serves 4
2oz (57g) raw pumpkin seeds
2oz (57g) flat-leaf parsley leaves

2oz (57g) basil leaves
2 garlic cloves, crushed
1 dessertspoon lemon juice
3fl oz (90ml) pumpkin seed oil (roasted if you can find it) *or*
   the same quantity of pumpkin seed butter instead of the
   separate seeds and oil (available from Health Products for
   Life – see page 479 in Resources)
2oz (57g) grated Parmesan

1 Place the pumpkin seeds in a small blender or food processor with the herbs, garlic, salt, lemon juice and Parmesan. Blitz until the mixture is blended but retains some texture.
3 Add the pumpkin seed oil or butter and mix until the pesto is an even consistency.

Sweet Potato Mash

A delicious and lower-Ⓖ version of mashed potatoes. Serve with meat, fish or tofu and vegetables.

1 sweet potato (unpeeled)
black pepper

1 Slice the sweet potato into thin circles, then steam for around 12 minutes until soft.
2 Season with pepper and mash with a fork.

Smoked Salmon Pâté

This could be a wonderful dinner-party starter. The cannellini beans provide great long-term energy and are a healthier alternative to the cream in most fish pâtés.

> 7oz (198g) smoked salmon
> 7oz (198g) canned cannellini beans, drained
> juice of ½ lemon
> a drizzle of water or olive oil (to loosen if the mixture is too thick)
> 1 tbsp chopped fresh parsley
> 1 tbsp chopped fresh dill
> black pepper

Blend all the ingredients in a food processor until the mixture is really smooth, adding a little oil or water to loosen the mixture if preferred, then chill and serve.

Smoked Trout Pâté

Another lower-fat pâté, this time using cream cheese instead of cream.

> 2 smoked trout fillets, skinned, boned and flaked
> 7oz (198g) low-fat cream cheese
> juice of ½ lemon
> black pepper
> 1 tsp horseradish sauce (optional)

Blend all the ingredients in a food processor or mash well with a fork. Serve with hot pitta bread triangles (5 🌀 per half-slice) and salad, or with rye bread (5 🌀 per slice).

Curry Roasted Celeriac

An unusual accompaniment to meat or fish.

½ a celeriac, peeled and chopped into 1in chunks
¼ tbsp mild or medium-strength curry powder
2 cloves garlic, unpeeled
2 tbsp olive oil
black pepper

1 Mix together the oil and curry powder. Toss the celeriac and garlic in the mixture and season with black pepper.
2 Roast in a roasting tray at 180°C/350°F/gas mark 4 for 40–50 minutes, shaking the tray halfway through to recoat the pieces.

Sardines on Toast

This may take you back to your childhood. Sardines are endowed with lashings of omega-3 fats, and make a fast, delicious meal served this way. Just add a big green salad.

3 slices rye bread
2 tbsp olive oil
2 tomatoes, sliced
6oz (170g) sardines in brine, drained
black pepper

1 Toast bread and drizzle with olive oil.
2 Place tomato slices and sardines on toast and season with black pepper.

Hot-Smoked Fish with Avocado

The avocado provides healthy mono-unsaturated fat, while the fish gives plenty of omega-3 oils – just don't eat this more than once a week, to keep within your fat limit.

> 2 fillets hot-smoked salmon or trout
> 2in (5cm) stick of cucumber, cut into bite-sized pieces
> ½ ripe medium-sized avocado
> juice of ½ lemon
> 1–2 tsp chopped dill or chives
> 1–2 tsp chopped flat-leaf parsley
> black pepper

1 Skin the fish and remove any bones, then flake into chunks. Place in a salad bowl with the cucumber.
2 Halve the avocado and cut one side into bite-sized pieces. (Leave the stone in the leftover half and drizzle this with lemon juice to prevent discoloration, then cover and place in the fridge for future use.) Add the avocado to the bowl along with the lemon and herbs.
3 Season with black pepper and gently mix together.

Fish in an Oriental-Style Broth

This dish is full of fresh, clean flavours and would be perfect for a special dinner.

¼pt (150ml) vegetable bouillon (Marigold Reduced Salt
    bouillon powder provides the best flavour for soup bases)
2 tbsp mirin (Japanese rice wine, available from supermarkets)
2 tbsp tamari
1 small chunk ginger, sliced
2 cloves garlic, crushed
2 slices lemon
2 fish fillets (haddock, plaice or cod)
2oz (57g) broccoli, broken into very small florets
4 spring onions, thinly sliced
2oz (57g) pak choi, finely shredded
2oz (57g) carrots, julienned (cut into matchstick size pieces)
½ tsp sesame oil

1 Place the stock, mirin, tamari, ginger, garlic and lemon in a wok and bring to the boil.
2 Measure the thickness of the fish fillets at their thickest points, then reduce the heat in the wok and slide the fish in. Poach for 10 minutes for every inch (2.5cm) of thickness, or until the flesh turns opaque and flakes easily.
3 Lift the fish out of the broth and remove the skin, then divide the flesh between 2 soup bowls, cover and keep warm.
4 Bring the broth back to the boil and add the vegetables in the following order, at 30-second intervals, cooking for a total of 2–3 minutes or until they are tender but still *al dente*: broccoli, carrots, pak choi, then spring onions. Remove the vegetables and add to the bowls.
5 Boil the broth for a further 30 seconds, then remove the ginger and lemon slices and stir in the oil. Ladle over the fish and vegetables and serve immediately.

Garlicky Butternut Squash and Aubergine

A wonderfully satisfying dish that goes well with anything from chicken to a simple Rocket and Watercress Salad with a good drizzle of Pumpkin Seed Pesto for protein.

½ a butternut squash, peeled and diced into 1in (2cm) pieces
½ a medium aubergine, diced into pieces the same size as the squash
6 cloves garlic, unpeeled
1 tsp cumin
1 tbsp olive oil
Solo sea salt
black pepper

1 Put the squash, aubergine and garlic into a bowl with the oil, cumin and seasoning, mixing until all the vegetables are covered.
2 Place the mix in a roasting tin and put into a preheated oven (180°C/350°F/gas mark 4) for 40–45 minutes, or until the vegetables soften and start to brown.
4 Do eat the roasted garlic if you like the taste, squeezing out the softened flesh with a fork, otherwise simply discard and enjoy the flavour that will have permeated the rest of the vegetables.

Smoked Salmon and Asparagus Omelette

A sophisticated light supper – or even breakfast in bed!

> 6 spears asparagus
> 4 eggs
> Solo sea salt
> black pepper
> 2 tsp olive oil
> 2oz (57g) smoked salmon slices
> 2 slices lemon
> 2 sprigs flat-leaf parsley

1 Steam the asparagus until just cooked, then refresh by plunging them into cold water, then drain and set aside.
2 Beat the eggs with the seasoning.
3 Heat a medium-sized frying pan and add the oil, allowing it to heat up and coat the whole pan. Pour the egg into the pan and gently move around using a wooden spoon, allowing all of the egg to be exposed to the heat until the underside cooks through and colours slightly. Reduce the heat, loosen the base with a spatula and flip over to cook the other side for a minute or so until just firm, then cut in half and tip each half onto a separate plate.
3 Lay the salmon on one half of each slice and place 3 asparagus spears on top, then fold the other half over to create a triangle. Top with a slice of lemon and sprig of flat-leaf parsley and serve immediately.

Main meals

From poached salmon to fajitas, there are enough delicious options here to keep you going through a year's worth of lunches, dinners and dinner parties. Vegetarian options are included for many, and meat eaters' options are also included for some of the vegetarian dishes. Generally speaking, the recipes are designed for easy adaptation, as far as protein is concerned. If the menu suggests a meal you prefer not to have, simply choose an alternative.

Recipes given are for two people unless otherwise stated. Some of these dishes can be prepared in advance and frozen.

ⒼⓁ scores:

Recipe	Page number	ⒼⓁ
Steam-fried Vegetables with …	340	6–8
Fatburner Sandwiches	341	11–12
Fatburner Baked Potato or Sweet Potato	342	10–12
Tuna Steak with Black-Eyed Bean Salsa	343	10
Sticky Mustard Salmon Fillets	344	1
Trout with Puy Lentils and Roasted Tomatoes on the Vine	344	11
Grilled Herring	345	0
Spicy Mackerel with Couscous	346	14
Thai Baked Cod	347	1
Cod Roasted with Lemon and Garlic	348	0
Poached Salmon	348	0
Borlotti Bean Bolognese	349	8
Pasta with Pumpkin Seed Pesto	350	8
Roasted Vegetables with Mediterranean Quinoa	350	15
Dhal (Lentil Curry)	352	6

Fast and easy

Steam-Fried Vegetables with ...

This is a healthier, lower-fat version of stir-frying. Versatility is the name of the game here. You can make this steam-fry with sauces ranging from Chinese to Mexican; throw in cauliflower and sugar snaps one night, carrots and mushrooms the next; use tempeh on Monday and chicken on Sunday – in short, anything goes. This is the perfect fallback recipe, using whatever's in the fridge and store cupboard for a truly tasty, convenient meal.

Vegetables
Spring onions and garlic, then choose from carrots, broccoli, courgettes, cauliflower, sugar snap peas, runner beans, water chestnuts, mushrooms, bean sprouts, peppers, bamboo shoots and so on, ensuring there's enough to fill half your plate.

Seasonings
Thai: fresh coriander, green curry paste and a dash of coconut milk
Chinese: tamari or soy sauce, ginger and garlic
Japanese: ginger, tamari or soy sauce, teriyaki or yakitori sauce (try Kikkoman's, available in supermarkets)
Mexican: fajita or enchilada dry seasoning, or tomato salsa
Mediterranean: ½ jar tomato passata with chopped basil and flat-leaf parsley, and a few chopped black olives if liked
Indian: tomatoes with coriander, cumin and chilli powder to taste

Protein-rich foods
11oz (312g) tofu, or tempeh, cubed
or 4oz (113g) chicken, off the bone and cubed
or 5oz (142g) filleted fish, cubed

1 Steam-fry onion and garlic in the chosen seasoning. Add protein-rich food and stir-fry until cooked.
2 Add your choice of vegetables, stir-fry briefly, then add a tablespoon of water and put on the lid. Steam until vegetables are cooked but still crunchy.

Fatburner Sandwiches

When it's lunchtime and you're starving, sometimes only a sandwich will do. To make this low-ⓖ version, top two slices of rye bread or fill a wholemeal pitta pocket with any one of the following combinations.

4oz (113g) cottage cheese, with cucumber slices and chopped chives

or 5oz (142g) hummus and lettuce

or 1 small roast chicken breast (skin removed) and 1 sliced tomato

or 1 small smoked trout or salmon fillet with a smear of low-fat cream cheese or Pumpkin Seed Pesto (see page 330) and watercress

or 2oz (57g) canned salmon or tuna in brine, with cucumber and cress

or egg 'mayonnaise' (made with 2 hard-boiled eggs, a tablespoon of cottage cheese, a chopped spring onion and Solo sea salt and black pepper)

Fatburner Baked Potato or Sweet Potato

Many diets give the humble spud short shrift, but a baked potato can be a great base for a satisfying lunch. It's also available at many city sandwich shops in case you've forgotten to bring anything to work with you. All you need to remember is to choose a small potato so you don't overdo the carbs. Do eat the skins since they're full of fibre. When making your own, cook them for as short a time as possible (around 50–60 minutes, at 220–230°C/425–450°F/gas mark 7–8), till done but still firm inside. Have them with any of the fillings below and a large salad or Coleslaw (see page 316). A sweet potato makes a delicious change.

2oz (57g) tuna in brine blended with a teaspoon of cottage cheese or natural yoghurt

4oz (113g) low-fat cottage cheese with chives and spring onions

5oz (142g) hummus with a sliced tomato

7oz (198g) baked beans

1 mug Dhal (see page 352)

1 small roast chicken breast (no skin) tossed in 1 tbsp yoghurt dressing (blended with paprika, black pepper and fresh chives, basil or parsley)

1 dessertspoon Pumpkin Seed Pesto (see page 330) with 2oz (57g) cottage cheese and chopped chives

Fish

Tuna Steak with Black-Eyed Bean Salsa

A robust summer dish. Vegetarians could substitute a thick slice of smoked tofu for the fish.

For the salsa
2 tomatoes, deseeded and chopped into bean-sized pieces
1 x 14 oz (397g) can black-eyed beans, rinsed and drained
1 red pepper, chopped finely
1 mild, fresh red chilli, deseeded and finely chopped
2 cloves garlic, crushed
juice of 2 limes
2 tsp olive oil
2 tsp sesame oil
2 tbsp fresh coriander or flat-leaf parsley, roughly chopped
black pepper

2 tuna fillets
1 tbsp olive oil for frying

1 Mix together the salsa ingredients. Set to one side while you cook the tuna steaks.
2 Heat a frying pan and spray or lightly drizzle with olive oil. When hot, add the fish and press firmly into the pan to sear on both sides, before reducing the heat and cooking for a further 1–3 minutes (until the flesh flakes easily).
3 Serve with the salsa on the side.

Sticky Mustard Salmon Fillets

Salmon not only provides plenty of protein but also is a source of essential fats. Try to go for wild salmon, as it's a healthier option than farmed fish. Again, vegetarians could marinate tofu slices instead of salmon.

> juice and zest of ½ orange
> 1 tsp runny honey
> 1 tsp wholegrain mustard
> 2 skinless, boneless salmon fillets

1 Preheat the oven to 180°C/350°F/gas mark 4.
2 Whisk the orange juice and zest into the mustard and honey and marinate the salmon in the mixture for 30 minutes or longer, in the fridge.
3 Bake for 20–25 minutes at 180°C/350°F/gas mark 4 (or according to pack instructions) and serve with steam-fried spinach and red or yellow peppers, and boiled baby new potatoes (5 ⒼⓁ per small) or brown basmati rice (5 ⒼⓁ per half-serving).

Trout with Puy Lentils and Roasted Tomatoes on the Vine

A simple but sophisticated dish that is perfectly balanced. Smart enough to serve at a supper party.

> 3oz (85g) dried Puy lentils, washed
> 1 tsp Marigold bouillon powder
> 1 tsp mixed dried herbs (such as *herbes de provence*)
> 2 trout fillets, fully prepared
> cherry tomatoes on the vine (half a bunch, or 5–6 tomatoes per person)

2 slices lemon
handful of fresh flat-leaf parsley
black pepper

1 Cover the lentils with cold water and bring to the boil, then simmer for 20 minutes or so until the water is more or less absorbed, adding the bouillon powder and mixed herbs when the lentils are soft to the bite. (Do not worry if the lentils seem hard – Puy lentils retain their shape and have a satisfyingly chewy texture even when cooked.)

2 Place the fish in a non-stick roasting tin and lay the tomatoes around them, then bake at 190°C/375°F/gas mark 5 for 12–15 minutes or according to the instructions for the fish.

3 Lay the fish on a dollop of lentils, with a slice of lemon and chopped parsley on each fillet and the tomatoes on the side. Sprinkle with black pepper.

Grilled Herring

Norwegians are onto something: herrings are one of the best fish for omega-3 essential fats as well as protein and vitamins. The flavour is strong, so it needs little enhancement.

1 prepared herring (5oz/142g)
half a lemon
black pepper

Squeeze lemon juice and grind black pepper over herring and place it under a medium grill for 20 minutes, turning halfway through cooking.

Spicy Mackerel with Couscous

The hint of North Africa in this spicy sauce is a wonderful complement to the rich taste of mackerel. It's partnered with couscous, an excellent source of carbohydrate which is very easy to prepare.

> 2 very small smoked mackerel fillets (skinned if preferred), or ½ a medium fillet each
> ¾pt (400ml) boiling water
> 4oz (113g) couscous
> 1 tsp Marigold vegetable bouillon
> 1 tbsp olive oil
> 1 small onion, finely chopped
> 1 clove garlic, crushed
> ¼ tsp chilli powder
> 1 tsp ground cumin
> 1 red pepper, chopped
> 1 courgette, sliced
> 1 tbsp tomato purée
> 1 tsp lemon juice

1 Pour the boiling water over the couscous, stir in the bouillon, cover and leave to stand for 15 minutes, to allow it to absorb the water. Then fluff up and separate the grains with a fork.
2 Meanwhile, put the oil in a sauté pan and steam-fry the onion, garlic, chilli powder and ground cumin for two minutes.
3 Add the red pepper and courgette and sauté for a further two minutes.
4 Add the tomato purée and lemon juice and steam-fry with the lid on until the vegetables are tender but still crisp.
5 Arrange each fillet on a mound of couscous and top with sauce.

Thai Baked Cod

This dish is permeated with classic Thai flavours, which are clean and sharp, yet subtle. You can use any white fish instead of cod if you prefer. It's even better if the fish is left to marinate in the sauce for a few hours before cooking. It goes very well with the Crunchy Thai Salad (see page 315) and soba (buckwheat) noodles (7 🌀 per small serving).

> juice and grated zest of 1 lime
> ½in (1cm) piece ginger root, grated
> 1 stick lemon grass, sliced finely
> 2 cloves garlic, crushed
> 1 tsp tamari or soy sauce
> 1 mild, fresh, red chilli, deseeded and finely chopped
> 3oz (85g) cod fillets

1 Mix together the lime juice, lime zest, ginger, lemon grass, crushed garlic, tamari and chilli. *Beware*: when you chop chilli, wash your hands immediately after, since the oil is an irritant.
2 Place the cod fillets in a baking dish.
3 Pour the lime mixture over the fish, turning it so it is well coated. Leave to marinate in the fridge if time.
4 Cover with lid or foil and bake in a preheated oven (180°C/350°F/gas mark 4) for around 20 minutes (or until cooked – this will depend on the thickness of the fish).

Cod Roasted with Lemon and Garlic

A delicious, no-fuss fish dish that is perfect for a light summer supper.

> ½ tbsp olive oil
> ½ tbsp chopped fresh parsley
> 2 garlic cloves, crushed
> Solo sea salt
> black pepper
> 2 cod fillets (or haddock or plaice)
> 1 lemon, sliced thinly

1 Mix together the oil, parsley, garlic and seasoning and rub over fish, setting aside to marinate for 10 minutes.
2 Place the fish on a baking try and arrange the lemon slices on top. Cook in a preheated oven at 180°C/350°F/gas mark 4 for 15–20 minutes or until just cooked (and the flesh flakes easily).
3 Serve with Tomato and Red Onion Salad (see page 316).

Poached Salmon

Salmon responds well to extremely simple treatments, as in this recipe. Fast food with a difference!

> 2oz (57g) salmon fillets
> 2 lemon wedges
> black pepper

1 Place salmon fillets in a shallow pan with just enough water to cover, and poach them gently for around 15 minutes, depending on the thickness of the fillets.
2 Season and serve garnished with lemon wedges.

Vegetarian

Borlotti Bean Bolognese

This is a mouthwatering vegetarian alternative to the classic 'spag bol'. It can be prepared in batches and frozen for convenience.

¾ x 14oz (397g) can of borlotti beans, drained and rinsed
1 onion, chopped
2 cloves garlic, crushed
4oz (113g) button mushrooms, sliced
1 tbsp olive oil
1 tsp mixed dried herbs
1 tsp vegetable bouillon powder
1 tbsp tomato purée
5oz (142g) canned tomatoes
Solo sea salt
black pepper

1 Sauté the onion and garlic in oil and herbs for 2 minutes, then add the mushrooms and cook till soft.
2 Add the vegetable bouillon powder, tomato purée, canned tomatoes and beans, then season and simmer for a few minutes.
3 Serve with wholegrain spaghetti or other wholegrain pasta.

Pasta with Pumpkin Seed Pesto

Sometimes at the end of a long day it is all you can do to boil the kettle for some pasta. Luckily, this dish is pretty instant, if you keep some Pumpkin Seed Pesto in the fridge. Serve with a Tomato and Red Onion Salad.

2 servings Pumpkin Seed Pesto (see page 330)
handful of fresh basil leaves
2 tsp pumpkin seeds (dry-roasted in a pan if time)
freshly ground black pepper
6oz (170g or ⅓ regular packet) wholewheat or buckwheat pasta

1 Cook the pasta according to pack instructions, then drain well and return to the pan.
2 Stir through the pesto and put on plates.
3 Top with basil, pumpkin seeds and black pepper.

Roasted Vegetables with Mediterranean Quinoa

Quinoa is amazingly versatile and very special, because it is packed full of protein. It's a great foil for these Mediterranean flavours.

For the roasted vegetables
1 handful of cherry tomatoes
1 medium courgette, cubed
1 red onion, sliced into wedges
1 red pepper, sliced
1 handful of button mushrooms
2 dessertspoons olive oil
Solo sea salt

For the quinoa
8oz (227g) quinoa
1pt (570ml) water
1 tsp vegetable bouillon or powder
4 stoned black olives (Kalamata ones are delicious), roughly
     chopped
1 tbsp fresh basil leaves, finely chopped
black pepper

1 Place all vegetables (except the cherry tomatoes) on a baking
   tray, lightly drizzle with the olive oil and lightly sprinkle with
   Solo sea salt.
2 Bake in a preheated oven (180°C/350°F/gas mark 4) for
   40–50 minutes. Remove twice during cooking and shake
   tray to turn and recoat the vegetables. Add the tomatoes the
   second time you shake the vegetables as they cook much
   more quickly.
3 Meanwhile, rinse the quinoa very well under cold, running
   water.
4 Put it in a saucepan with the bouillon powder and the water,
   bring to the boil, cover and simmer for 13 minutes or until
   water has boiled away and the grains are light and fluffy.
5 Allow the quinoa to cool, and mix through the basil and
   olives with a fork.
6 Serve a mound of the quinoa topped with vegetables. Add
   freshly ground black pepper.

Dhal (Lentil Curry)

This dish is a variation on a recipe given to me by a lady from Goa, and is one of my favourites. It always goes down well with meat-eaters as well as vegetarians. This is incredibly moreish, and leftovers can be kept in the fridge and eaten with a baked potato for lunch the following day, or frozen.

Serves 4

11oz (312g) orange lentils
1pt (570ml) water
1 medium onion, chopped
4 cloves garlic, crushed
1 x 14oz (397g) can tomatoes
1 heaped tsp curry powder
4 tsp Marigold Reduced Salt vegetable bouillon powder

1 Rinse the lentils well in cold, running water until the water runs clear.
2 Place in a saucepan with the water, onion, garlic and bouillon powder.
3 Bring to the boil and simmer for 10 minutes.
4 Add tomatoes and curry powder and stir well. Cover and leave to simmer for a further 20 minutes, stirring occasionally to make sure the mixture does not stick to the bottom. If it starts to get too thick, add a little water, or, if it seems too watery, leave uncovered. The lentils should form a porridge-like paste.

Chickpea Curry

Nutty-tasting and firm in texture, chickpeas appear in the cuisines of Spain, Mexico, southern Europe, the Middle East and India. You can buy them dry, soak overnight and cook them yourself (follow the pack instructions), although this can take a while depending on the age of the chickpeas. I've used tinned chickpeas for ease in this recipe, however.

1 x 14oz (397g) can chickpeas, drained and rinsed
1 large white onion, chopped
1 stick celery, chopped finely
1 medium carrot, chopped
2 tsp olive oil
2 tbsp tomato purée
1pt (570ml) vegetable stock
2 cloves garlic, crushed
1 tsp cumin
½ tsp turmeric
½ flat tsp mild or medium curry powder (according to taste)
1 tsp ground ginger
½ tsp Solo sea salt

1 Gently heat the oil in a large frying pan and fry the garlic for a minute.
2 Add the onion and dry spices and cook for a further 2 minutes.
3 Toss in the vegetables and steam-fry in 2 tablespoons of the stock for a couple of minutes.
4 Add the chickpeas, the tomato purée and the rest of the stock and let the curry simmer uncovered until the vegetables are tender and the sauce has thickened slightly (around 30 minutes).

Grilled Goat's Cheese on Portabella Mushrooms

A full-flavoured supper that will please anyone from vegetarians to hardened meat-eaters. Serve with a mixed salad, perhaps with a light dressing of walnut oil and balsamic vinegar or lemon juice.

> 6 portabella mushrooms, cleaned with a dry brush or kitchen towel
> 4 round slices goat's cheese (each about ¼in/½cm thick)
> 1 tbsp sun-dried tomato paste
> 6 large basil leaves, torn
> 1 tbsp walnuts, roughly chopped
> 1 dessertspoon olive oil
> black pepper

1 Spread sun-dried tomato paste on the undersides of the mushrooms, then gently fry them in olive oil until the mushrooms start to go brown, taking care when you turn them over not to dislodge too much of the sun-dried tomato paste.
2 Place mushrooms bottom side up on a grill pan and top each with a slice of goat's cheese. Grill gently till the cheese starts to bubble and turn golden on top.
3 Remove from the heat and place on a bed of mixed salad (pre-dressed if using dressing), then scatter the walnuts and basil on top and serve immediately.

Sesame Steamed Vegetables with Quinoa

Steaming vegetables brings out their individual delicate flavours, but the dressing in this recipe adds real pizzazz, turning them into a light, delicious feast.

For the quinoa
8oz (227g) quinoa
1pt (570ml) water
1 tsp vegetable bouillon or ½ stock cube

For the dressing
2 tsp sesame oil
2 tsp tamari
1 tbsp sesame seeds, toasted in a dry pan until golden
squeeze of lemon juice

For the vegetables
4 broccoli florets, chopped
handful of baby corn
2 handfuls of mangetout
2 spring onions, chopped

1 Rinse the quinoa very well under cold, running water. Put it in a saucepan with the water and stock, bring to the boil, cover and simmer for 13 minutes or until water is absorbed. Then fluff up the grains using a fork.

2 Mix the dressing ingredients in a cup.

3 Place the broccoli in a vegetable steamer and steam for around 4½ minutes before throwing in the mangetout and baby corn for a further 2 minutes or so, until the vegetables are just lightly cooked.

4 Serve the vegetables on a mound of quinoa and pour the dressing over the top, then sprinkle with chopped spring onions.

Chestnut and Mushroom Pilaf

The flavours in this dish go together beautifully. To add a bit of colour, serve with steamed savoy cabbage or leeks.

6oz (170g) peeled, cooked chestnuts (vacuum-packed or tinned)
1 tbsp olive oil
2oz (57g) brown basmati rice
1 small onion, chopped
2 cloves garlic, crushed
¼pt (150ml) Marigold vegetable bouillon made up into stock
4oz (113g) shiitake or button mushrooms, sliced
1in (2.5cm) root ginger, peeled and finely chopped
2 tsp tamari or soy sauce
2oz (57g) frozen peas

1 Gently heat the oil in a heavy frying pan and fry the rice in it until it's pale brown (this will take around 3–4 minutes). Add garlic and ginger, stirring for 30 seconds, then add the onion, cooking for a further 3 minutes. Lastly, add mushrooms and cook for 3 minutes.

2 Stir in the bouillon and chestnuts, then cover and simmer until liquid is absorbed and rice just tender (takes around 35 minutes).

3 Stir in the frozen peas at the end and allow to cook gently and turn bright green.

Stuffed Peppers

You don't have to stop at peppers: aubergines and larger courgettes are excellent stuffed, too. Adding pine nuts makes a more
interesting stuffing than the usual cheese and rice. Serve with
salad.

2 large red peppers
1 tbsp olive oil
1 medium onion, finely chopped
2 cloves garlic, crushed
1 tbsp pine nuts
1 tsp Marigold vegetable bouillon powder
2–3 tbsp water
4oz (113g) brown basmati rice, cooked
6oz (170g) mushrooms, sliced
handful of fresh basil leaves, chopped
black pepper
1 tsp olive oil to grease tray

1 Cut top off peppers, remove seeds and pith and slice off the
 bulbous bit inside the pepper that sits below the stalk and
 contains most of the seeds. Reserve lid.
2 Put oil in a sauté pan and fry onion and garlic in it for 2 minutes. Add the chopped mushrooms and bouillon and fry for
 a further 2–3 minutes.
3 In a large bowl, combine cooked mixture with the rice, pine
 nuts and basil and season with black pepper.
4 Stuff peppers with the mixture and place tops back on.
5 Place on a lightly oiled baking tray and bake in a preheated
 oven (200°C/400°F/gas mark 6) for 35 minutes.

Grilled Burgers *

Here is a homemade vegetarian alternative to the hamburger. Alternatively, many supermarkets now stock good ready-made vegetarian burgers and sausages, but you need to choose the ones without hydrogenated fat or additives.

> 8oz (227g) tofu, mashed
> 4 tbsp tamari or soy sauce
> 1 medium carrot, grated
> 1 garlic clove, crushed
> 1 small spring onion, chopped
> 2 slices rye bread, toasted and crumbed
> 1 tbsp tomato purée
> 1 medium free-range egg
> black pepper
> 1 tbsp fresh coriander, chopped
> 1 tbsp olive oil

1 Mix the tofu and soy sauce in a bowl, leave for 20 minutes, then squeeze out and discard any excess moisture.
2 In a bowl, mix the prepared tofu with all the rest of the ingredients except the oil and form into 4 burgers. Chill for 20 minutes.
3 Lightly brush the burgers with oil and grill under a medium grill for 15 minutes, turning frequently.
4 Serve between slices of rye bread with sliced tomato and lettuce.

* Courtesy of Cauldron Foods

Sweet Potato and Red Onion Tortilla

An interesting variation on traditional potatoes, with a lower ⓖⓛ score. Cut this tasty Spanish-style tortilla into wedges and serve with a side salad or steamed broccoli.

> 1 large sweet potato, peeled and sliced horizontally into thin circles
> 1 tbsp olive oil
> 2 large red onions, chopped
> 2 cloves garlic, crushed
> 4 medium eggs
> Solo sea salt
> black pepper

1 Steam the sweet potato for 10 minutes or so or until tender, then slice thinly.
2 Heat half the oil in a pan and cook the onion and garlic over a very low heat for 12–15 minutes, covered, and stir occasionally until soft. Then remove from the heat to cool.
4 Beat the eggs and stir in the sweet potato and half the cooked onion. Season with Solo sea salt and black pepper.
5 Heat the remaining oil in a shallow, non-stick frying pan until hot, then add the reserved onion. Pour in the egg mixture and cook over a very low heat for 6 minutes or until the bottom is golden and the mixture looks set.
6 If the top is set at this point, simply take a spatula and loosen the edges of the tortilla so that you can slide it onto a plate and serve. However, if the top is still runny when the base has set, slide the tortilla onto a plate, and then tip it back into the pan topside down, to cook the top quickly before serving.

Japanese Noodles

Soba (buckwheat) noodles complement this Japanese sauce and steam-fry perfectly.

For the sauce
4 tbsp of dashi (Japanese stock made from bonito flakes, available from Oriental supermarkets)
1 tbsp of tamari or soy sauce
1 tsp of mirin (Japanese rice wine, available from supermarkets)
1 tsp grated ginger
4 finely sliced shiitake mushrooms
1 tsp cornflour mixed with 2 tsp water to form smooth paste (optional)

For the tofu mixture
11oz (312g) smoked tofu, cut into bite-sized pieces
Finely sliced vegetables, choosing from carrots, bean sprouts, sugar snap peas, mangetout, broccoli pieces or green pepper
113g soba noodles

1 Combine the sauce ingredients and simmer in a saucepan. If preferred, add the cornflour to thicken the sauce slightly.
2 Lightly grill tofu until it begins to brown, turning to colour both sides.
3 Add the grilled tofu, along with the vegetables, to the sauce and simmer for a few minutes until the vegetables have softened slightly.
4 Cook the soba noodles according to the pack instructions (they take almost no time), and toss the steam-fry through the noodles.

Chilli

This wonderful dish – just the thing for a crisp autumn evening – has fooled many a hardy meat-eater. You can prepare this in double quantities and freeze it. It works well with brown basmati rice, on a small baked potato, or in a toasted tortilla wrap.

> 1 small onion, sliced
> 2 cloves garlic, crushed
> ½ green pepper, sliced
> 1 tbsp olive oil
> ½ tsp chilli powder
> 1 tsp paprika
> 1 tsp ground cumin
> 1 tsp ground coriander
> 2oz (57g) dried soya mince (pre-soaked)
> *or* 6oz (170g) Quorn mince
> 7oz (198g) canned tomatoes, chopped
> 1 tbsp tomato purée
> 4oz (113g) canned kidney beans, drained

1 Steam-fry onion, garlic and pepper in oil with chilli powder, paprika, cumin and coriander.
2 Add pre-soaked soya mince or Quorn mince and stir for 2 minutes.
3 Add tomatoes, tomato purée and kidney beans. Mix well and leave to simmer for at least half an hour, stirring occasionally to prevent it from sticking or burning. If the mixture becomes too thick, add a little water.

Meat

Chicken Tandoori

It's the end of the week and you fancy some spicy food. What better than this fabulous Chicken Tandoori recipe? (For vegetarians, tofu would work just as well.) Even better, the herbs and spices in this dish lend it anti-inflammatory properties. Serve with brown basmati rice and steamed vegetables.

2 chicken breasts, skinned and chopped into bite-sized chunks
3oz (85g) natural yoghurt
handful of flaked almonds
½ tbsp lemon juice
2 garlic cloves, crushed
½ tsp grated fresh ginger root
½ tsp ground cumin
½ tsp ground coriander
¼ tsp ground turmeric
pinch of cayenne pepper
black pepper

1 Place the chicken pieces in a shallow casserole.
2 Mix together the rest of the ingredients and spread over the chicken, then cover the dish and place it in the fridge to marinate for at least an hour.
3 Bake the chicken in the marinade at 200°C/400°F/gas mark 6 for 35–40 minutes until meat is cooked thoroughly. Do not turn.

Chicken Chermoula

Chermoula is a North African spice and herb mix that makes a wonderful marinade for chicken or tofu.

½ tbsp olive oil
1 ½ tbsp lemon juice
2 cloves garlic, crushed
1 tbsp fresh parsley, chopped
½ tbsp fresh coriander, chopped
½ tsp ground coriander
½ tsp cayenne pepper
½ tsp ground cumin
½ tsp paprika
black pepper
2 skinned, boned chicken breasts

1 Mix all ingredients except for the chicken together in a bowl to make the marinade.
2 Cut several slashes in each chicken breast and rub the marinade into the meat. Cover the chicken and place in the fridge for 2 hours.
3 Take out and grill at a medium heat for around 10–15 minutes or until the meat is cooked and the juices run clear, turning the chicken over halfway through.
4 Slice the breasts and spread on top of couscous or the Quinoa Tabbouleh (page 320), or serve with Coleslaw (3 **GL**) (page 316) and Sweet Potato Mash (7 **GL**) (see page 331).

Garlic and Lemon Roast Chicken

Organic, free-range chicken is the best available. Once you've roasted the chicken, remove the skin before eating. Leftover meat can be used to make sandwiches or salads (as above) the next day.

> ½ lemon
> 1 tsp olive oil
> 4 cloves garlic, 2 crushed, 2 whole and unpeeled
> 1 medium chicken
> Solo sea salt
> freshly ground black pepper

1 Mix together the juice of the lemon, oil and crushed garlic and rub all over the chicken, then sprinkle with freshly ground black pepper and Solo sea salt. Place the squeezed lemon and whole garlic cloves inside the cavity.

2 Put the chicken on a rack in a roasting dish (to allow the fat to drain) and bake in a preheated oven at 180°C/350°F/gas mark 4, calculating 20 minutes per 1lb (454g) plus an extra 20 minutes. Baste 2–3 times during cooking.

Chicken with Roasted Courgettes and Red Onion

Roasting vegetables with chicken is a great idea, as the veg absorb the flavour of the chicken. This version uses a Mediterranean-inspired mix of aubergine, courgette, new potatoes and red onion.

2 courgettes, cut into chunks
2 red onions, cut into wedges
6 small baby new potatoes
1½ tbsp olive oil
1–2 tbsp balsamic vinegar, depending upon preference
4 sprigs fresh thyme
2 cloves garlic, unpeeled
pinch of Solo sea salt
2 skinless chicken breasts
black pepper

1 Put the vegetables into a small roasting tin, pour over 1 tbsp of the oil and half of the vinegar and add a pinch of salt and the thyme. Toss together and place the chicken breasts on top, pressing them into the mixture so that they nestle between the vegetables.

2 Drizzle the remaining vinegar and oil over the chicken and season.

3 Roast for 40–45 minutes at 180°C/350°F/gas mark 4, shaking the vegetables around to recoat with oil and vinegar halfway through, and turning the chicken, making sure that it doesn't dry out on top.

Spiced Turkey Meatballs

A leaner alternative to beef meatballs with a spicy kick, these patties go down well with teenagers and are brilliant for barbecues. (If you do barbecue them, avoid charring the meat, because this promotes the development of harmful free radicals.)

Serves 4
2 large cloves garlic, crushed
1 large green chilli, deseeded and finely chopped
large pinch ground cumin
1 tbsp olive oil
14oz (397g) lean minced turkey
Solo sea salt and black pepper

1 Gently fry the garlic, chilli and cumin in the oil for a couple of minutes and leave to cool.
2 Add to the turkey, season with a little Solo sea salt and pepper and mix thoroughly through the mince. Shape the mixture into 4 patties.
3 Grill for 10 minutes or until cooked thoroughly, turning halfway through.
4 Serve with baked beans and grilled mushrooms and tomatoes, or wholegrain spaghetti (if using spaghetti, place lightly grilled courgette pieces on top before topping with the meatballs: slice the courgettes lengthways and drizzle with a little oil and Solo sea salt – and lightly grill, turning halfway through).

Ratatouille Sausage Bake

A no-fuss, warming dish, superb as a mid-week supper. This seems like a lot of vegetables but they cook down quite a lot and any leftovers are delicious on a baked potato. Vegetarians could simply omit the sausages and add half a can of kidney beans with a pinch of chilli powder per person to the ratatouille, and serve with baby new potatoes.

> 4 lean, good-quality sausages (venison are the leanest,
>   otherwise opt for lean pork or beef)
> 4 red, green, yellow and/or orange peppers
> 2 red onions, sliced
> 2 courgettes, sliced
> 1 x 14 oz (397g) can chopped tomatoes
> 2 tbsp tomato purée
> 2 cloves garlic, crushed
> 2 tsp dried mixed Italian herbs
> black pepper

1 Place peppers, onions and courgettes in a shallow casserole or roasting tin and mix in the tomatoes, tomato purée, garlic and herbs, combining well so that the tomato sauce has coated everything.
2 Place the sausages on top of the vegetable base.
3 Place in a preheated oven for around an hour at 180°C/350°F/gas mark 4.
4 Grind black pepper on top when ready to serve.

Nick's Beef Burgers

Created by a cavalry officer friend, this burger recipe will satisfy an army and is seriously delicious served with the Mexican Bean Dip (4 🟢) (see page 328) and lettuce in a toasted pitta bread (5 🟢 per half-slice).

> 8oz (227g) extra-lean beef mince
> 1 tbsp tamari or soy sauce
> 1 tsp Worcester sauce
> 1 tbsp finely chopped fresh coriander
> ¼ red onion, finely chopped
> ½ egg, beaten
> ½ tsp Solo sea salt
> ½ tsp black pepper

1 Mix all other ingredients together, then add to the mince.
2 Knead the mixture thoroughly, then divide into 4 patties and flatten into a burger shape.
3 Place on a plate and cover, before putting in the fridge to firm for approximately 10 minutes or until required.
4 Grill under a medium heat for approximately 7 minutes per side or to taste.

Fajitas

Here's a low-fat take on this ever-popular Tex-Mex dish. Double or triple the recipe to make a fun family supper, or a great informal meal for friends. Substitute a can of black-eyed beans if you do not eat meat.

For the fajitas
2 onions, sliced
1 clove garlic, crushed

1 red and 1 yellow pepper, topped, seeded and sliced
   lengthways
olive oil
2 chicken breasts, skinned and cut into slices
⅔ tbsp Old El Paso Fajita Seasoning
2 tortillas

For the tomato salsa
2 plum tomatoes, chopped
2 spring onions, finely chopped
1 clove garlic, crushed
2 tbsp fresh coriander, finely chopped
1 tbsp lime juice
1 tbsp olive oil
pinch Solo sea salt and black pepper

1 Steam-fry the onion, garlic and peppers in the oil.
2 Rub the seasoning into the chicken and grill until cooked.
3 Mix into the vegetables. (If you are using black-eyed beans,
  add the fajita seasoning to the steam fry and cook for a further few minutes, then stir the beans through and remove
  from the heat.)
4 To make the salsa, stir the ingredients together in a large
  bowl, then spoon onto each tortilla and add the chicken and
  vegetable or bean mixture and roll up.

Chicken Dumplings with Chilli Dipping Sauce

These Oriental-flavoured dumplings are steamed, making them much lower in fat than traditional fried meatballs. Turkey is equally tasty in this recipe.

> 2 skinless, boneless chicken breasts, cut into chunks
> 1 tbsp tamari
> 1 red chilli, deseeded and chopped finely
> ¾in chunk fresh ginger, peeled and finely grated
> 4 spring onions, roughly chopped
> 1 clove garlic, finely grated
> 1 tbsp fresh coriander, roughly chopped
> 2 tbsp sweet chilli dipping sauce

1 Place the meat, tamari, chilli, ginger, spring onions, garlic and coriander in a food processor and pulse until the mixture is coarsely chopped and combined.
2 Using your hands, shape the mix into 12 balls, then cover and chill for at least 20 minutes (and up to 8 hours).
3 When you are ready to cook the dumplings, place them in a steamer for 20 minutes, checking that the chicken is thoroughly cooked through, with no pink flesh showing inside.
4 Serve with Crunchy Thai Salad (4 **GL**) (see page 315) and soba (buckwheat) noodles (7 **GL** per small serving).

Thai Green Curry

The aromatic blend of spices and creamy coconut milk in this dish suits a number of protein-rich foods, so you can adapt this recipe whether you eat meat or not (simply add tofu chunks or prawns as directed). Green curry paste, fish sauce and kaffir lime leaves are now widely available in most supermarkets. If you can't find the last two, the curry will still be delicious.

> 1 small onion, chopped
> 2 cloves garlic, crushed
> 2 heaped tsp Thai green curry paste
> 1 tbs olive oil
> 1 small chicken breast, cubed
> *or* 11oz (312g) firm tofu, cubed
> *or* 6oz (170g) peeled prawns
> 1 dessertspoon fish sauce
> ¾pt (400ml) canned coconut milk
> 2 kaffir lime leaves
> 1 large courgette, chopped
> handful of fresh basil leaves

1 Steam-fry onions, garlic and curry paste in oil for 2 minutes.
2 Add chicken, tofu or prawns – whichever you choose – and fry for a further 5 minutes.
3 Add fish sauce, coconut milk and kaffir lime leaves. Stir well, cover and leave to simmer for at least half an hour.
4 5–10 minutes before serving, add courgettes and basil leaves and continue simmering.

Indian Spiced Chicken

This dish should liberate you to experiment with different combinations of spices, although you can always just use a ready-made curry powder. Either way, it's irresistible.

> juice of 1 lemon
> 1 clove garlic, crushed
> ½ tsp turmeric powder
> ½ tsp ground cumin
> 1 tsp ground coriander
> dash of cayenne pepper
> 2oz (57g) chicken breasts

1 Blend the lemon juice, garlic and spices.
2 Place rinsed chicken in a dish and toss it in the spice blend so it is well coated. Leave to marinate for at least 30 minutes, or ideally several hours.
3 Place under a medium grill for 15 minutes (or until cooked – this will depend on the thickness of the chicken), turning once, halfway through cooking.

Coronation Chicken Salad

A good leftovers meal. Full of crunch with a slightly sweet, spicy flavour. Perfect for packed lunches or picnics.

> 1 gem lettuce, torn into bite-sized pieces
> cold meat from ½ small roast chicken, skin removed
> ½ medium eating apple, cubed
> 1 stick celery, chopped
> 1½ tbsp low-fat mayonnaise
> 1½ tbsp low-fat yoghurt

2 tsp mango chutney
1 tsp tomato purée
1 tsp paprika

1 Create a bed of lettuce on a large plate.
2 Mix together the mayonnaise, yoghurt, mango chutney, tomato purée and paprika.
3 Combine the sauce with the chicken, apple and celery.
4 Pile on top of the lettuce and serve either on oatcakes or in pitta bread, or with any leftover boiled potatoes.

Tarragon and Lemon Roast Chicken Breast

Tarragon and lemon lend extra flavour to roast chicken.

1 clove garlic, sliced
2 sprigs fresh tarragon
2 small chicken breasts (with skin)
1 dessertspoon olive oil
1 clove garlic, sliced
2 sprigs fresh tarragon
½ lemon

1 Place garlic slices and tarragon under chicken skin.
2 Place chicken breasts in a baking dish and drizzle with olive oil and lemon juice.
3 Place in an oven preheated to 190°C/375°F/gas mark 5 and bake for 15–20 minutes or until cooked (this will depend on the thickness of the chicken). Before eating, remove the skin.

Spicy Pork Loin

A delicious way to serve pork, which should prevent it from drying out. Serve with steam-fried greens and Sweet Potato Mash (7 ⒼⓁ) (see page 331).

> 12oz (340g) pork loin (fillet), fat trimmed
> 1 tbsp olive oil
> 3 tbsp tamari or soy sauce
> 2 tsp tomato purée
> 1in (2.5cm) chunk root ginger, peeled
> 1 large mild, red chilli, deseeded
> 1 garlic clove, peeled
> 2 tsp honey or dark muscovado sugar

1 In a blender, blitz the tomato purée, garlic, tamari or soy, chilli, ginger and honey or sugar, until it forms a smooth paste.
2 Lightly boil the mixture in a pan for a couple of minutes, then cool.
3 Rub the marinade all over the pork, then cover and place in the fridge for around 20–30 minutes or until needed.
4 Bake the pork on a rack in a roasting tin for 30–35 minutes at 180°C/350°F/gas mark 4, marinating again halfway through. Remove from the oven when cooked and rest for 5 minutes under tin foil before serving.

Venison Stroganoff

Venison is very tasty, is leaner than beef and is not farmed intensively, making it less likely to be contaminated with chemical residues. Replace with extra mushrooms (allowing

2 handfuls per person) if you want a vegetarian version, and serve with quinoa instead of rice to make sure you get adequate protein.

> 1 tbsp olive oil
> 3oz (85g) chestnut mushrooms, wiped clean and cut in half
> 1 onion, sliced
> 1 clove garlic, chopped
> Solo sea salt and black pepper
> 7oz (198g) venison rump, trimmed of fat and sliced into 2cm (¾in) strips
> 2fl oz (50ml) water
> 2oz (57g) yoghurt mixed with 1 rounded tsp cornflour
> ½ rounded tbsp chopped fresh tarragon
> ¼ tsp paprika

1 Heat half the oil in a frying pan and gently sauté the mushrooms, onion and garlic for about 10 minutes. Season and place in a bowl.
2 Increase the heat to high, add the rest of the oil and put in the meat, quickly sealing it and stirring occasionally. When it is cooked, add to the reserved mushroom mixture, leaving any juices in the pan.
3 Add the water to the pan and heat gently for 5 minutes to reduce, stirring to mix in all the juices. Add the yoghurt mixture and cook for another minute to allow the sauce to thicken.
4 Add in the precooked ingredients together with the herbs.
5 Serve with Sweet Potato Mash (7 **GL**) (see page 331) or 70g brown basmati rice (7 **GL** per small serving), sprinkled with paprika, and with steamed green beans on the side.

Desserts

This section is all about people who think life is sweet – and want to celebrate that, not succumb to seesawing blood sugar. You don't have to give up desserts on the Holford Diet. As you can see, cakes, flapjacks, pies and puddings all have a part to play. Once your fatburning capabilities have reached their stride, have one of these a week if you like – or perhaps two, on the maintenance diet. Once your blood sugar is balanced, you can *really* enjoy desserts, because they're not ruling your life.

Ⓖ scores:

Recipe	Page number	Ⓖ
Individual Berry Cheesecake	376	5
Chocolate Coconut Cookies	378	5
Kiwi and Coconut Pudding	378	6
Cinnamon Steamed Pears with Summer Berry Purée	379	5
Almond Macaroons	380	2
Apple Flapjack Crumble	381	11
Almond Rice Pudding	382	5
Coconut Quinoa Pudding	382	6
Ginger Stewed Apricots	383	4
Fruit Kebabs	384	7
Raspberry Mousse	384	2
Baked Apple with Spiced Blackberry Stuffing	385	6
Chocolate Ice Cream	386	6

Individual Berry Cheesecake

The base of this cheesecake uses chopped fruit and nuts for a much lower Ⓖ score. An easy-to-prepare pudding that can be made in advance.

For the base

¾oz (21g) chopped walnuts and pecans (or other nuts)

4 dried apricots

½ tsp walnut oil

For the cheese

7oz (198g) very low-fat plain cream cheese

2 tbsp lemon juice

zest of ½ lemon

3 tsp xylitol

For the topping

4 tbsp berries (for example, raspberries, blueberries or
    blackberries)

1 tbsp apple juice or water

1 Place nuts and apricots with oil in small blender and process until broken into very small pieces and sticking together. Press into the bottom of 2 ramekins and chill.

2 In a bowl add the lemon juice to the xylitol and stir to allow the granules to dissolve.

3 Mix the dissolved xylitol and lemon juice and zest into the cream cheese until smooth and thoroughly combined, then spoon into the prepared ramekins, level off the top and return to the fridge.

4 Place the berries in a small pan and gently stew them in apple juice or water until they soften and begin to burst. Remove from heat and cool before pouring onto cheesecakes.

5 Chill the cheesecakes once finished, until ready to serve.

Chocolate Coconut Cookies

These miniature biscuit bars are absolutely scrummy served after a meal. A healthier version of a well-known chocolate bar!

Makes 12 (serves 4)
5oz (142g) desiccated coconut
3 egg whites
3 tbsp xylitol
1 tsp lime or lemon juice
1 tbsp cornflour
3 small squares of good-quality dark chocolate, such as Green and Black's

1 Combine the coconut, egg white, xylitol, cornflour and lime or lemon juice and mix well into a stiff paste.
2 Divide into 12 walnut-sized balls and shape into rectangles (like a piece of sushi rice) or flattish circles. Place on a lined baking tray and bake at 180°C/350°F/gas mark 4 for 10 minutes, then reduce the heat to 150°C/300°F/gas mark 2 for a further 5 minutes. Remove from the oven.
3 Melt the chocolate over a *bain marie* or in a microwave oven, then dip one half of each coconut bar into the chocolate and lay on a lightly greased or lined plate and chill in the fridge to set. Alternatively drizzle the melted chocolate over the bars.

Kiwi and Coconut Pudding

The easiest pudding ever, yet special enough for entertaining. This can be made in advance and kept in the fridge until needed.

2 ripe kiwi fruits, peeled and cut into thin slices, crossways
4 tbsp Rachel's Organic Coconut Greek Style Live Yoghurt

1 Divide the kiwi slices between two bowls or ramekins (glass dishes look best, because you can see the different layers of the finished pudding).

3 Spoon the yoghurt on top of both bowls.

Cinnamon Steamed Pears with Summer Berry Purée

Steaming is much easier than poaching these pears, which are lovely served with puréed summer berries.

> 2 ripe pears
> ½ tsp cinnamon
> 1 tsp xylitol
> 2 heaped tbsp summer berries

1 Slice the bottom off each pear, so that they can stand unaided, then remove the core using either a melon-ball scoop or a teaspoon.

2 Mix together the cinnamon and the xylitol, then sprinkle into the hollow of each pear, where the core has been removed from.

3 Lay them in a steamer pan and steam for about 8–10 minutes, turning halfway through, until they are soft when pierced with a knife. (Do not stand them up or all of the sweet juices from inside will escape.)

4 While the pears are steaming, purée the summer berries in a blender or stew slightly in a tablespoonful of water until they burst and release some juice.

5 Serve the pears still warm, with a dollop of the fruit purée.

Almond Macaroons

These chewy little biscuits will fill the spot if you have a carb craving, but, being made of egg and nuts, have a low ⒼⓁ.

> **Makes 12 miniature biscuits (serves 3)**
> 1 egg white
> 2oz (57g) ground almonds
> 2oz (57g) xylitol
> ½ tsp ground ginger
> a few flaked almonds

1 Line a baking tray with rice paper.
2 Whisk the egg white until it forms stiff peaks.
3 Gently fold the ginger, ground almonds and xylitol into the egg white with a metal spoon, taking care not to beat out all of the air.
4 Place teaspoonfuls of the mixture onto the baking tray and lightly press a flaked almond onto the top of each macaroon.
5 Place in a preheated oven (180°C/350°F/gas mark 4) and bake for 15–20 minutes, until firm to the touch.
6 When cooked and cooled, remove from the trays and peel or trim the rice paper from the edges of each macaroon. Store in an airtight container.

Apple Flapjack Crumble

Serve this to family and friends and I promise you no one will guess that you are on a diet. Experiment by adding different dried fruit and nuts, or pumpkin and sunflower seeds, to the crumble instead of walnuts.

For the flapjack crumble
6oz (170g) oat flakes
2oz (57g) chopped walnuts
2 tbsp olive oil
2 tbsp xylitol

For the apple
2 Bramley (cooking) apples, cored and diced
¼ tsp ground ginger or ½ tsp cinnamon
1 tsp xylitol
1 tsp lemon juice

1 Gently melt the 2 tablespoonfuls of xylitol and oil together in a saucepan until the granules have dissolved, then add the dry crumble ingredients and mix well, stirring so that the oats just start to go crisp and become golden (around 3 minutes). Set to one side.

2 Place the apple, lemon juice and teaspoonful of xylitol in a new saucepan and gently stew until the apples soften and start to disintegrate, keeping them moving so that they do not stick.

3 Divide the apple between two ramekins and cover with the flapjack crumble topping. Serve still warm.

Almond Rice Pudding

This delicious, warming pudding is comfort food at its best, but the brown basmati rice, soya milk, nuts and xylitol reduce the Ⓖ considerably. This is a very flexible recipe – simply add more or less milk, and cook for more or less time to achieve the texture and consistency you prefer.

Serves 4
3oz (80g) brown basmati rice
1¼ pints (25fl oz/700ml) soya milk (sweetened)
1½oz (40g) xylitol
3oz (85g) ground almonds
2 drops of vanilla essence
4 handfuls of flaked almonds, lightly toasted

1 Put half of the milk, the rice, vanilla essence and xylitol into a saucepan and bring to the boil. Cover and leave to simmer for around 40 minutes (the rice will still be quite hard at this stage).

2 Add the rest of the milk and simmer without the lid on for another 30 minutes or so, until the mixture is soft and fairly gooey.

3 Stir through the ground almonds and cook for a further couple of minutes (add a bit more soya milk or some water if the mixture is too thick or sticking to the bottom at this stage).

4 Spoon into 4 bowls and sprinkle flaked almonds on each one before serving.

Coconut Quinoa Pudding

A high-protein, low-Ⓖ version of the comfort food classic rice pudding. This is not a glamorous-looking pudding but it does taste delicious, especially served alongside a spoonful of the Ginger Stewed Apricots (see opposite).

4oz (113g) quinoa, rinsed
¼pt (150ml) semi-skimmed milk or soya milk
1 tbsp desiccated coconut
2 tsp xylitol

Place all the ingredients in a saucepan and bring to the boil, then reduce the heat, cover and simmer until the quinoa is cooked (the grains will look light and fluffy, and will be soft to the bite).

Ginger Stewed Apricots

A spicy, warming pudding that goes beautifully with the Coconut Quinoa Pudding (see above) or simply a spoonful of crème fraîche.

4 ripe apricots, halved and stoned
1 tbsp xylitol
¼ tsp ground ginger
1 tbsp orange juice or water

Stew the apricot halves in a saucepan with the other ingredients until they are soft but still retain their shape.

Fruit Kebabs

Just the thing for a late-summer barbecue, and a favourite with all ages.

> 1 apple
> lemon juice
> 1 orange
> 4 black grapes
> 7oz (198g) natural yoghurt
> 1 tsp honey

1 Cube the apples and coat with a little lemon juice to prevent them from going brown.
2 Peel the orange, removing all the pith, and cut into chunks.
3 Halve the grapes and remove the pips.
4 Put the fruit onto skewers and grill under a high grill or on a barbecue.
5 Blend the yoghurt with honey and use as a dipping sauce.

Raspberry Mousse

This fruit fool tastes equally good made with strawberries or blackcurrants.

> 8oz (227g) raspberries (fresh or frozen and thawed)
> 4oz (113g) low-fat fromage frais
> 1–2 tsp honey
> handful of fresh mint leaves

1 Blend raspberries, fromage frais and honey.
2 Pour into individual serving dishes.
3 Garnish with a sprig of mint.

Baked Apple with Spiced Blackberry Stuffing

A warming, fibre-rich pudding for autumn and winter. Alternatively you could use blueberries.

> 2 tsp xylitol
> ¼ tsp cinnamon or ginger
> 1 heaped tbsp blackberries
> 2 Bramley (cooking) apples, cored to create a fairly large hole
>   inside

1 Mix the cinnamon or ginger and xylitol through the berries.
2 Place apples on an ovenproof dish or plate and stuff with the berry mixture.
3 Bake in a preheated oven at 180°C/350°F/gas mark 4 for around 35–40 minutes, or until soft right the way through (test by inserting a skewer) but still standing (overcooking will cause the apples to collapse).

Chocolate Ice Cream

This luscious ice cream shines if made with the highest-quality cocoa powder.

> 2¾oz (80g) xylitol
> 8fl oz (225 ml) milk
> 1 egg, beaten
> 1½oz (40g) dark chocolate cocoa powder
> 16fl oz (450ml) cream
> 1 tsp vanilla extract

1 Mix the xylitol, milk and egg together in a bowl, then pour into a small pan and cook over a medium low heat, stirring constantly, until the mixture thickens – this takes about 10 minutes. Take care not to let it boil.
2 Remove from the heat and add the cocoa powder, stirring until the cocoa dissolves and is mixed in well.
3 Allow to cool for 15 minutes at room temperature before adding the cream and vanilla extract and placing in the freezer for at least 2½ hours. Remove five minutes before serving.

Drinks

The following drinks can be drunk without limit throughout the day:

● still mineral water
● herbal teas
● dandelion coffee, Barley Cup, Caro, Teeccino

The following drinks are best limited to a glass a day:

● Aqua Libra

- Amé
- other sugar-free juice blends (best diluted)

Also, you can have one of these a day (within your 5🅖🅛 allowance for drinks, sweets and desserts):

- Fruit juices diluted 50 per cent with water (see page 230 for quantities)

If you're prone to overindulging in alcohol, you'll need to stop drinking it for two weeks to a month at the start of the diet for maximum fatburning. Thereafter, limit your consumption of alcohol to a maximum of three units a week. A unit is:

- a small glass of wine
- a half-pint of beer or lager
- a measure of spirits

Snacks

As we saw in Chapter 15, you need never be bored at snack time. Have your snacks mid-morning and mid-afternoon, away from main meals.

- You can have a piece of fruit, plus five almonds or a dessertspoon of pumpkin seeds. Choose from apples, pears, plums, cherries, berries, peaches, grapefruit and oranges. You can eat an entire punnet or even more of strawberries (see the table on page 212), but avoid bananas; although they're fine with Get Up & Go for breakfast, they have too high a 🅖🅛 to be eaten as an additional snack.

- Low-🅖🅛 bread and oatcakes with protein spreads and dips are a good savoury option. Try one thin slice of rye, pumpernickel, sourdough or other low-Ⓖ bread, *or* two oatcakes, with either half a small tub of cottage cheese, half a small tub of hummus, *or* a tablespoon of sugar-free peanut butter. You could substitute a raw carrot or a selection of crudités for the bread or oatcakes.

● If you like, you can have a small, plain, low-fat bio yoghurt (5oz/142g), or half a small tub of cottage cheese, with berries.

These should keep you going strong through the day.

Here's another delicious idea – if you bring them to work, you may have to hide them from your colleagues!

Spiced Chickpea Chews

A low-fat, savoury snack rich in combined protein and carb.

> **Serves 3 (keep some in an airtight container for a ready snack)**
> 1 can chickpeas, rinsed and drained
> 1 tsp olive oil
> 1 tbsp lemon juice
> 1 tsp paprika or cayenne pepper
> pinch of Solo or sea salt and black pepper

1 Toss the chickpeas in the oil and place in a preheated oven (150°C/300°F/gas mark 2) for 1 hour until crisp, shaking them around in the tin from time to time.
2 Take out, drizzle with lemon juice and sprinkle the paprika or cayenne pepper and seasoning over the top.
3 Shake the chickpeas in the tray to coat thoroughly and then leave to cool.

PART FIVE

Hidden Benefits

29

Vitality Plus

Newton's Third Law of Thermodynamics, applied to what you eat, says that all the energy you consume as calories must go somewhere. You've been putting some of it down into storage as fat.

But, as we've now amply seen, on the Holford Diet three things are going to happen. You'll start to burn off fat, you'll find yourself eating less without even trying, and your energy levels will shoot up.

When I first came into the field of nutrition, I was deeply impressed by the work of a then maverick called Dr Roy Walford, professor of pathology at the UCLA School of Medicine in Los Angeles, who claimed he had discovered the secret of eternal youth. Dr Walford (who sadly died of a rare genetic neurological disease called ALS), now respected as one of the truly pioneering gerontologists of our time, had proved how to increase the lifespan of any animal by up to 30 per cent!

Walford fed laboratory animals food that had slightly fewer calories, but was of very high quality, with high levels of vitamins and minerals and a low glycemic load. These lucky animals clocked the equivalent of 130 human years! But what really impressed me was seeing them. His diet hadn't just added years to their life: it had clearly added life to their years. Compared with the 'normal' animals, they looked healthy and lean, and were very active and inquisitive.

I started following the human equivalent of his diet, which was very close to today's Holford Diet. And I've stayed lean, and physically and mentally active, ever since. The research Dr Walford started is now being tested on humans in a long-term study, and so far all the signs are good. His lucky volunteers have all the same positive characteristics that the animals displayed on his diet and are bang on course for reaching 100 with the health of a 60-year-old. It's looking more and more as if you really can turn back the clock.

Energy, or the lack of it, is the bane of the twenty-first century. When ION conducted Britain's biggest ever health survey in 2002, a staggering 76 per cent of people said they felt tired much of the time. We also found that the more overweight a person was, the more likely they were to complain of fatigue. It's ironic that an overweight person should feel tired when their body is a storehouse packed full of energy-giving fat.

As I've shown, the trouble is that food is going straight to fat rather than straight to energy. When you change your body's metabolism to use the energy in your food more efficiently, you'll be off and running.

But don't take my word for it. I invited four magazines, the *Sunday Times Magazine*, *Time Out*, *She* and *Woman's Realm*, to find volunteers and put my original Fatburner Diet diet to the test over a three-month period.

Woman's Realm tested it out on three people – Sabine, Ian and Tina. Here's what they said:

❛ *Sabine complained of erratic weight and constant lack of energy. She's tried loads of diets that only ever gave temporary and limited success. It was her ambition to get down to eight stone (112lb) and stay there, plus regain some of her get-up-and-go in the process!*

Sabine reached her target weight in just a few months. Her food weaknesses – mid-morning nibbles on crisps and chocolate – have completely gone. "Once I got used to eating lots of fruit, my craving for sugar and chocolate disappeared." Sabine now says her whole attitude to food has changed. "I'm no longer obsessed with eating and automatically reach for healthy things when I shop and cook." Sabine says it's wonderful to feel so relaxed around food. ❜

Sabine lost 10lb in those three months – and gained energy, in leaps and bounds.

❛ *Ian's weight had hovered stubbornly around the 15 stone (210lb) mark. He was also drinking and smoking heavily and wanted to reduce both significantly.*

Now only a few pounds off his target weight, Ian has managed to give up smoking and drastically reduce his alcohol consumption – a daunting task on top of his highly pressurised job as a theatre producer/actor. Ian started gradually, cutting out tea and coffee then reducing his red-meat/fried-food intake. Soon he was following the diet rigorously. Once he'd lost a stone (14lb) in weight, Ian started to reduce his alcohol consumption – from two bottles of wine to two glasses per day – and eventually felt ready to stop the cigarettes – that he did overnight. Ian's comments: "I was very apprehensive at the beginning – I had a lot of vices to conquer. But once I got over my craving for caffeine it was easier to crack the weight problem." ❜

Ian lost 19lb, and all his addictions.

> *Gina's problem was willpower. Having a huge appetite and a sweet tooth for chocolate and puddings, she admitted to eating throughout the day whether she was hungry or not!*
>
> *First of all she reduced her tea and coffee intake and substituted fruit or healthy snacks for chocolate. Gradually, as she ate fewer foods high in saturated fat (like red meat), and more fruits and vegetables, her craving for sugar and sweet things lessened.*

Gina lost 10lb and continues to lose 1–2lb a week.

She magazine selected 10 volunteers. This is what they reported:

> *Increased alertness was a significant benefit. By the third day, everybody felt well – alert on rising, and three of us (including me) were bounding about full of the joys of spring. Two out of ten felt hungry, but the rest said that, as far as hunger was concerned, it was a comparatively easy diet to stick to. Mrs Kilby noted by day four that her concentration had improved, and this was backed up by comments from other testers. Nobody had that weak and wobbly feeling associated with dieting. By the end of the week, everyone had stayed the course. Weight loss over the week varied from 3lb to 7lb, 4–5lb being the average.*

The *Sunday Times Magazine* selected one volunteer. This is what they said:

> *After the first few days I began to feel wonderful – alert and fit and thoroughly detoxified with no more puffy eyes staring back from the bathroom mirror. There's no shortage of recipe ideas. I lost 10lb in a month and regained 2lb on holiday, but will whittle that off by eating sensibly.*

This was *Time Out*'s comment:

> ❮ *Weight loss: 4lb to 7lb in four weeks. Verdict: Makes you look and feel good. Side effects: None.* ❯

In the early days, when we put people on this diet, 86 per cent reported a definite improvement in energy. The average 'energy' score using our checklist was 7, and, three to six months later, the average score was 3. (Remember, the lower your score the better in this case.)

Now it's your turn to check your energy score. And in truth, you can expect even better results than the ones above from people on the prototype Fatburner Diet. That's because the Holford Diet incorporates new findings in obesity research, as well as even more feedback from thousands of volunteers over the years.

Energy levels are intimately linked to insulin resistance and blood sugar balance, as we've seen throughout this book. So, to figure out your energy score, go back to the insulin-resistance checklist on page 56.

If you answer yes to seven or more questions, you are struggling to keep your blood sugar level even, and you probably have serious energy slumps or feel exhausted much of the time.

If you answer yes to between seven and ten questions, you are beginning to show signs of a sugar sensitivity, which needs to be addressed. You may have several dips in energy a day.

If you answer yes to fewer than four questions, you are unlikely to have a blood sugar problem, and your energy level is on the up and up or consistently high.

Make a note of your score, then retest yourself in three months.

It's not all right to feel just 'all right'. I want you to feel full of energy, however old you are. Are you ready for it?

30

Warning: This Diet Will Seriously Undamage Your Health

As we've seen, extra energy is definitely on the agenda if you follow the Holford Diet. But I've hardly touched on the other side benefits – and they are something:

- better skin;
- younger looks;
- more even mood;
- sharper memory and concentration; and
- reduced risk for diabetes, heart disease, cancer and arthritis.

This is a diet where you don't only lose weight. You look great and feel great – clear-headed, calm, glowing, and knowing that you are getting healthier as each week passes.

Eat yourself beautiful

Did you know your skin is new every 20 days? We are literally making new skin cells every day, and the healthier your diet, the healthier your skin. I know because, as I mentioned at the start of this book, I suffered for seven years with bad acne, and saw numerous specialists whose advice ranged from special cleansing routines to creams and antibiotics. Some of these substances made a mild difference, but none really worked. Then I discovered optimum nutrition and within one month the spots were gone. Within three months, the scarring was visibly reduced. Why?

There are six secrets to having great skin, and all of them are fulfilled by following the Holford Diet.

Inner balance

The first, and most important, is to keep your blood sugar level even. When your blood sugar level peaks to high, which is the fate of the insulin-resistant, the skin also receives excess sugar. Bacteria in the skin feed off sugar, and they are what causes spots. When the blood sugar level dips too low, the body produces adrenalin. This increases the production of sebum, an oily secretion in the skin, which in excess can block pores and cause an isolated pocket of infection to grow.

The reason excess sebum can block pores, as well as make the skin oily, is that the sebum gets oxidised, making it hard. The skin is always being bombarded with free radicals, rogue molecules that are sometimes called *oxidants*.

Major baddies as far as your skin and your health are concerned, oxidants originate from anything burned, especially fats. So they're in cigarette smoke (there are a trillion in each puff), fried food, burned meat and exhaust fumes, as well as the air itself, since particles become damaged by the sun's burning rays. In truth, you are exposed to something like a bucketful of oxidants each year. These are damaging your skin every day and that is why people who live near the equator, or at high altitudes, and are therefore exposed to stronger sunlight, have much older-looking skin.

There are only two things you can do to minimise oxidant skin damage: either limit your exposure to strong sunlight or rub on a sunscreen when you do, and take in more antioxidant nutrients through diet and supplements.

> **TOP TIP**
>
> You can feed the skin with antioxidants from the outside. The best two skin products I know of are Environ and Dermalogica. Both have antioxidant capsules that you pierce and rub on your skin. The results are amazing. (See page 476 for details.)

Essential antioxidants

The Holford Diet is naturally full of antioxidants, partly by luck and partly by design. Some of the all-time best, low-ⓖⓛ fruits and vegetables also have the highest levels of antioxidants. To stay young and healthy you need to eat antioxidant-rich foods every day.

When I first came into the field of nutrition we used to measure the amount of antioxidant nutrients in food, including vitamin A, betacarotene, vitamin C, vitamin E, selenium, zinc, glutathione and co-enzyme Q10. We then started to discover more and more plant-based antioxidants. Examples of these phytonutrients are anthocyanidins in berries and allicin in garlic.

A method for measuring a food's total anti-ageing antioxidant power was then invented, called the *ORAC score* of a food

(ORAC stands for 'oxygen radical absorption capacity'). The ORAC score of a food is the single best measure of a food's anti-ageing potential. To give you some examples I've listed below and overleaf some of the top common fruits and vegetables, starting with those with the highest ORAC scores.[1] I've also listed their ⓖⓛ for a 100g serving.

Top anti-ageing fruits

	ORAC per 100g	ⓖⓛ per serving
Prunes	5,770	17
Raisins	2,830	46
Blueberries	**2,400**	**1**
Blackberries	**2,036**	**1**
Strawberries	**1,540**	**1**
Raspberries	**1,220**	**1**
Plum	**949**	**5**
Orange	**750**	**5**
Grapes, red	739	7
Cherries	**670**	**2**
Kiwi fruit	610	5
Grapefruit, pink	**495**	**3**
Cantaloupe melon	250	4
Banana	210	10
Apple	207	5
Apricot	175	4
Peach	170	4

While raisins and prunes have the highest ORAC rating, they also send your blood sugar soaring. Remember, the ⓖⓛ limit for a snack on the Holford Diet is five points. I've put the best all-rounders in this list – berries, plums, oranges, cherries and pink grapefruit – in bold, because these fruits will both help you lose weight and keep your skin healthy.

Be aware, however, that these are the scores for the whole fruit, not the juice. While an orange is the equivalent of 5 🅖🅛 points, and therefore a perfect snack for the diet, a 250ml glass of orange juice, which normally contains the juice and the sugar of between two and three oranges, has a 🅖🅛 of 13 points. That's too much.

In the chart below I've picked out the best vegetables, both for their ORAC score and their 🅖🅛, highlighted in bold.

Top anti-ageing vegetables

	ORAC per 100g	🅖🅛 per serving
Kale	**1,770**	**1**
Garlic clove	**1,662**	**1**
Spinach	**1,260**	**1**
Tenderstem	**1,183**	**2**
Pumpkin/squash	**1,150**	**3**
Brussels sprouts	**980**	**2**
Broccoli	**890**	**2**
Beetroot	840	5
Avocado	**782**	**1**
Beans, baked	503	7
Beans, kidney	460	7
Onion	450	2
Sweetcorn	400	9
Peas, frozen	375	3
Potato	300	16
Sweet potato	295	17
Carrot	200	3
String beans	200	2
Tomato	195	3

As you can see in the chart opposite, the best antioxidant vegetables are also the best fatburning vegetables, with a low ⒼⓁ score. I recommend you have a serving of one of these top scorers every day, with the exception of avocado – don't have more than three a week.

Of all the antioxidant nutrients, the two most important for the skin are vitamins A and C. Vitamin A is what protects your skin from sun damage. Vitamin C makes collagen, a substance that's a bit like 'glue' holding your cells together. When you lack vitamin C, your skin loses its tone and wrinkles develop. On the Holford Diet I not only recommend that you eat foods naturally rich in these nutrients, but I also recommend that you supplement with a multivitamin containing at least 1,500 mcg of vitamin A, plus 1,000g (or even 2,000g) of vitamin C, which is the optimal amount for both fatburning, anti-ageing and boosting your immune system.

Fats and flexibility

The third secret for healthy skin is to eat the right fats. Essential fats, found in seeds and fish, are vital for your skin and, without them, it can look dry and old. Skin cells contain these essential fats, which not only keep skin looking young and flexible but also are needed to reduce skin inflammation. Omega-3 fats are very powerful anti-inflammatory agents which can reduce redness and swelling in conditions such as eczema.

The Holford Diet recommends that you eat foods naturally high in essential fats, such as oily fish, seeds and nuts. These essential fats not only help your skin, they also help you to burn fat. You may also choose to use them as supplements, as I do every day. I take a supplement that contains a combination of EPA and DHA, which are the most powerful omega-3 fats, and GLA, the most powerful omega-6 fat. (See also Chapter 8.)

Liquid loveliness

The final secret for healthy skin is to drink enough water – and that means eight glasses a day. The body is 66 per cent water and you need to keep it topped up with water to function properly, from the cellular and chemical levels up. Here, essential fats are invaluable, helping to maintain perfect water balance in the body by keeping the right amount of it inside your cells.

Drinking enough water to stay hydrated is not only good for your health. It also helps to reduce your appetite, as we often mistake thirst for hunger.

The calorie connection

Skin cells are not much different from other cells in your body and, for this reason, those four secrets for healthy skin – balance your blood sugar, eat an antioxidant-rich diet, get enough essential fats and drink eight glasses of water a day – are also the top tips for staying young and slowing down the ageing process. And there are two more.

In the last chapter I told you about the excellent research of Dr Roy Walford, who proved that if you cut down on calories you live longer. Calorie restriction, however, is not the same as malnutrition. It is about giving the body exactly what it needs and no more.

That's exactly what the Holford Diet is all about. Many foods in today's diet provide 'empty' calories. That is, they provide sugar or saturated fat, but none of the micronutrients needed to process them. These foods are out if you want to lose weight and extend your lifespan. Nutrient-dense foods such as fish, beans, nuts and seeds provide as many nutrients as calories, plus, in the case of fresh fruit and vegetables, plenty of essential and calorie-free water.

Since the first animal experiments in 1935, studies on several species have shown that animals eating 30 to 40 per cent fewer calories can extend their lifespan by a third to (in the case of fish) a half. However, it isn't just about limiting calories. These animals were given optimum nutrition as well as fewer calories, with good intakes of antioxidants.

There's every reason to assume the same principle applies to humans. Consider the islanders of Okinawa in Japan. They eat 17 to 40 per cent fewer calories than other Japanese and have more centenarians than any other population. According to Dr Walford, 'You can extend longevity by restricting food even after full adulthood and middle age.'

Having a high-quality diet with minimal calories also means minimal oxidative stress on the body. You are giving yourself exactly what you need and no more. But how much is that? Dr Walford said that you can extend lifespan by cutting calories by 10 to 25 per cent. He ate between 1,500 and 2,000 calories a day, compared with the average intake of 2,500 to 3,000 calories. And that is exactly what I recommend you do. The recipes in the Holford Diet, and the menus based on them, are designed to be less calorific, yet fill you up and satisfy your appetite in the healthiest way possible.

Life insurance companies know well the correlation between weight and longevity. Based on these statistics, weight charts give an ideal weight range for your height. You can see one of these in Appendix 1. Generally, the ideal weight for increased life expectancy is the low end of this range. Even more important, as we've seen in this book, is keeping your body fat percentage down, which can also be greatly helped by a regular exercise regime. Appendix 1 also shows you how to calculate this percentage.

The homocysteine factor

Homocysteine is a toxic amino acid (a building block of protein) found in the blood. You may not have heard of it yet, but you certainly will.

Your homocysteine level is a stronger predictor of having a heart attack or stroke than your cholesterol level. This is quite literally the most important medical breakthrough of the twenty-first century and I can't do it justice here – which is why I've written a book, *The H Factor*, with Dr James Braly, an expert on this subject. No fewer than 6,000 medical studies have linked high levels of this amino acid to about 100 medical conditions, including obesity.

A comprehensive research study at the University of Bergen in Norway, published in 2001 in the *American Journal of Clinical Nutrition*,[2] measured the homocysteine levels of 4,766 men and women aged 65 to 67 in 1992, and then recorded any deaths over the next five years. During this time, 162 men and 97 women died. The researchers then looked at the risk of death in relation to their homocysteine levels. This is what they found: 'A strong relation was found between homocysteine and *all* causes of mortality.' They discovered that the chances of a 65- to 67-year-old dying from any cause increased by almost 50 per cent for every five-unit increase in homocysteine!

So, how can you lower levels of this toxic amino acid? It all hinges on something called SAMe.

Put simply, if you have a high homocysteine level, it means you've got a blockage in your body's ability to turn protein into one of the most important anti-ageing nutrients of all, s-adenosyl methionine. SAMe is what's called a *methyl donor*. Every single second of your life there are a billion chemical reactions in your body, in which one chemical is turned into another by adding on what's called a methyl group. The regulation of insulin, adrenalin and serotonin, three body chemicals that are vital to weight control, all depend on methyl reactions.

If you've got fully functional methyl reactions, you will be very healthy, happy and 'connected'. I call this having a high 'methyl IQ', and this is indicated by a low homocysteine level in your blood. If you have a high homocysteine level that means you have a poor methyl IQ and are likely to gain weight easily, have insulin resistance and suffer from depression and are at greater risk of developing diabetes, heart disease, strokes and Alzheimer's later in life.

The average 'H' score is 10 to 11 units. The ideal is 6. I often see patients with levels of 20 or more. With every 5-unit drop in your H score, you almost halve your risk of dying prematurely. If, for example, your H score was 16, and you drop it to six or less and maintain it there, you can probably add around 10 years to your life!

High-homocysteine and methylation problems, on the other hand, literally age your cells faster, drain vitality from you and make you feel old far beyond your years. Homocysteine ages the body directly. If, for example, you expose the cells that line arteries throughout your body to homocysteine, the cells get older much more quickly.[3]

So finally we are discovering that the reason we age is twofold. Cells, and their replacement 'instructions', get increasingly damaged by poor methylation and excessive oxidation, both of which are reflected by your homocysteine score.

This is great news because it's easily remedied. The right diet and supplements can rapidly reverse both poor methylation and excessive oxidation, bringing your homocysteine level into the superhealthy range below 6 units. This is important because it means you really can measure where you are regarding homocysteine, and adjust your diet and supplements accordingly. By the way, you can measure your own homocysteine level using a home test kit (see www.thehfactor.com or call 01904 410410 for a kit).

The key homocysteine-busting nutrients are vitamins B2 and B6, folic acid, vitamin B12, zinc and magnesium. The high-strength multivitamin I recommend taking, along with the Holford Diet, provides optimum amounts of these. In fact, the diet is the perfect way to lower your homocysteine level and improve your health.

Eat to beat the blues

Being overweight and feeling blue are connected in more ways than one. Being overweight can be depressing in its own right – you don't look as good as you could, you may be tired, it may be harder to walk up stairs or run for the bus. However, scientists are discovering a much closer connection between these two conditions after looking at what happens in the brains of those prone to depression and weight gain.

A consistent finding is that both overweight people and depressed people have low levels of serotonin in the brain. This is the brain's 'happy' chemical and it also controls your appetite. SSRI antidepressants help promote serotonin in the brain and not only relieve depression in up to 50 per cent of people, but also reduce appetite.

However, the side effects of SSRIs are in themselves depressing, so much so that most SSRI drugs are now banned in children up to the age of 18 and are under review for adults. Although there are more than 25 reported side effects, the main concern is that something like one in ten adolescents was found to develop suicidal tendencies as a result of taking these drugs. Talk about out of the frying pan into the fire!

Protein and serotonin

Serotonin is made directly from a nutrient that you and I eat every day. It's an amino acid called *tryptophan*, found in protein foods. If you take tryptophan out of a person's diet, two things will happen. First, they'll become depressed, and secondly, they'll crave carbohydrates.

When you eat protein foods such as chicken or fish you will raise blood levels of tryptophan. Tryptophan then turns into 5-hydroxytryptophan (5-HTP), small amounts of which are also present in beans, fish and other protein foods, and then into serotonin. The body stores 5-HTP in the platelets in the blood before passing it to the brain.

Now, you might logically think that a high-protein diet, for example bacon and eggs for breakfast rather than a high-carbohydrate choice such as a croissant, toast or cereal, would increase the brain's levels of serotonin best. It doesn't. Research by Professor Richard Wurtman and Judith Wurtman at the Massachusetts Institute of Technology (MIT) has consistently shown that meals containing carbohydrate, rather than protein, raise serotonin best.[4]

The reason for this apparent anomaly is that tryptophan in the bloodstream competes very badly with all the other amino acids in protein, so little gets across into the brain. However, when you eat a carbohydrate food such as an apple, this causes some insulin to be released into the bloodstream, which carries the tryptophan and 5-HTP into the brain, and causes serotonin levels to rise.

This may be why many depressed people crave sweet foods to give them a lift. So, if you find sugar makes you feel happier, you are probably low in serotonin. The trouble is, a vicious cycle lies this way: most carbohydrate snacks are high in refined sugar and fat, and make you fat, which is depressing.

Judith Wurtman, who directs the Program in Women's Health at the MIT Clinical Research Center, says that when you stop eating carbohydrates on a high-protein diet, your brain stops regulating serotonin, leading to low mood and food cravings.

'When serotonin is made and becomes active in your brain, its effect on your appetite is to make you feel full before your stomach is stuffed and stretched,' she says. 'Serotonin is crucial not only to control your appetite and stop you from overeating; it's essential to keep your moods regulated.'

Carbohydrate cravings

This explains the common craving of high-protein dieters (especially women) for carbohydrates. Women have much less serotonin in their brains than men, so a serotonin-depleting diet will make women feel irritable. Some people feel down in the afternoon or early evening and crave carbohydrate.

According to Wurtman's clinical studies, if the carbohydrate craver eats protein instead, he or she will become grumpy, irritable or restless. Furthermore, filling up on fatty foods such as bacon or cheese makes you tired, lethargic and apathetic. This is another reason why I don't favour high-protein/low-carbohydrate diets.

One way to guarantee healthy serotonin levels is to supplement with 5-HTP. This not only improves your mood, but also will reduce your appetite, especially for sugary foods. And aside from all the problems with sugar we've seen – unstable blood sugar, exhaustion and weight gain – it has even been implicated in aggressive behaviour,[5, 6, 7, 8, 9, 10] anxiety,[11, 12] hyperactivity and attention deficit,[13] depression,[14] eating disorders,[15] fatigue,[16] learning difficulties[17, 18, 19, 20] and PMS. So it's a good idea to ditch the stuff, and the best way of doing that is by following the Holford Diet.

A sharper mind

The effect of nutrition on the brain is a matter of keen interest these days. We now know that memory and concentration, as well as mood, depend hugely on what we put in our digestive systems. Keeping an even blood sugar level is key, as is an optimal intake of essential fats and antioxidants.

To illustrate just how vital these essential Fatburner nutrients are, consider these studies. One measured the amount of DHA, an omega-3 fat, in the umbilical cord of newborn babies and found those with higher levels were faster thinkers eight years later. Another gave infants extra DHA for the first four months and found that they thought faster six years later. These benefits of essential fats are seen at both ends of the age spectrum. A person's risk of developing Alzheimer's falls by 60 per cent if they eat a diet high in omega-3 fats, especially DHA, according to recent research by Dr Martha Morris at Chicago's Rush Institute for Healthy Aging. Vitamins E and C, both in diet and in supplements, have also been shown to cut the risk of age-related memory problems by more than 60 per cent![21, 22, 23]

Then there's the homocysteine factor (see above). Dropping your homocysteine level by five points halves the risk for Alzheimer's, according to a study published in the *New England Journal of Medicine*.[24] You'll be getting all of these nutrients – B vitamins, antioxidants, vitamins E and C, plus essential fats – on the Holford Diet.

Staying cool

We had a look at the effect stress has on mind and body in Chapter 7. A mild dose of stress can actually stimulate memory and mental alertness, but long-term stress is definitely bad news: it puts too much of the hormone cortisol into circulation, and this literally damages the brain. Another factor that causes too much of the stress hormone cortisol is blood sugar peaks and troughs. When your blood sugar level crashes, the body produces more cortisol. It thinks you are being starved and goes into panic mode.

Raised levels of cortisol have been linked to poorer memory and a shrinking of the brain's memory-sorting centre. This is probably why either high stress or high sugar worsens memory and concentration. After only two weeks of the raised cortisol levels of stress, the dendrite 'arms' of brain cells, which reach out to connect with other brain cells, start to shrivel up, according to research carried out at Stanford University in California by Robert Sapolsky, professor of neuroscience.

The good news is that such damage isn't permanent. Stop the stress and the dendrites grow back. And one way to reduce your stress levels is to reduce your intake of sugar and stimulants. The more dependent on stimulants you are, and the more your blood sugar levels fluctuate, the more you are likely to react stressfully to life's inevitable challenges.

With the right nutrition and the right attitude, age-related memory loss doesn't need to happen to you. You can build new brain cells at any age. Research clearly shows that healthy, well-educated elderly people can show no decline in mental function right up to death, and no increased rate of brain shrinkage even after 65. It's a 'use it or lose it' situation.

Fighting disease

If you have heart disease, diabetes, breast cancer, osteoporosis or arthritis, or any of your close family members (mother, father, sister or brother) has suffered from any of these conditions, especially early in their life, the Holford Diet may literally be a lifesaver for you.

The principles upon which it is based – the product of the results of 20 years of research at ION, reviewing thousands of scientific studies, testing our ideas out with more than 100,000 now healthy volunteers – can reverse most major life-threatening illnesses. Let's examine a few.

Diabetes. Since the Holford Diet is specifically designed to stabilise blood sugar levels, I hardly need say that it is the diet of choice for diabetics. Professional diabetes associations around the world are adopting ⒼⓁ-counting as an essential part of managing diabetes. Hundreds of studies now prove that a low-ⒼⓁ diet helps to improve blood sugar balance and hence reduce the need for medication. These are well summarised in a recent review article in the *Journal of the American Medical Association* for those who want the science.[25]

In Chapter 21 you'll see that I recommend supplementing with the mineral chromium, at least for the first three months of the Holford Diet. Chromium not only helps reduce your appetite, but it also improves the symptoms or diabetes and reduces the need for medication.

Heart disease and strokes. Just about every vital statistic of the Holford Diet is good news for your heart and arteries. If your blood pressure or your cholesterol, homocysteine or triglyceride levels are high, you can expect them to come down.

Here's what happened to Mike:

❨ *In mid-April I had my blood checked and found my cholesterol to be 6.5. I do eat really healthily and felt that my condition was due to hereditary cholesterol rather than dietary factors. A friend had reduced theirs through the supplements recommended in your book, so I thought it was worth a try.*

> *Five weeks later I went for a second blood test to find my choles-terol had dropped to 5.1. My GP couldn't believe it! He would not wholeheartedly acknowledge the success, but he didn't knock it either, saying, 'Whatever you're taking is working – come back in a year!'*

Valerie, aged 73, is another case in point. She had suffered from high blood pressure for over 30 years, as well as a touch of arthritis. Her doctor had given her two drugs, Captopril and a junior aspirin every day. They had helped a bit, but her blood pressure was still high, often as high as 160/80.

She decided to have a homocysteine test. Her homocysteine score was 42.9, putting her in the very high-risk category, so she went on my diet and the supplement programme recom-mended in my book *The H Factor*. After two months she retested and her H score had dropped by 88 per cent to a healthy 5.1. Her blood pressure has also dropped and stabilised at 132/80 and she no longer needs medication. Her arthritis has improved, causing her much less joint pain and she feels alto-gether better in herself.

Take a look at the chart below, which shows the kind of risk reduction you can expect by normalising your levels of homo-cysteine, cholesterol and triglycerides, and your blood pres-sure, as well as correcting any insulin resistance.

Medical statistics	Estimated potential risk reduction
High blood cholesterol (low HDL, low LDL)	60 per cent
High blood fats (triglycerides)	30 per cent
High blood pressure	30 per cent
High blood homocysteine	60 per cent
Insulin resistance	30 per cent

Diet and lifestyle changes

Reducing saturated fat, increasing omega-3 fats	30 per cent
Reducing alcohol	30 per cent
Quitting smoking, increasing antioxidants	50 per cent
Upping B vitamins	30 per cent
Less sodium, more potassium, magnesium and calcium	30 per cent
Increasing exercise	30 per cent
Decreasing weight	30 per cent
Reducing stress (cortisol)	30 per cent

Ten good trials have shown that eating low-ⓖⓛ foods alone will lower your cholesterol, especially the 'bad' LDL cholesterol, and triglycerides.[26] In a study involving 75,000 nurses, those with a high-glycemic-load diet doubled their risk of heart disease.[27] Then there are the beneficial effects of reducing oxidants and increasing antioxidants, reducing saturated fat and increasing essential fats, having more B vitamins and taking more exercise. The National Heart Forum estimates that if you could normalise your cholesterol and blood pressure, do some exercise on a regular basis, quit smoking and lose weight, that alone would reduce your risk by almost a third.[28] Couple this will the proven benefits of a low-ⓖⓛ diet high in essential fats, plus supplementing with antioxidants and homocysteine-lowering B vitamins, and there's a good chance you could eradicate your risk completely.

Cancer. Most people are still not aware that the primary risk factor for cancer is diet. When the World Cancer Research Fund examined more than 5,000 studies on diet and cancer, they concluded that you could halve the risk of cancer by changing your diet.[29] Many people mistakenly think that cancer is largely genetic. It isn't, and the following study, which involved 45,000 pairs of twins, will show you why I can say this with confidence.

This study, published in the *New England Journal of Medicine*, looked at whether people with the same genes had the same risk of cancer. What they found was that cancer is more likely to be caused by diet and lifestyle choices than by genes. Identical twins, who are genetically the same, had no more than a 15 per cent chance of developing the same cancer. This suggests that the cause of most cancers is about 85 per cent environmental – that is, down to factors such as diet, lifestyle and exposure to toxic chemicals. This study concluded that diet, smoking and (lack of) exercise accounted for up to 82 per cent of cancers studied.[30]

To some extent you can divide cancer into two kinds. First there are cancers of the lungs and digestive tract – oesophagus, stomach, colorectal cancer. These are strongly linked to diet, with alcohol, smoking, hot drinks and meat the major culprits. Burnt meat is by far the worst offender – eating burned or browned meat every day significantly increases your risk.

The other kind are hormonal cancers, most notably breast and prostate cancer. Both of these, and especially breast cancer, are linked to 'oestrogen dominance' and to high-🍬 diets. Oestrogen is the hormone that encourages breast and uterine cell growth, and an excess of oestrogen signals (or a lack of progesterone, which counters the effects of oestrogen) can trigger breast cancer.

Ten years ago I went public with my views on HRT, saying that it was an unacceptable risk factor for breast cancer, a view that is finally being accepted by government bodies around the world. But many women's diets are also to blame. The reason is twofold.

First, as you start to lose blood sugar balance, and become overweight and insulin-resistant, the resulting excess fat produces oestrogen. Yes, fat cells – not just the ovaries – produce oestrogen. This leads to a lifetime of extra exposure to oestrogen. That's risk number one.

Here's risk number two. Increased consumption of high-GL foods leads, as we've seen, to insulin resistance, present in the majority of overweight people and 25 per cent of those not overweight. Insulin resistance in its turn can lead to polycystic ovary syndrome (PCOS). With this condition, women have more and more cycles in which they don't ovulate. Only if a woman ovulates is progesterone produced, so oestrogen, unopposed by progesterone, can then trigger breast cancer. (If you want to go deeper into this subject read my book *Say No to Cancer*.)

The Holford Diet is a perfect diet in all respects for preventing both digestive cancers and hormonal cancers. Once again, the low-GL foods, high in antioxidants, essential fats and B vitamins, all help to keep your body fighting fit. The emphasis on fresh, organic foods wherever possible is important here, too. In fact, in all its essentials this diet matches the recommendations of the World Cancer Research Fund for reducing cancer risk. Supplementing with a good high-strength multivitamin, plus 1 or 2 grams of vitamin C, further boosts your body's natural immunity.

I have seen this approach not only keep thousands of women free from breast cancer, but even reverse the cancer in women who have it. That's what happened to Betty, who first consulted me in 1986. Here's what she says:

> ❝ *I feel moved to tell you I consulted you in 1986 with a recurrence of breast cancer. Now, 13 years later, I am pleased to tell you I have just celebrated my seventy-fifth birthday and am fit and well, taking no medication and attending no clinics. I am sure this is in large part due to the advice I received from you.* ❞

Arthritis. If you've got aching joints, welcome to the club. Nine out of ten people have arthritis by the time they're 60. I want to make sure you're one of the one in ten who don't. It's a vicious circle because once you develop aching joints you don't want to exercise, and then weight gain is just around the corner.

However, you will be pleased to hear that the principles of the Holford Diet work extremely well at repairing arthritic joints. That is because the five main causes of inflammation and damage to joints are all reversible. These are:

- glycation, which means damage caused by sugar;
- inflammation caused by a lack of essential fats;
- too much oxidation, not enough antioxidants;
- allergy; and
- lack of joint-building minerals and nutrients such as glucosamine.

Glycation is inflammation caused by glucose imbalance and insulin resistance. Glucose can damage joints in the same way it damages arteries. That's why there is a strong link between diabetes and arthritis. While ordinarily the adrenal hormone cortisol – the body's best anti-inflammatory agent – can handle such problems, out-of-control blood sugar results in adrenal exhaustion. So it's far better to restore blood sugar balance to avoid the damage in the first place. Reducing your use of stimulants such as caffeine and nicotine also helps.

The next cause of inflammation is a lack of what are called prostaglandins, the hormone-like substances made from essential fats, especially omega-3 fats. A diet high in meat and dairy products, which are high in saturated fats, promotes pain and inflammation, while a diet high in fish and seeds, high in essential fats, reduces it. That's what the Holford Diet achieves.

Then there are free radicals, or oxidants. In much the way that oxidants from exhaust fumes or cigarettes damage your skin, oxidants in the bloodstream damage joints. That's why a diet high in antioxidants, backed up by supplements, helps to reduce inflammation.

The final common cause of arthritis is having unidentified food allergies. John is a case in point. He could barely walk 100 yards without pain and had to go up the stairs on his hands and knees, despite being on a lot of medication. He took York Test's IgG allergy test and discovered he was allergic to certain foods. Once he eliminated these from his diet he began to feel less pain. He gradually reduced his medication and now needs none. He no longer experiences pain and he has regained his moblility.

Once inflammation is under control, joints can and do repair themselves. This, of course, requires a good supply of bone-building minerals such as calcium, magnesium and zinc, all abundant in wholefoods I recommend you eat on the Holford Diet. Seeds are an especially good source of these nutrients, as well as an excellent source of essential fats. When you put all this together with appropriate supplements, you have an incredibly powerful anti-arthritis strategy.

Take Ed. I met him after he had retired from a highly successful business career. He had the money, he had the time, but he could barely walk without pain, let alone pursue his passion for golf. I advised him on how to change his diet and what supplements to take. It took him three months to become pain-free. Here's what he said:

> ❝ I used to have constant pain in my knees and joints, could not play golf or walk more than ten minutes without resting my legs. Since following your advice my discomfort has decreased 95–100 per cent. It is a different life when you can travel and play golf every day. I never would have believed my pain could be reduced by such a large degree, and no return, no matter how much activity in a day or week. ❞

If you'd like to find out more specifically about arthritis, I recommend you read my book *Say No to Arthritis*.

I know you just want to lose weight – and you will. But I hope I have convinced you that the diet you are about to start will change your life for the better. Not only will you feel the benefits in the next few weeks, but you will live the benefits for years to come. The Holford Diet is a diet for living your life to the full.

- If you choose to eat low-**GL** foods that are also high in antioxidants you will improve your skin. These include berries, plums, grapefruit and oranges, as well as kale, spinach, Tenderstem, broccoli, beetroot, Brussels sprouts and avocados.

- You need some carbohydrate to make serotonin in the brain, which keeps you happy and reduces your appetite.

- By controlling your blood sugar and providing brain-friendly nutrients the Holford Diet helps sharpen your memory and concentration.

- You can slow down the ageing process and extend your lifespan by following the Holford Diet because you'll be eating less quantity (calories) and more quality (optimum nutrition).

- The Holford Diet also helps to lower many vital statistics that mean greater risk for disease, including your cholesterol, triglycerides, homocysteine and blood pressure.

- The Holford Diet helps to prevent heart disease, cancer, diabetes, Alzheimer's and arthritis and is consistent with the cutting-edge science of disease prevention through nutrition.

References

1 Agricultural Research, November 1996, pp. 4–8 (see ORAC Chart and the Watsons' approach to optimal health and longevity at http://optimal-health.cia.com.au/OracLevels.htm); Ronald Prior et al., Jean Mayer USDA Human Nutrition Research Center on Aging at Tufts, Boston, MA, in *Journal of Agriculture and Food Chemistry*, Vol 46 (1998), pp. 2686–93, and *American Society for Horticultural Science* (1999); *Journal of Agriculture and Food Chemistry*, Vol 49(11) (2001), pp. 5165–70

2 S. E. Vollset et al., 'Plasma total homocysteine and cardiovascular and non-cardiovascular mortality: the Hordaland Homocsyteine Study', *American Journal of Clinical Nutrition*, Vol 74(1) (2001), pp. 130–6

3 D. Xu, R. Neville and T. Finkel, 'Homocysteine accelerates endothelial cell senescence', Federation of European Biochemical Societies letter, Vol 470 (2000), pp. 20–4

4 R. Wurtman and J. Wurtman, 'Carbohydrates and depression', *Scientific American*, Vol 260(1) (1989), pp. 68–75

5 D. Benton et al., 'Mild hypoglycaemia and questionnaire measures of aggression', *Biological Psychology*, Vol 14(1–2) (1982), pp. 129–35

6 A. Roy et al., 'Monoamines, glucose metabolism, aggression toward self and others', *International Journal of Neuroscience*, Vol 41(3–4) (1988), pp. 261–4

7 A. G. Schauss, *Diet, Crime and Delinquency*, Parker House (1980)

8 M. Virkkunen, 'Reactive hypoglycaemic tendency among arsonists', *Acta Psychiatrica Scandinavica*, Vol 69(5) (1984), pp. 445–52

9 M. Virkkunen and S. Narvanen, 'Tryptophan and serotonin levels during the glucose tolerance test among habitually violent and impulsive offenders', *Neuropsychobiology*, Vol 17(1–2) (1987), pp. 19–23

10 J. Yaryura-Tobias and F. Neziroglu, 'Violent behaviour, Brain dysrythmia and glucose dysfunction: A new syndrome', *Journal of Orthomolecular Psychiatry*, Vol 4 (1975), pp. 182–5

11 M. Bruce and M. Lader, 'Caffeine abstention and the management of anxiety disorders', *Psychological Medicine*, Vol 19 (1989), pp. 211–14

12 W. Wendel and W. Beebe, 'Glycolytic activity in schizophrenia', in D. Hawkins and L. Pauling (Eds), *Journal of Orthomolecular Psychiatry* (1973)

13 R. Prinz and D. Riddle, 'Associations between nutrition and behaviour in 5 year old children', *Nutrition Reviews*, Vol 43 (1986), suppl

14 L. Christensen, 'Psychological distress and diet – effects of sucrose and caffeine', *Journal of Applied Nutrition*, Vol 40(1), 1988, pp. 44–50

15 D. Fullerton et al., 'Sugar, opionoids and binge eating', *Brain Research Bulletin*, Vol 14(6) (1985), pp. 273–80

16 L. Christensen 'Psychological distress and diet-effects of sucrose and caffeine', *Journal of Applied Nutrition*, Vol 40 (1988), pp. 44–50

17 M. Colgan and L. Colgan, 'Do nutrient supplements and dietary changes affect learning and emotional reactions of children with learning difficulties? A controlled series of 16 cases', *Nutrition and Health*, Vol 3 (1984), pp. 69–77

18 J. Goldman et al., 'Behavioural effects of sucrose on preschool children', *Journal of Abnormal Child Psychology*, Vol 14(4) (1986), pp. 565–77

19 M. Lester et al., 'Refined carbohydrate intake, hair cadmium levels and cognitive functioning in children', *Nutrition and Behaviour*, Vol 1 (1982), pp. 3–13

20 S. Schoenthaler et al., 'The impact of low food additive and sucrose diet on academic performance in 803 New York City public schools', *International Journal of Biosocial Research*, Vol 8(2) (1986), pp. 185–95

21 M. Morris et al., 'Vitamin E and vitamin C supplement use and risk incident Alzheimer disease', *Alzheimer's Disease and Associated Disorders*, Vol 12 (1998), pp. 121–6

22 M. Morris et al., 'Dietary intake of antioxidant nutrients and the risk of incident AD', *Journal of the American Medical Association*, Vol 287(24) (2002), pp. 3230–7; see also pp. 3223–61

23 M. Sano et al., 'A controlled trial of selegiline, alpha tocopherol or both as treatment of AD', *New England Journal of Medicine*, Vol 336 (1997), pp. 1216–22

24 S. Seshadri et al., 'Plasma homocysteine as a risk factor for dementia and AD', *New England Journal of Medicine*, Vol 346(7) (2002), pp. 476–83

25 D. S. Ludwig, 'The Glycemic Index', *Journal of the American Medical Association*, Vol 287 (18) (2002), pp. 2414–23

26 Ibid

27 S. Liu et al., 'A prospective study of dietary glycemic load, carbohydrate intake, and risk of coronary heart disease in US women', *American Journal of Clinical Nutrition*, Vol 71(6) (2000), pp. 1455–61

28 'Nutritional Aspects of Cardiovascular Disease', Department of Health (1994)

29 World Cancer Research Fund, 'Food, Nutrition and the Prevention of Cancer: A global perspective' (1997)

30 P. Lichenstein et al., 'Environmental and heritable factors in the causation of cancer', *New England Journal of Medicine*, Vol 343(2) (2000), pp. 78–85

APPENDICES

Appendix 1

Ideal Weight, Body Mass Index and Body Fat Percentage

Weight in relation to height

The following table gives you your ideal weight range depending on your height and sex.

Your ideal weight for height

Men aged 25 and over

Height (ft/m)	Weight (lb/st/kg)
5' 1"/1.55m	112–129lb/8–9st 3lb/51–59kg
5' 2"/1.57m	115–133lb/8st 3lb–9st 7lb/52–60kg
5' 3"/1.6m	118–136lb/8st 6lb–9st 10lb/54–62kg
5' 4"/1.63m	121–139lb/8st 9lb–9st 13lb/55–63kg
5' 5"/1.65m	124–143lb/8st 12lb–10st 3lb/56–65kg
5' 6"/1.68m	128–147lb/9st 2lb–10st 7lb/58–67kg
5' 7"/1.70m	132–152lb/9st 6lb–10st 12lb/60–69kg
5' 8"/1.73m	136–156lb/9st 10lb–11st 2lb/62–71kg
5' 9"/1.75m	140–160lb/10st–11st 6lb/64–73kg
5' 10"/1.78m	144–165lb/10st 4lb–11st 11lb/65–75kg
5' 11"/1.80m	148–170lb/10st 8lb–12st 2lb/67–77kg
6' 0"/1.83m	152–175lb/10st 12lb–12st 7lb/69–79kg
6' 1"/1.85m	156–180lb/11st 2lb–12st 12lb/71–82kg
6' 2"/1.88m	160–185lb/11st 6lb–13st 3lb/73–84kg
6' 3"/1.90m	164–190lb/11st 10lb–13st 8lb/74–86kg

Women aged 25 and over

Height (ft/m)	Weight (lb/st/kg)
4' 8"/1.42m	92–107lb/6st 8lb–7st 9lb/42–49kg
4' 9"/1.45m	94–110lb/6st 10lb–7st 12lb/43–50kg
4' 10"/1.47m	96–113lb/6st 12lb–8st 1lb/44–51kg
4' 11"/1.50m	99–116lb/7st 1lb–8st 4lb/45–53kg
5' 0"/1.52m	102–119lb/7st 4lb–8st 7lb/46–54kg
5' 1"/1.55m	105–122lb/7st 7lb–8st 10lb/48–55kg
5' 2"/1.57m	108–126lb/7st 10lb–9st/49–57kg
5' 3"/1.60m	111–130lb/7st 13lb–9st 4lb/50–59kg
5' 4"/1.63m	114–135lb/8st 2lb–9st 9lb/52–61kg
5' 5"/1.65m	118–139lb/8st 6lb–9st 13lb/54–63kg
5' 6"/1.68m	122–143lb/8st 10lb–10st 3lb/55–65kg
5' 7"/1.70m	126–147lb/9st–10st 7lb/57–67kg
5' 8"/1.73m	130–151lb/9st 4lb–10st 11lb/59–68kg
5' 9"/1.75m	134–155lb/9st 8lb–11st 1lb/61–70kg
5' 10"/1.78m	138–159lb/9st 12lb–11st 5lb/63–72kg

Body mass index

Even better than knowing your ideal weight for your height is to calculate your body mass index, or BMI, a measure of fat based on your height and your weight. Your BMI is a reliable indicator of total body fat. The score is valid for both men and women, but does have some limits:

- It may overestimate body fat in athletes and others who have a muscular build.

- It may underestimate body fat in older people and those who have lost muscle mass.

Your BMI can be used to work out whether you are overweight or obese. Here are the scores:

Underweight = 18.5 or less
Normal weight = 18.5–24.9
Overweight = 25–29.9
Obese = 30 or more

Body Mass Index table

BMI	Normal							Overweight				Obese										Extreme obesity														
Height (inches)	19	20	21	22	23	24	25	26	27	28	29	30	31	32	33	34	35	36	37	38	39	40	41	42	43	44	45	46	47	48	49	50	51	52	53	54
															Body weight (pounds)																						
58	91	96	100	105	110	115	119	124	129	134	138	143	148	153	158	162	167	172	177	181	186	191	196	201	205	210	215	220	224	229	234	239	244	248	253	258
59	94	99	104	109	114	119	124	128	133	138	143	148	153	158	163	168	173	178	183	188	193	198	203	208	212	217	222	227	232	237	242	247	252	257	262	267
60	97	102	107	112	118	123	128	133	138	143	148	153	158	163	168	174	179	184	189	194	199	204	209	215	220	225	230	235	240	245	250	255	261	266	271	276
61	100	106	111	116	122	127	132	137	143	148	153	158	164	169	174	180	185	190	195	201	206	211	217	222	227	232	238	243	248	254	259	264	269	275	280	285
62	104	109	115	120	126	131	136	142	147	153	158	164	169	175	180	186	191	196	202	207	213	218	224	229	235	240	246	251	256	262	267	273	278	284	289	295
63	107	113	118	124	130	135	141	146	152	158	163	169	175	180	186	191	197	203	208	214	220	225	231	237	242	248	254	259	265	270	278	282	287	293	299	304
64	110	116	122	128	134	140	145	151	157	163	169	174	180	186	192	197	204	209	215	221	227	232	238	244	250	256	262	267	273	279	285	291	296	302	308	314
65	114	120	126	132	138	144	150	156	162	168	174	180	186	192	198	204	210	216	222	228	234	240	246	252	258	264	270	276	282	288	294	300	306	312	318	324
66	118	124	130	136	142	148	155	161	167	173	179	186	192	198	204	210	216	223	229	235	241	247	253	260	266	272	278	284	291	297	303	309	315	322	328	334
67	121	127	134	140	146	153	159	166	172	178	185	191	198	204	211	217	223	230	236	242	249	255	261	268	274	280	287	293	299	306	312	319	325	331	338	344
68	125	131	138	144	151	158	164	171	177	184	190	197	203	210	216	223	230	236	243	249	256	262	269	276	282	289	295	302	308	315	322	328	335	341	348	354
69	128	135	142	149	155	162	169	176	182	189	196	203	209	216	223	230	236	243	250	257	263	270	277	284	291	297	304	311	318	324	331	338	345	351	358	365
70	132	139	146	153	160	167	174	181	188	195	202	209	216	222	229	236	243	250	257	264	271	278	285	292	299	306	313	320	327	334	341	348	355	362	369	376
71	136	143	150	157	165	172	179	186	193	200	208	215	222	229	236	243	250	257	265	272	279	286	293	301	308	315	322	329	338	343	351	358	365	372	379	386
72	140	147	154	162	169	177	184	191	199	206	213	221	228	235	242	250	258	265	272	279	287	294	302	309	316	324	331	338	346	353	361	368	375	383	390	397
73	144	151	159	166	174	182	189	197	204	212	219	227	235	242	250	257	265	272	280	288	295	302	310	318	325	333	340	348	355	363	371	378	386	393	401	408
74	148	155	163	171	179	186	194	202	210	218	225	233	241	249	256	264	272	280	287	295	303	311	319	326	334	342	350	358	365	373	381	389	396	404	412	420
75	152	160	168	176	184	192	200	208	216	224	232	240	248	256	264	272	279	287	295	303	311	319	327	335	343	351	359	367	375	383	391	399	407	415	423	431
76	156	164	172	180	189	197	205	213	221	230	238	246	254	263	271	279	287	295	304	312	320	328	336	344	353	361	369	377	385	394	402	410	418	426	435	443

Source: Adapted from Clinical Guidelines on the Identification, Evaluation, and Treatment of Overweight and Obesity in Adults: The Evidence Report.

Body Mass Index table – metric version

Height (cms)	Normal						Overweight					Obese										Extreme obesity														
BMI	19	20	21	22	23	24	25	26	27	28	29	30	31	32	33	34	35	36	37	38	39	40	41	42	43	44	45	46	47	48	49	50	51	52	53	54
																		Body weight (kgs)																			
147	41	43	45	48	50	52	54	56	58	61	63	65	67	69	72	74	76	78	80	82	84	87	89	91	93	95	98	100	102	104	106	108	111	112	115	117
150	43	45	47	49	51	54	56	58	60	63	65	67	69	72	74	76	78	81	83	85	88	90	92	94	96	98	101	103	105	108	110	112	114	117	119	121
152	44	46	49	51	54	56	58	60	63	65	67	69	72	74	76	79	81	83	86	88	90	93	95	98	100	102	104	107	109	111	113	116	118	121	123	125
155	45	48	50	52	55	57	60	62	65	67	69	72	74	77	79	82	84	86	89	91	94	96	98	101	103	106	108	110	113	115	117	120	122	125	127	129
158	47	49	52	54	57	59	62	64	67	69	72	74	77	79	82	84	86	89	92	94	97	100	102	105	107	109	112	114	117	119	121	124	126	129	131	134
160	49	51	54	56	59	60	64	66	69	72	74	77	79	82	84	87	89	92	94	97	100	102	105	108	110	113	115	117	120	122	126	128	130	133	136	138
163	50	53	55	57	60	63	66	68	71	74	77	79	82	84	87	89	93	95	98	100	103	105	108	111	113	116	119	121	124	126	128	132	134	137	140	142
165	52	54	57	60	63	65	68	71	73	76	79	82	84	87	90	93	95	98	101	104	106	108	112	114	117	119	122	125	127	130	133	136	139	142	144	147
168	54	56	59	62	65	67	70	73	76	78	81	84	87	90	93	95	98	101	104	107	110	112	115	118	120	123	126	129	131	135	137	140	143	146	149	152
170	55	58	61	64	66	69	72	75	78	81	84	87	90	93	96	98	101	104	107	110	113	116	118	122	124	127	130	133	136	139	142	145	149	150	153	156
173	57	59	62	66	68	71	73	76	78	80	83	86	89	92	95	98	101	104	107	110	113	117	119	122	125	128	131	134	137	139	142	145	149	153	158	161
176	58	61	64	68	71	73	75	78	80	83	86	89	92	95	98	101	104	107	110	113	116	119	122	125	128	131	134	137	140	143	146	149	153	156	158	161
178	60	63	66	69	73	76	79	82	85	88	91	94	97	100	103	107	110	113	116	119	123	126	129	132	136	139	142	145	148	152	155	158	161	164	167	170
180	62	65	68	71	75	78	81	84	87	91	94	97	100	104	107	110	113	117	120	123	126	130	133	137	140	143	146	150	153	156	160	162	165	169	172	175
183	64	67	70	74	77	80	83	87	90	93	96	100	103	107	110	113	117	120	123	127	130	133	137	140	143	147	150	153	157	160	164	167	171	173	177	180
185	65	68	72	75	79	83	86	89	93	96	99	103	106	110	113	116	120	123	127	130	133	137	141	144	147	151	154	158	161	165	168	171	175	178	182	185
188	67	70	74	78	81	84	88	92	95	99	102	106	109	113	116	120	123	127	130	134	137	141	145	148	152	156	159	162	166	169	173	177	180	183	187	190
191	69	73	76	80	84	87	91	95	98	102	106	109	112	116	120	123	126	130	134	137	141	145	148	152	156	160	163	166	170	173	177	181	185	188	192	196
193	71	74	78	82	86	89	93	97	100	104	108	112	115	119	123	127	130	134	138	142	145	149	152	156	160	163	167	171	175	179	182	186	190	193	197	201

Measuring percentage of body fat

A more important statistic than your BMI is your body fat percentage. Overleaf is an equation to work out an approximation of this percentage. (Your local gym may offer a service for measuring your body fat percentage more accurately using callipers or testing equipment.) An ideal percentage of fat for a man is less than 15 per cent; for a woman it's less than 22 per cent. You can reduce your body fat percentage by around 10 per cent a month on the Holford Diet.

Step 1

Find your body weight (BW) on the chart and write down the corresponding conversion factor. For every pound over the figures given, add 1.08 to the conversion factor.

So: if you weigh 175lb, your conversion factor is 189.36.

If you weigh 132lb, your conversion factor is 142.83 (140.67 plus 2 x 1.08).

Step 2

Find your waist girth on the chart and write down the corresponding conversion factor.

So: if you have a 35in waist, your conversion factor is 145.26.

Step 3

Subtract the waist conversion factor from the body weight conversion factor.

So: 189.36 − 145.26 = 44.1.

Step 4

To the result, add 98.42 for men or 76.76 for women. This gives you your lean body weight (LBW).

So: 44.10 + 98.42 = 142.52.

Step 5

To calculate your fat weight (FW), subtract the LBW from the BW:

BW – LBW = FW.

So: 175 – 142.52 = 32.48.

Step 6

To determine the actual percentage of your body fat, divide FW by BW and multiply by 100:

FW / BW x 100 = %BF.

So: 32.48/175 x 100 = 19%.

Body fat percentage calculation chart

Body weight	Conversion factor	Waist girth	Conversion factor
100	108.21	25	103.75
105	113.62	25.5	105.83
110	119.03	26	107.9
115	124.44	26.5	109.98
120	129.85	27	112.05
125	135.26	27.5	114.13
130	140.67	28	116.2
135	146.08	28.5	118.28
140	151.49	29	120.35

continues ▶

Body weight	Conversion factor	Waist girth	Conversion factor
145	156.9	29.5	122.43
150	162.31	30	124.51
155	167.72	30.5	126.58
160	173.13	31	128.66
165	178.54	31.5	130.73
170	183.95	32	132.81
175	189.36	32.5	134.88
180	194.77	33	136.96
185	200.18	33.5	139.03
190	205.59	34	141.11
195	211	34.5	143.18
200	216.41	35	145.26
205	221.82	35.5	147.33
210	227.23	36	149.41
215	232.64	36.5	151.48
220	238.05	37	153.56
225	243.46	37.5	155.63
230	248.87	38	157.71
235	254.28	38.5	159.78
240	259.69	39	161.86
245	265.1	39.5	163.93
250	270.51	40	166.01
255	275.92	40.5	167.08
260	281.33	41	170.16
265	286.74	41.5	172.23
270	292.15	42	174.31
275	297.56	42.5	176.38
280	302.97	43	178.46
285	308.38	43.5	180.53
290	313.79	44	182.61

Appendix 2

The Complete Glycemic Load of Foods

GLYCEMIC INDEX

The glycemic index is about the *quality* of the carbohydrate within a food, not the *quantity*. In other words, the glycemic index (GI) of a food remains the same whether you eat 10 grams or 100 grams. It is a comparison of how one type of carbohydrate (for example that in bread) compares with another type of carbohydrate (for example sugar). It's worked out by feeding volunteers however much of the food in question they would need to eat to consume 50 grams of 'available' carbohydrate. (Some carbohydrate, such as fibre, is not available to the body for its energy needs.)

If, for example, a food contains half available carbohydrate, the volunteers would be fed 100 grams of the food to obtain 50 grams of the available carbohydrate. The extent to which this raises blood sugar levels (see figure on page 93), compared with the extent to which 50 grams of glucose does, determines its GI score. Glucose, by definition, scores 100 on the GI Index. So, if a food creates half the increase in blood sugar compared with glucose, it's GI score will be 50. This means that you could eat twice as much carbohydrate in the form found in this food to match the effect of glucose on your blood sugar level.

GLYCEMIC LOAD

The glycemic load of a food (**GL**) is basically the GI of a food multiplied by the serving size. So, the **GL** actually tells you what that specific serving, biscuit or slice of bread will do to your blood sugar.

The **GL** of a food is worked out as follows:

GI score divided by 100 multiplied by the available carbohydrate (carbohydrates minus fibre) in grams.

So, in our example above this would be:

50 (GI score)/100 x 50 (50 grams of carbohydrate in 100 gram serving) = 25

So a 100 gram serving of our example food has a **GL** of 25

Take watermelon as another example. Its glycemic index (GI) is pretty high, about 72. According to the calculations by the people at the University of Sydney's Human Nutrition Unit, in a serving of 120 grams it has 6 grams of available carbohydrate per serving, so its glycemic load is pretty low, $72/100 \times 6 = 4.32$ (rounded to 4).

So, as long as you know the glycemic index of a food, the size of the serving you wish to use, and the amount of available carbohydrate in the food, you can calculate the **GL** yourself. However, I have calculated the **GL** for a comprehensive range of foods, which can be found in the chart on pages 434–50.

Please note that the glycemic index for some foods has not been published. In these instances we have estimated the **GL** based on the GI for very similar foods. These foods are marked 'E'.

The most accurate way to gauge whether or not you should eat a food is the glycemic load of a food, which is a calculation based on both the quantity of carbohydrate in a food, and the quality of that carbohydrate.

A 🅖🅛 of 10 or less is good, **shown in bold**

A 🅖🅛 of 11–14 is OK, shown in normal text

A 🅖🅛 of 15 or more is bad, *shown in italics*

However, even this is only a guide, because the amount of a food you eat will obviously alter its effect on your blood sugar, and hence your weight. So, while generally I say liberally eat the **bold** foods with low 🅖🅛, limit the normal-text foods and avoid the *italic* foods, what is most important is to limit the total glycemic load of your diet.

If you want to lose weight and feel great, eat no more than 40 🅖🅛 a day. This means roughly 10 for breakfast, 10 for lunch, 10 for dinner and 5 each for your two snacks, mid-morning and mid-afternoon. You can also drink 5 🅖🅛, so your total daily intake from food and drink is 45 🅖🅛. If you choose the good, low-🅖🅛 foods you'll be able to eat more food. If you choose the bad high-🅖🅛 foods you'll be eating much less.

In the chart below mainly select from the bold foods, then use the right-hand column to work out how much to eat for 5 🅖🅛, which is the serving for a snack, or 10 🅖🅛, which is a serving for a main meal. If you are not sure what a 'serving' means, look at the amount of grams for 5 🅖🅛 and check the grams on the packet of the food in question. Foods containing no carbohydrate, composed entirely of protein or fat (meat, fish, eggs, cheese, mayonnaise) have, in effect, a 🅖🅛 of 0, and are not included in this chart.

Remember that foods marked with an 'E' have an estimated value, while other foods have measured values. As the 🅖🅛 of more foods are calculated, this table will be expanded on www.theholforddiet.com.

The glycemic load of common foods

Bakery Products

Item	Serving size (in g)	GLs per serving	10GLs	5GLs	5 GLs
Muffin – apple, made without sugar	**60**	**9**	**1 muffin**	**½ muffin**	**33g**
Muffin – apple muffin, made with sugar	60	13	1 small muffin	Small ½ muffin	23g
Crumpet	50	13	1 crumpet	½ crumpet	19g
Muffin – apple, oat, sultana, made from packet mix	50	14	1 small muffin	Small ½ muffin	18g
Muffin – bran	57	15	½ muffin	¼ muffin	18g
Muffin – blueberry	57	17	½ muffin	¼ muffin	17g
Muffin – banana, oat and honey	50	17	½ muffin	¼ muffin	15g
Muffin – carrot	57	20	½ muffin	¼ muffin	14g
Banana cake, made without sugar	80	16	1 small slice	half a small slice	25g
Croissant	57	17	½ croissant	¼ croissant	17g
Doughnut	47	17	½ doughnut	¼ doughnut	14g
Sponge cake, plain	63	17	½ slice	¼ slice	19g

Breads

Item	Serving size (in g)	GLs per serving	10GLs	5GLs	5 GLs
Rye kernel (pumpernickel) bread	30	6	2 slices	1 slice	25g
Sourdough rye	30	6	2 slices	1 slice	25g
Volkenbrot, wholemeal rye bread	30	7	2 slices	1 slice	21g
Rice bread, high-amylose	30	7	2 small slices	1 small slice	21g
Rice bread, low-amylose	30	8	2 thin slices	1 thin slice	19g
Wholemeal rye bread	30	8	2 thin slices	1 thin slice	19g
Wheat tortilla (Mexican)	50	8	1½ tortillas	Less than 1 tortilla	31g
Chapatti, white wheat flour, thin, with green gram	50	8	1½ chapattis	1 chapatti	31g
White, high-fibre	30	9	1 thick slice	1 thin slice	17g
Wholemeal (wholewheat) wheat flour bread	30	9	1 thick slice	1 thin slice	17g
Gluten-free fibre-enriched,	30	9	1 thick slice	Half a thick slice	17g
Gluten-free multigrain bread	30	10	1 slice	Half a slice	15g
Light rye	30	10	1 slice	Half a slice	15g
White wheat flour bread	30	10	1 slice	Half a slice	15g

Item	Serving size (in g)	GLs per serving	10GLs	5GLs	5 GLs
Pitta bread, white	30	10	1 pitta	Half a slice	15g
Wheat flour flatbread	30	10	1 slice	Half a slice	15g
Breads					
Gluten-free white bread	30	11	1 slice	Half a slice	14g
Corn tortilla	50	12	1 tortilla	Half a tortilla	21g
Middle Eastern flatbread	30	15	2/3 slice	1/3 slice	10g
Baguette, white, plain	30	15	1/20 baton	1/40 baton	10g
Bagel, white, frozen	70	25	1/2 bagel	1/4 bagel	14g
Breakfast Cereals					
Fatburner Muesli (see page 308) E	30	1	As much as you like	As much as you like	100g
Porridge made from rolled oats	30	2	As much as you like	1 very large bowl	75g
Get Up & Go with strawberries and 1/2 pint of milk E	30	5	1/2 pint drink	1/4 pint drink	5fl oz/ 150ml
All-Bran™	30	6	2 small servings	1 small serving	25g

Item	Serving size (in g)	GLs per serving	10GLs	5GLs	5 GLs
Muesli, gluten-free	30	7	2 small servings	1 small serving	21g
Muesli (Alpen)	**30**	**10**	**1 serving**	**½ serving**	**15g**
Muesli, Natural	**30**	**10**	**1 serving**	**½ serving**	**15g**
Raisin Bran™ (Kellogg's)	30	12	1 small serving	½ serving	13g
Weetabix™	30	13	2 biscuits	1 biscuit	12g
Bran Flakes™	30	13	1 small serving	½ serving	12g
Sultana Bran™ (Kellogg's)	30	14	1 small serving	½ serving	11g
Special K™ (Kellogg's)	30	14	1 small serving	½ serving	11g
Shredded Wheat	*30*	*15*	*1 biscuit*	*½ serving*	*10g*
Cheerios™	*30*	*15*	*1 very small serving*	*½ serving*	*10g*
Frosties™, sugar-coated cornflakes (Kellogg's)	*30*	*15*	*1 very small serving*	*½ serving*	*10g*
Grapenuts™	*30*	*15*	*1 very small serving*	*½ serving*	*10g*
Golden Wheats™ (Kellogg's)	*30*	*16*	*1 very small serving*	*½ serving*	*9g*
Puffed Wheat	*30*	*16*	*1 very small serving*	*½ serving*	*9g*
Honey Smacks™ (Kellogg's)	*30*	*16*	*1 very small serving*	*½ serving*	*9g*
Cornflakes, Crunchy Nut™ (Kellogg's)	*30*	*17*	*1 very small serving*	*½ serving*	*9g*
Coco Pops™ (cocoa-flavoured puffed rice)	*30*	*20*	*½ serving*	*¼ serving*	*8g*

Item	Serving size (in g)	GLs per serving	10GLs	5GLs	5 GLs
Rice Krispies™ (Kellogg's)	30	21	½ serving	¼ serving	7g
Cornflakes™ (Kellogg's)	30	21	½ serving	¼ serving	7g
Cereal Grains					
Semolina	150	6	1 very large serving	1 small serving	125g
Taco shells, cornmeal-based, baked (Old El Paso)	0	8	2 shells	1 shell	13g
Quinoa	150	8	1½ cups	⅔ cup	94g
Cornmeal	150	9	1 very large serving	1 small serving	83g
Kamut E	150	9	1 very large serving	1 small serving	83g
Pearl barley	150	11	1 serving	½ serving	68g
Cracked wheat (bulgur/bourghul)	150	12	1 serving	½ serving	63g
Brown basmati rice	150	13	1 small serving	½ serving	58g
Buckwheat	150	16	1 small serving	⅓ serving	47g
Rice, brown	150	18	1 small serving	⅓ serving	42g
Rice, long-grain, white, precooked, microwaved 2 min. (Express Rice, Uncle Ben's)	150	19	½ serving	¼ serving	39g

Item	Serving size (in g)	GLs per serving	10GLs	5GLs	5 GLs
Rice, basmati, white, boiled	150	22	½ serving	¼ serving	34g
Couscous	150	23	½ serving	¼ serving	33g
Rice, white	150	23	½ serving	¼ serving	33g
Rice, long grain, boiled	150	23	½ serving	¼ serving	33g
Millet, porridge	150	25	½ serving	¼ serving	30g

Crispbreads/Crackers

Item	Serving size (in g)	GLs per serving	10GLs	5GLs	5 GLs
Oatcake	**25**	**8**	**4 oatcakes**	**2 oatcakes**	**16g**
Digestive	**25**	**10**	**1 biscuit**	**½ biscuit**	**13g**
Cream cracker	25	11	2 biscuits	1 biscuit	11g
Rye crispbread	25	11	2 biscuits	1 biscuit	11g
Water cracker	25	17	2 biscuits	1 biscuit	7g
Puffed rice cake	25	17	2 biscuits	1 biscuit	7g

Dairy Products and Alternatives

Item	Serving size (in g)	GLs per serving	10GLs	5GLs	5 GLs
Plain yoghurt (no sugar)	200	3	3 small pots	½ small pot	333g
Non-fat yoghurt (plain, no sugar)	200	3	3 small pots	½ small pot	333g

Item	Serving size (in g)	GLs per serving	10GLs	5GLs	5 GLs
Milk, full-fat	250	3	833ml	416ml	416ml
Milk, skim (Canada)	250	4	625g	312g	312g
Soya yoghurt (Provamel)	200	7	2 small pots	1 small pot	150g
Soya milk (no sugar)	250	7	2 small cups	1 small cup	178ml
Dairy Products and Alternatives					
Custard, homemade from milk	100	7	1 small cup	½ cup	71ml
Ice cream, regular	50	8	2 scoops	1 scoop	31ml
Soya milk (sweetened with apple juice concentrate)	250	8	2 small cups	1 small cup	156ml
Soya milk, reduced-fat (1.5%), 120mg calcium	250	8	2 small cups	1 small cup	156ml
Soya milk (sweetened with sugar)	250	9	1½ cups	⅔ small cup	138ml
Low-fat yoghurt, fruit, sugar, (Ski™)	200	10	1½ small pots	⅔ small pot	100g
Rice milk E	250	14	1 small cup	½ cup	90g
Milk, condensed, sweetened (Nestlé)	*50*	*17*	*1 tsp*	*½ tsp*	*14g*

Item	Serving size (in g)	GLs per serving	10GLs	5GLs	5 GLs
Fruit and Fruit Products					
Blackberries E	120	1	2 large punnets	1 large punnet	600g
Blueberries E	120	1	2 large punnets	1 large punnet	600g
Raspberries E	120	1	2 large punnets	1 large punnet	600g
Strawberries, fresh, raw	120	1	2 large punnets	1 large punnet	600g
Cherries, raw	120	3	2 punnets	1 punnet	200g
Grapefruit, raw	120	3	1 large	1 small	200g
Pear, raw	120	4	2 large pears	1 large pear	150g
Melon/cantaloupe, raw	120	4	1 small melon	½ small melon	150g
Watermelon, raw	120	4	2 big slices	1 big slice	150g
Peach, raw (or canned in natural juice)	120	5	2 peaches	1 peach	120g
Apricots, raw	120	5	8 apricots	4 apricots	120g
Orange, raw	120	5	2 large	1 large	120g
Plum, raw	120	5	8 plums	4 plums	120g
Apple, raw	120	6	2 small	1 small	100g
Kiwi fruit, raw	120	6	2 kiwis	1 kiwi	100g
Pineapple, raw	120	7	2 thin slices	1 thin slice	85g

Item	Serving size (in g)	GLs per serving	10GLs	5GLs	5 GLs
Grapes, raw	**120**	**8**	20 grapes	10 grapes	75g
Mango, raw	**120**	**8**	½ mango	1 slice	75g
Apricots, dried	**60**	**9**	6 apricots	3 apricots	33g
Fruit Cocktail, canned (Delmonte)	**120**	**9**	1 small can	½ small can	66g
Pawpaw/papaya, raw	**120**	**10**	½ small papaya	1 slice	60g
Prunes, pitted	**60**	**10**	6 prunes	3 prunes	30g
Apple, dried	**60**	**10**	6 rings	3 rings	30g
Banana, raw	120	12	1 banana	½ banana	50g
Fruit and Fruit Products					
Apricots, canned in light syrup	120	12	Less than 1 small tin	½ small tin	50g
Lychees, canned in syrup and drained	120	16	½ can	¼ x 200g can	37g
Figs, dried, tenderised, Dessert Maid brand	60	16	2 figs	1 fig	19g
Sultanas	60	25	20	10	12g
Raisins	60	28	20	10	11g
Dates, dried	60	42	2 dates	1 date	7g

Item	Serving size (in g)	GLs per serving	10GLs	5GLs	5 GLs
Jams/Spreads					
Pumpkin seed butter E	16	1	3 large pots	1½ large pots	765g
Peanut butter (no sugar) E	16	1	3 large pots	1½ large pots	765g
Blueberry spread (no sugar) E	30	4	6 dsp	3 dsp	21g
Apricot fruit spread, reduced sugar	30	7	4 dsp	2 dsp	21g
Orange marmalade	30	9	4 dsp	2 dsp	17g
Strawberry jam	30	10	3 dsp	1 heaped dsp	15g
Legumes and Nuts					
Hummus (chickpea dip)	30	1	4 large tubs	4 small tubs	765g
Soya beans	150	1	6 cups	3 cups	750g
Peas, dried, boiled	150	2	3 cups	1½ cups	375g
Pinto beans, boiled in salted water	150	4	2 cups	1 cup	187g
Borlotti beans, boiled, canned	150	4	1½ cans	⅔ can	187g
Lentils	150	5	2 cups	1 cup	150g
Butter beans	150	6	1½ cups	⅔ cup	125g

Item	Serving size (in g)	GLs per serving	10GLs	5GLs	5 GLs
Split peas, yellow, boiled 20 min.	150	6	1½ cups	⅔ cup	125g
Baked beans, canned	150	7	½ tin	¼ tin	107g
Kidney beans	150	7	¾ tin	⅓ tin	107g
Chickpeas (garbanzo beans, Bengal gram), boiled	150	8	1½ cups	⅔ cup	94g
Chickpeas, canned in brine	150	9	¾ tin	⅓ tin	83g
Chestnuts, cooked E	150	8	1½ cups	⅔ cup	94g
Flageolet beans, canned in brine E	150	8	¾ tin	⅓ tin	83g
Haricot/Navy beans	150	12	½ tin	¼ tin	62g
Black-eyed beans, boiled	150	13	1 cup	½ cup	58g

Pasta and Noodles

Item	Serving size (in g)	GLs per serving	10GLs	5GLs	5 GLs
Ravioli, durum wheat flour, meat filled, boiled	90	7.5	½ packet	1 small serving	60g
Vermicelli, white, boiled	90	8	1 large serving	½ large serving	56g
Spaghetti, wholemeal, boiled	90	8	1 large serving	½ large serving	56g
Pasta, wholemeal, boiled	90	8	1 large serving	½ serving	56g
Fettuccine, egg, boiled	90	9	1 serving	½ serving	50g

Item	Serving size (in g)	GLs per serving	10GLs	5GLs	5 GLs
Spirali, durum wheat, white, boiled to *al dente* texture	90	9	1 serving	½ serving	47g
Spaghetti, white, boiled	90	9	1 serving	½ serving	47g
Instant noodles	90	9	1 serving	½ serving	47g
Spaghetti, durum wheat, boiled 10–15 min.	90	10	1 serving	½ serving	43g
Gluten-free pasta, maize starch, boiled 8 min.	90	11	1 small serving	½ small serving	41g
Macaroni, plain, boiled	90	11	1 very small serving	½ very small serving	39g
Rice noodles, dried, boiled	90	11	1 very small serving	½ very small serving	39g
Udon noodles, plain (buckwheat/wheat), boiled	90	15	⅔ serving	½ serving	30g
Corn pasta, gluten-free (62.5g serving size)	90	16	*1 small serving*	*½ small serving*	*28g*
Gnocchi, boiled	90	16	*1 very small serving*	*½ small serving*	*27g*
Rice pasta, brown, boiled 16 min.	90	17	*1 very small serving*	*½ small serving*	*26g*

Snack Foods (Savoury)

Olives, in brine E	50	1	4 cups	2 cups	270g
Peanuts	50	1	1 large pack	1 medium or 2 small packs	250g
Cashew nuts, salted	50	3	1½ small packs	Less than 1 small pack	83g

Item	Serving size (in g)	GLs per serving	10GLs	5GLs	5 GLs
Popcorn, salted, no sugar	**20**	**8**	**1 small pack**	**½ small pack**	**12g**
Potato crisps, plain, salted	50	11	1½ small packs	⅔ small pack	23g
Pretzels, oven-baked, traditional wheat flavour	30	16	8	4	9g
Corn chips plain, salted	50	17	13 chips	7 chips	15g
Snack Foods (Sweet)					
Fruitus apple cereal bar E	**35**	**5**			**35**
Rebar fruit and veg bar E	**50**	**8**	**1 bar**	**½ bar**	**25**
Muesli bar containing dried fruit	30	13	Less than 1 bar	Less than ½ bar	12g
Chocolate, milk, plain (Mars/Cadburys/Nestlé)	50	14	Less than ½ bar	Less than ¼ bar	18g
Apricot fruit bar (dried apricot filling in wholemeal pastry)	50	17	1 bar	½ bar	15g
Twix ® Cookie Bar, caramel (M&M/Mars, USA)	60	17	1 stick	½ stick	18g
Snickers Bar ®	60	19	⅔ bar	⅓ bar	16g
Polos – peppermint sweets	30	21	8	4	7g
Jellybeans, assorted colours	30	22	4 jellybeans	2 jellybeans	7g
Pop Tarts™, double choc	50	24	21	10g	10g

Item	Serving size (in g)	GLs per serving	10GLs	5GLs	5 GLs
Mars Bar ®	*60*	*26*	*½ bar*	*¼ bar*	*13g*
GoodCarb Real Belgian Chocolate Brownie (all 3 varieties)	45	3	3 brownies	1½ brownies	75g
GoodCarb Original Granola	50	5	2 servings	1 serving	50g
Soups					
Tomato	**250**	**6**	**1 can**	**½ can**	**208g**
Minestrone	**250**	**7**	**1 can**	**½ can**	**179g**
Lentil, canned	**250**	**9**	**⅔ can**	**⅓ can**	**139g**
Split pea	*250*	*16*	*½ can*	*¼ can*	*78g*
Black bean	*250*	*17*	*½ can*	*¼ can*	*74g*
Green pea, canned	*250*	*17*	*½ can*	*¼ can*	*74g*
Sugars					
Xylitol	**20**	**2**	**6 tbsp**	**3 tbsp**	**50g**
Blue agave cactus nectar (liquid sweetener in drinks)	**20**	**2**	**100ml**	**50ml**	**50g**
Fructose	**20**	**4**	**3 tbsp**	**5 tsp**	**25g**

Item	Serving size (in g)	GLs per serving	10GLs	5GLs	5 GLs
Sucrose	20	14	3 tsp	1½ tsp	7g
Honey	20	16	2 tsp	1 tsp	6g
Glucose	20	20	2 tsp	1 tsp	5g
Maltose (malt)	20	22	2 tsp	1 tsp	5g
Vegetables					
Tomato E	70	2	5 medium	2½ medium	175g
Broccoli E	100	2	5 handfuls	2½ handfuls	250g
Kale E	75	1	10 handfuls	5 handfuls	375g
Avocado E	190	1	10 medium	5 medium	950g
Onion E	180	2	5 medium	2½ medium	450g
Asparagus E	125	2	5 handfuls	2½ handfuls	315g
Green beans E	75	1	10 handfuls	5 handfuls	375g
Carrots	80	3	2 carrots	1 carrot	133g
Green peas	80	3	5 tbsp	2–3 tbsp	133g
Pumpkin	80	3	267g	1½ servings	133g
Beetroot	80	5	4 small	2 small	80g

Item	Serving size (in g)	GLs per serving	10GLs	5GLs	5 GLs
Swede	**150**	**7**	½ swede	1 small serving	107g
Banana/plantain, green	**120**	**8**	1 small	½ small	**75g**
Broad beans	**80**	**9**	2 tbsp	1 tbsp	**44g**
Sweetcorn	**80**	**9**	1 serving	½ serving	**44g**
Parsnip	80	12	1 small	½ small	33g
Yam	150	13	1 small serving	½ small serving	58g
Boiled potato	150	14	2 small	1 small	53g
Microwaved potato	150	14	2 small	1 small	53g
Mashed potato	*150*	*15*	*2 tbsp*	*1 tbsp*	*50g*
New potato, unpeeled and boiled 20 min.	*150*	*16*	*4 very small*	*2 very small*	*47g*
Instant mashed potato	*150*	*17*	*2 dsp*	*1 dsp*	*44g*
Sweet potato	*150*	*17*	*1 small*	*½ small*	*44g*
Baked potato, white, baked in skin	*150*	*18*	*1 large*	*⅔ medium*	*42g*
French fries	*150*	*22*	*8–10*	*4–5 fries*	*34g*
Baked potato, baked without fat	*150*	*26*	*½ medium*	*¼ medium*	*29g*

The glycemic load of common drinks

Item	Serving size (in ml)	GLs per serving	10GLs in ml	5GLs	5 GLs in ml
Drinks					
Tomato juice, canned, no added sugar	**250**	**4**	**1 pint**	**½ pint**	**315**
Yakult®, fermented milk drink with *Lactobacillus casei*	**65**	**6**	**1⅓ x 65ml bottle**	**⅔ x 65ml bottle**	**30**
Smoothie drink, soy, banana	**250**	**7**	**1⅓ x 250ml carton**	**⅔ x 250ml carton**	**175**
Smoothie drink, soy, chocolate hazelnut	**250**	**8**	**250ml carton**	**½ 250ml carton**	**150**
Carrot juice, freshly made	**250**	**10**	**⅖ pint or ⅔ cup**	**⅕ pint or ⅓ cup**	**125**
Grapefruit juice, unsweetened	250	11	⅖ pint or ⅔ cup	⅕ pint or ⅓ cup	115
Apple juice, pure, unsweetened	250	12	⅓ pint or ⅔ cup	⅙ pint or ⅓ cup	105
Orange juice	250	13	⅓ pint or ⅔ cup	⅙ pint or ⅓ cup	95
Cordial, orange, reconstituted	250	13	⅓ pint or ⅔ cup	⅙ pint or ⅓ cup	95
Smoothie, raspberry	250	14	250ml carton	½ 250ml carton or ⅓ cup	90
Pineapple juice, unsweetened	*250*	*16*	*½ pint or 1 cup*	*¼ pint or ½ cup*	*80*
Cranberry juice drink, Ocean Spray®	*250*	*16*	*½ pint or 1 cup*	*¼ pint or ½ cup*	*80*

Item	Serving size (in ml)	GLs per serving	10GLs in ml	5GLs	5 GLs in ml
Drinks					
Coca Cola®, soft drink/soda	250	16	⅔ x 330ml can	⅓ x 330ml can	80
Fanta®, orange soft drink	250	23	½ pint or ⅔ cup	¼ pint or ⅓ cup	50
Lucozade®, original	250	40	¼ pint or ½ cup	⅛ pint or ¼ cup	30

The GL values of foods listed here are derived from research published in 2002 by K. Foster-Powell, S. H. Holt, J. C. Brand-Miller in 'International table of glycemic index and glycemic load values: 2002', *American Journal of Clinical Nutrition*, Vol 76(1) (2002), pp. 5–56.

Notes

Serving size notes:

All pasta serving sizes are for cooked food. For the equivalent of dry weight, halve the score – so, if you're cooking spaghetti and the serving size is 120g, that means you put 60g in the saucepan.

Portion guide at a glance (all servings provide 7 Ⓖ):

Food	Dry weight (g)	Looks like	Looks like when cooked
Rice	40	1½ tbsp	2½ tbsp
Pasta	40	2 handfuls	4 handfuls
Quinoa	68	3 tbsp	4 rounded tbsp
Potato (boiled new)	70	3–4 small	3–4 small
Couscous	25	1 tbsp	3 handfuls

Appendix 3

The Dangers of High-Protein Diets

There are big problems with high-protein diets, especially in the long term, that I'd like you to know about. While I agree that high-protein diets do help balance your blood sugar, and hence cause weight loss, the reason I'm not a fan of this approach is that I believe the risks and the restrictions outweigh the benefits. The most famous high-protein diet is the Atkins Diet. Headlines the world over have issued warnings of heart and cancer risk, kidney damage and bone mass loss – and quite rightly so. Let's examine these causes of concern.

Kidney problems. Protein produces breakdown products that are hard work for the kidneys. If your kidneys are healthy and your protein excess isn't too high, no problem. But how far can you push it? Researchers found that about 30 per cent of women between the ages of 42 and 68 had a mild kidney problem. They also found that, in women who had normal kidney function, there was no link between high protein intakes and a decline in renal function.

However, those who already had a mild kidney problem and ate a high-protein diet – particularly one high in meat protein – showed some deterioration. Interestingly, dairy and vegetable proteins were not associated with worsening kidney function. And the parameters here for 'high protein' were much narrower than for what you'd normally eat on the Atkins Diet. Ironically, one of the first signs of poor kidney function is water retention (see Chapter 9), which leads to weight gain. However, the consequences are much more serious as kidney function starts to decline, leading to the need for dialysis.

Bone problems. Protein is acidic, and excess amounts need to be neutralised. The Nurse's Health Study, conducted in the US and analysed by the Harvard School of Public Health, recently found that women who consumed 95g of protein a day, as compared with those who consumed less than 68g a day, had a 22 per cent greater risk of forearm fractures.[1] In another study, eating more than 80g of protein a day, which is equivalent to bacon and eggs for breakfast and a steak for dinner, was found to increase your risk of osteoporosis.[2]

This happens because protein is made of amino acids. Too much acid is neutralised by the body's release of calcium, an alkaline mineral, from the bones – a finding that has been confirmed by 'metabolic ward' studies in which people are kept in a controlled environment, fed precise diets and measured for their calcium loss. Such studies have found that a negative calcium balance is created when 95g of protein is consumed while a person eats 500mg of calcium. The calcium intake must be raised to 800mg before calcium balance is achieved – that is to say, when the calcium entering the body is the same as the amount leaving.

Dr Shalini Reddy from the University of Chicago conducted a six-week study on ten healthy adults eating a low-carb diet. Volunteers lost an average of 9lb over the course of the study – that's 1½ lb a week.

That's the good news. The bad news is that the acid excretion in the urine, which is an indication of acid levels in the blood, rose by 90 percent in some volunteers. There was also a sharp rise in the amount of calcium excreted in the urine during the low-carbohydrate, high-protein diets, and even during the 'maintenance' diets for these regimes, despite only a slight decrease in calcium intake. This means the people were losing calcium from the body. Also, urinary citrate, a compound that inhibits kidney-stone formation, decreased, implying an increased risk of kidney-stone formation.[3]

According to Dr Reddy, 'Consumption of a low-carbohydrate, high-protein diet for six weeks delivers a marked acid load to the kidney, increases the risk for stone formation, decreases estimated calcium balance, and may increase the risk for bone loss.' These studies all suggest that such high-protein diets may increase the risk of bone loss over the long term. Of course, we are going to have to wait a while to find out, but I'd rather you weren't the guinea pig.

Breast and prostate cancer risk. After reviewing thousands of studies on diet and cancer, the World Cancer Research Fund states that there is an unequivocal link between high meat consumption and cancer incidence, especially for breast, colon and prostate cancer.[4] For breast and prostate cancer the link is strongest in relation to high dairy and dairy meat (beef) consumption. People in countries where beef and dairy products are not eaten have a fraction of the risk. In China, for example, the chances of a woman's dying from breast cancer are 1 in 10,000, while her chance in the UK is 1 in 10. For prostate cancer the difference is even greater. In rural China the incidence is 0.5 in 100,000, yet it is estimated that, by 2015, 1 in 4 men in the UK will have a diagnosis of prostate cancer at some point in his life! Why?

The main likely cause of prostate and breast cancer is that these hormone-sensitive cells go into overgrowth due to exposure to abnormal levels of hormones or hormone-like substances, which include many of the man-made pollutants, from pesticides to PCBs, and dioxins to DDT. These tell a cell to continue growing. The hormone oestrogen does this too, which is why oestrogen HRT increases the risk of developing breast cancer.

Milk is high in oestrogen, but it's also high in other growth-stimulating chemicals, which, as we've seen, is hardly surprising, since milk is designed to make baby calves grow massively. It's called insulin-like growth factor. There are different types – IGF-1, IGF-2 and so on, although much of the focus is on IGF-1, which is very abundant in milk and beef. The amount in modern milk is double this, partly because cows have been selectively reared to produce milk during pregnancy. On top of that, in the US cows are treated with BST (bovine somatotrophin), a growth hormone capable of further increasing milk yield by about 12 per cent.

All this means a cow's daily milk production has gone up from 3 to 30 litres. Not surprisingly, this milk has 2 to 5 times the amount of IGF-1, while the beef from a BST-treated animal has about double the IGF. Casein, the protein in milk, then helps to carry the IGF into us.

But what does IGF-1 do and why is it a strong candidate for increasing the risk of cancer? We make IGF, but very little in adulthood. It's produced mainly in childhood to stimulate growth. Normally, it is produced by the liver, especially during puberty. In girls it stimulates the growth of breast tissue, encouraging cells to divide and grow. In boys it stimulates growth of the prostate. There's nothing wrong with IGF-1, just as there's nothing wrong with oestrogen. It's a perfectly normal hormone. It's just that we aren't designed to be eating sources of it in adulthood. And that makes me very worried when a nation of dieters starts living off meat and cheese.

When levels in the blood increase by 8 per cent, the risk for prostate cancer increases seven times. Levels of IGF are, on average, 9 per cent higher in meat-eating omnivores and dairy-eating vegetarians than in vegans. Recent research from Shangai, China, has found that the higher a woman's IGF-1 levels, the higher her risk for breast cancer. This study found that women in the top 25 per cent of IGF-1 scores had two to three times the risk of women in the bottom 25 per cent of IGF-1 levels.[5]

A study from York University in the UK on the link between IGF and prostate cancer risk in men found a similar result. Men in the top 25 per cent of IGF levels had three times the risk of prostate cancer.[6] These are just two of a dozen trials finding a strong link between circulating levels of IGF-1 and prostate cancer. There are many more linking IGF with breast cancer, with the combination of being insulin-resistant and having high IGF and excessive levels of oestrogen increasing the risk most greatly.[7,8,9] The way to reverse this risk is to correct insulin resistance by eating low-Ⓖ carbohydrates, reduce your consumption of milk and beef, eat organic where possible and stay away from HRT.

Underactive thyroid. What's more, high-protein diets can lead to an underactive thyroid. Just two weeks without carbo-hydrates suppresses the body's production of thyroxine, which controls your metabolic rate. It also promotes the stress hormone cortisol, which makes you even more insulin-resist-ant (see pages 56–9). This, in turn, even further reduces thyroxine production, the major symptom of which is weight gain. Thyroxine is now the second most commonly prescribed drug in the US. So don't be surprised if your metabolism slows down, and you experience rebound weight gain after being on a high-protein, very low-carb diet.

Other problems. Cancer is not the only disease associated with this type of high-protein, high-meat and high-dairy diet. Other research strongly suggests that high consumption of meats and dairy products can lead, or at least contribute to, heart disease, type II diabetes, gall-bladder disease, osteoporosis, kidney failure, kidney stones, multiple sclerosis, rheumatoid arthritis, constipation, diverticulosis, haemorrhoids and hiatal hernia.[10] Recent research in mice has also shown substantial reduction in the ability to conceive in females placed on high-protein diets.[11]

Dr Atkins argued, justifiably, that, if you can correct blood sugar problems, you can reduce your risk for many of these diseases. And, while you *can* correct blood sugar problems with a high-fat/high-protein diet, unless caution is exercised you may put yourself at risk of all of the negative effects associated with such a diet. The fact is, you can control your blood sugar just as well, if not better, by eating with the right kinds of carbohydrate, the right kinds of fat, plus sufficient – not excessive – protein and less saturated fat. That's what I'm recommending to you in the Holford Diet because I believe it's safer, tastier, easier and more effective.

Ironically, if you follow the development of the Atkins Diet, you'll see that it is edging in this direction. The earliest version was really low on carbs, while the latest version ends up with 30 per cent carbohydrates, 30 per cent protein, and 40 per cent fat. In my opinion, this still falls short of the ideal diet for painless weight loss, weight maintenance and overall lifelong health.

The other argument sometimes given in favour of high-protein, high-fat diets is that they mimic the diets of our hunter-gather ancestors. I would dispute this – even in the most carnivorous phases of our evolution, our ancestors would never have eaten the amount of fat advised on a conventional high-protein, high-fat diet. Why? Because it wasn't in the meat. Today's animals are fattened up. Almost all meat you buy is marbled with fat, even if you buy the lean stuff. Real meat, as our ancestors ate, was real *lean* meat. However, our ancestors really thrived when they switched from the higher-protein 'hunter-gatherer' diets to the lower-protein, higher-carbohydrate 'peasant farmer' diet. That's when humanity multiplied and become dominant. Of course, these diets were also low-ⒼⓁ.

Appendix 4

Keeping Track and Contributing to the Research

Follow the instructions in Chapter 23 to monitor your progress week by week using the Fatburner progress report on the following pages. There's a progress report for each of the first four weeks, and a spare progress report for subsequent weeks.

The Fatburner progress reports

WEEK No. 1   Starting date: /   /   Ending date: /   /

THIS WEEK

Initial weight _____ Bust/chest _____ Waist _____ Hips _____ Thighs _____

Final weight _____ Bust/chest _____ Waist _____ Hips _____ Thighs _____
(at end of week)

Target weight _____ Bust/chest _____ Waist _____ Hips _____ Thighs _____

PROGRESS THIS WEEK

Weight lost _____ Total inch loss _____

How many aerobic sessions? _____ How many toning sessions? _____

How well did you follow the diet? _____ % the exercises? _____ %

PROGRESS TO DATE

Initial weight _____ Initial total inches _____
(at start of diet)   (bust+waist+hips+thighs)

Weight lost to date _____ Inches lost to date _____

WEEK No. 2   Starting date: /   /   Ending date: /   /

THIS WEEK

Initial weight _____ Bust/chest _____ Waist _____ Hips _____ Thighs _____

Final weight _____ Bust/chest _____ Waist _____ Hips _____ Thighs _____
(at end of week)

Target weight _____ Bust/chest _____ Waist _____ Hips _____ Thighs _____

PROGRESS THIS WEEK

Weight lost _____ Total inch loss _____

How many aerobic sessions? _____ How many toning sessions? _____

How well did you follow the diet? _____ % the exercises? _____ %

PROGRESS TO DATE

Initial weight _____ Initial total inches _____
(at start of diet) (bust+waist+hips+thighs)

Weight lost to date _____ Inches lost to date _____

WEEK No. 3   Starting date: / /   Ending date: / /

THIS WEEK

Initial weight _____ Bust/chest _____ Waist _____ Hips _____ Thighs _____

Final weight _____ Bust/chest _____ Waist _____ Hips _____ Thighs _____
(at end of week)

Target weight _____ Bust/chest _____ Waist _____ Hips _____ Thighs _____

PROGRESS THIS WEEK

Weight lost _____ Total inch loss _____

How many aerobic sessions? _____ How many toning sessions? _____

How well did you follow the diet? _____ % the exercises? _____ %

PROGRESS TO DATE

Initial weight _____ Initial total inches _____
(at start of diet)   (bust+waist+hips+thighs)

Weight lost to date _____ Inches lost to date _____

WEEK No. 4 Starting date: / / Ending date: / /

THIS WEEK

Initial weight _____ Bust/chest _____ Waist _____ Hips _____ Thighs _____

Final weight _____ Bust/chest _____ Waist _____ Hips _____ Thighs _____
(at end of week)

Target weight _____ Bust/chest _____ Waist _____ Hips _____ Thighs _____

PROGRESS THIS WEEK

Weight lost _____ Total inch loss _____

How many aerobic sessions? _____ How many toning sessions? _____

How well did you follow the diet? _____ % the exercises? _____ %

PROGRESS TO DATE

Initial weight _____ Initial total inches _____
(at start of diet) (bust+waist+hips+thighs)

Weight lost to date _____ Inches lost to date _____

WEEK No. ☐   Starting date: / /   Ending date: / /

THIS WEEK

Initial weight _____ Bust/chest _____ Waist _____ Hips _____ Thighs _____

Final weight _____ Bust/chest _____ Waist _____ Hips _____ Thighs _____
(at end of week)

Target weight _____ Bust/chest _____ Waist _____ Hips _____ Thighs _____

PROGRESS THIS WEEK

Weight lost _____ Total inch loss _____

How many aerobic sessions? _____ How many toning sessions? _____

How well did you follow the diet? _____ % the exercises? _____ %

PROGRESS TO DATE

Initial weight _____ Initial total inches _____
(at start of diet)   (bust+waist+hips+thighs)

Weight lost to date _____ Inches lost to date _____

Fatburner research

You can help with ongoing Fatburner research. If you've completed the diet for four or more weeks, let us know your results by filling in this simple questionnaire, answering as many questions as you can and sending or faxing it to Fatburner Research, Holford and Associates, Carters Yard, London SW18 4JR (fax: +44 (0)20 8874 5003). Alternatively, you can complete the feedback questionnaire online at www.theholforddiet.com.

Fatburner research questionnaire

Your full name: _____

Address: _____

_____

_____

Contact number: _____

What was your initial weight?_____ lb/kg

How many weeks have you been following/did you follow the Holford Diet? _____

What was your final weight?_____ lb/kg

Bust/chest _____ in/cm   Waist _____ Hips _____ Thighs _____

Body fat percentage _____ (if known)

How well did you follow the diet indications? _____ per cent

How well did you follow the exercise indications? _____ per cent

How easy was the diet to stick to? Easy/reasonable/hard/very hard (circle answer)

How were the recipes? Excellent/good/fair/not good (circle answer)

Did you mainly follow the rules or the recipes? _____ per cent (half and half would be 50/50)

How did you feel while on the diet?_____

_____

_____

Did you notice any other changes to your health? _____

_____

_____

What do you think made the biggest difference? _____

_____

_____

Any other comments? _____

_____

_____

_____

_____

Appendix 5

Working Out Your Training Heart Rate Zone

The best way to know that you are exercising at an intensity that will burn fat and boost your metabolism is to measure your pulse while exercising. If it is within your training heart rate zone for 15 minutes or more then your exercising is having a fatburning effect.

To find your training heart rate zone, you need to subtract your age from 220, then calculate 65% of this amount for the lower end of your training zone and 80% for the upper limit:

$$220 - \text{age} \_\_ \times .65 = \text{lower limit}$$
$$220 - \text{age} \_\_ \times .80 = \text{upper limit}$$

For example, for a 30-year-old:

$$220 - 30 = 190 \times .65 = \text{lower limit} = 124 \text{ beats per min}$$
$$220 - 30 = 190 \times .80 = \text{upper limit} = 152 \text{ beats per min}$$

To find your pulse rate, you will need a watch with a second hand. There are several points at which the pulse can be felt easily: the neck (the carotid pulse) on either side of the Adam's apple; or the wrist (the radial pulse). To find your pulse, apply light pressure with your fingers. Normally, for medical examinations your pulse is taken for 60 seconds. But to find your pulse while exercising, stopping for this long would lower your pulse and give you a false reading. So taking your pulse for only 10 seconds and multiplying the result by 6 will give you the number of beats in one minute without giving your heart rate a chance to slow down. This will be your exercising pulse rate.

When you first embark on your aerobic exercise sessions, you will need to stop briefly every 10–15 minutes to monitor your pulse. After a while you will become familiar with how the correct pulse feels for you. See the chart below to find your exercise heart rate for your age.

Training heart rate zone (while exercising)

Age	65–80% of maximum heart rate (beats in 1 minute)	(beats in 10 sec.)
20	130–160	22–27
22	129–158	22–26
24	127–157	21–26
26	126–155	21–26
28	125–154	21–26
30	124–152	21–25
32	122–150	20–25
34	121–149	20–25
36	120–147	20–25
38	118–146	20–24
40	117–144	20–24
45	114–140	19–23
50	111–136	19–23
55	107–132	18–22
60	104–128	17–21
65	101–124	17–21
70	98–120	16–20

The centre column shows how many beats you should have in one minute. Beginners should aim for the lower figure on the left-hand side (that is, 65% of their maximum heart rate for their age), then slowly increase to 80% of their maximum heart rate. Do not exceed this higher level. The column on the far right gives you how many beats you should have in a 10-second pulse count. Beginners should stay at the lower end of their exercise range.

References: Appendices

1 E. Knight et al., 'The effect of dietary protein intake on kidney function in women with normal or mildly abnormal kidneys', *Annals of Internal Medicine*, Vol 138(6) (2003), pp. 460–7

2 D. Feskanich et al., 'Protein consumption and bone fractures in women', *American Journal of Epidemiology*, Vol 143(5) (1996), pp. 472–9

3 L. Allen et al., 'Protein-induced hypercalcuria: a longer-term study', *American Journal of Clinical Nutrition*, Vol 32 (1979), pp. 741–9; C. Anand et al., 'Effect of protein intake on calcium balance of young men given 500mg calcium daily', *Journal of Nutrition*, Vol 104 (1974), pp. 695–700

4 S. Reddy et al., 'Effect of low-carbohydrate high-protein diets on acid-base balance, stone-forming propensity, and calcium metabolism', *American Journal of Kidney Diseases*, Vol 40 (2002), pp. 265–74

5 'Food, Nutrition and the Prevention of Cancer', World Cancer Research Fund, American Institute for Cancer Research (1997)

6 A. Malin et al., 'Evaluation of the synergistic effect of insulin resistance and insulin-like growth factors on the risk of breast carcinoma', *Cancer*, Vol 100(4) (2004), pp. 694–700

7 S. E. Oliver et al., 'Screen-detected prostate cancer and IGF', *International Journal of Cancer*, Vol 108(6) (2004), pp. 887–92

8 H. Seeger, D. Wallwiener and A. O. Mueck, 'Influence of stroma-derived growth factors on the estradiol-stimulated proliferation of human breast cancer cells', *European Journal of Gynaecological Oncology*, Vol 25(2) (2004), pp. 175–7

9 D. W. Voskuil et al., 'Insulin-Like Growth Factor (IGF)-System mRNA Quantities in Normal and Tumor Breast Tissue of Women with Sporadic and Familial Breast Cancer Risk', *Breast Cancer Research and Treatment*, Vol 84(3) (2004), pp. 225–33

10 A. Malin et al., 'Evaluation of the synergistic effect of insulin resistance and insulin-like growth factors on the risk of breast carcinoma', *Cancer*, Vol 100(4) (2004), pp. 694–700

11 S. B. Sondike et al., 'Effects of a low-carbohydrate diet on weight loss and cardiovascular risk factor in overweight adolescents', *Journal of Pediatrics*, Vol 142(3), pp. 253–8

12 D. Gardner, presentation at European Society of Human Reproduction and Embryology, awaiting publication

Recommended Reading

CHAPTER 2
Cannon, Geoffrey, *Dieting Makes You Fat*, Sphere (1984).
Plant, Jane, *The Plant Diet*, Virgin (2003).

CHAPTER 4
Haynes, Antony, *The Insulin Factor*, Thorsons (2004).
Steward, Leighton, et al., *Sugar Busters*, Ballantine Books
　(1995).

CHAPTER 6
Holford, Patrick, *Beat Stress and Fatigue*, Piatkus (1999).

CHAPTER 7
Holford, Patrick, *Say No to Arthritis*, Piatkus (1999).
Holford, Patrick, and Braly, James, *The H Factor*, Piatkus (1999).

CHAPTER 8
Holford, Patrick, *The Optimum Nutrition Bible*, Piatkus (1997,
　rev. 2004).
Holford, Patrick, *Optimum Nutrition for the Mind*, Piatkus
　(2003).

CHAPTER 9
Leeds, Anthony, et al., *The GI Factor*, Hodder & Stoughton (1996).

CHAPTER 10

Erasmus, Udo, *Fats That Heal, Fats That Kill*, Alive Books (1987, rev. 1994).

CHAPTER 11

Braly, James, *The Food Allergy and Nutrition Revolution*, Keats Publishing, Inc. (1992).

Braly, James, and Hoggan, Ron, *Dangerous Grains*, Avery Publishing Group (2002).

CHAPTER 12

Holford, Patrick, *The Optimum Nutrition Bible*, Piatkus (1997, rev. 2004).

CHAPTER 13

Ichazo, Oscar, *Master Level Exercise: Psychocalisthenics*, Sequoia Press (1993).

Sharkey, Brian, *Fitness and Health*, Human Kinetics Europe Ltd, (2003).

CHAPTER 19

Durrant-Peatfield, Barry, *The Great Thyroid Scandal and How to Survive It*, Barons Down Publishing (2003).

Neil, Kate, and Holford, Patrick, *Balancing Hormones Naturally*, Piatkus (1998).

Thomas, Gloria, *Apples and Pears*, Orion (1998).

CHAPTER 22

Holford, Patrick, *The Optimum Nutrition Cookbook*, Piatkus (2001).

CHAPTER 25

Neil, Kate, and Holford, Patrick, *Balancing Hormones Naturally*, Piatkus (1998).

Holford, Patrick, *The Optimum Nutrition Cookbook*, Piatkus (2001).

Resources

Eating disorders

If you have a concern about eating disorders I recommend you contact the Eating Disorders Association at 1st Floor, Wensum House, 103 Prince of Wales Road, Norwich NR1 1DW. Adult helpline: +44 (0)8456 341 414; Youthline: +44 (0)8456 347 650 or go to www.edauk.com.

Institute for Optimum Nutrition (ION)

ION runs the Homestudy Course and the three-year Nutrition Therapists' Diploma course. For details on courses, consultations and publications send a stamped, addressed envelope to ION, Blades Court, Deodar Road, London SWI5 2NU. Phone: +44 (0)20 8877 9993; fax: +44 (0)20 8877 9980 or visit www.ion.ac.uk.

Natural Progesterone Information Society (NPIS)

NPIS provides women and their doctors with details of how to obtain natural progesterone information packs for the general public and health practitioners, and books, tapes and videos relating to natural hormonal health. For an order form and prescribing details (for doctors) please write with a stamped, addressed envelope to NPIS, BCM Box 4315, London WC1N 3XX.

Nutrition consultations

For a personal referral by Patrick Holford to a nutritional therapist in your area, visit www.patrickholford.com and select 'consultations' for an immediate online referral. This service gives details on whom to see in the UK as well as internationally. If there is no one available nearby, you can always do an online assessment – see below.

Nutrition assessment online

You can have your own personal health and nutrition assessment online using the MyNutrition questionnaire. This gives you a personalised assessment of your current health, and what you most need to change in order to lose weight and feel great. Visit www.patrickholford.com and select 'consultations'.

Psychocalisthenics

Psychocalisthenics is an excellent exercise system that takes less than 20 minutes a day, develops strength, suppleness and stamina, and generates vital energy. The best way to learn it is to do the Psychocalisthenics Training. See www.patrickholford.com (seminars) for details on these, or call +44 (0)20 8871 2949. Also available is the book *Master Level Exercise: Psychocalisthenics*, and the *Psychocalisthenics* CD and DVD. For further information please visit www.pcals.com.

Salt alternatives – Solo Low Sodium Sea Salt

The average person gets far too much sodium because we eat too much salt (sodium chloride) and salted foods, and not enough potassium and magnesium, found in fruits and vegetables. Not all salt, however, is bad for you. Solo Low Sodium Sea Salt contains 60 per cent less sodium than ordinary salt and is high in the essential minerals magnesium and potassium. Solo Low Sodium Sea Salt is sold in UK, Ireland, Spain, the Netherlands, Singapore, Hong Kong, Japan, Bahrain, Saudi Arabia, United Arab Emirates, Jordan, Baltic States and United States of America. Visit their website: www.soloseasalt.com for more information or call their international helpline on: +44 (0)8451 304 568.

Sugar alternatives – xylitol

While it is best to avoid sugar and sugar alternatives as much as possible there are two natural sugars that have the lowest ⓖⓛ score. These are blue agave syrup, which is used to sweeten healthier drinks, and xylitol. Xylitol has a ⓖⓛ score of one-seventh of that of regular sugar and tastes the same. Therefore, if you need to sweeten a food or drink use xylitol. Xylitol is available from Health Products for Life on +44 (0)20 8874 8038, or visit www.healthproductsforlife.com.

Skincare products

Environ products were developed by the cosmetic surgeon Dr Des Fernandes to prevent skin cancer and address the damaging effects of the environment on our skin. Formulated with scientifically proven active ingredients, including Vitamin A and antioxidant vitamins C, E and betacarotene, which are used in progressively higher concentrations, Environ will maintain a normal healthy skin or effectively treat and prevent the signs of ageing, pigmentation, problem skin and scarring.

Environ products can be purchased by contacting Health Products for Life on: +44 (0)20 8874 8038, or going to www.healthproductsforlife.com. For international enquiries call +27 21 683 1034 or email environc@iafrica.com.

Water filters

There are many water filters on the market. One of the best is offered by the **Fresh Water Filter Company**, who produce mains-attached water-filtering units. For details visit www.healthproductsforlife.com or call +44 (0)20 8874 8038.

Tests

Food allergy and intolerance
YorkTest sell a home test kit for food allergies and intolerances that requires a pinprick blood sample. You don't have to go to your doctor. YorkTest Laboratories will test you for sensitivity to up to 113 foods, including gluten, wheat and yeast. Call Health Products for Life on +44 (0)20 8874 8038 to order, or visit www.healthproductsforlife.com.

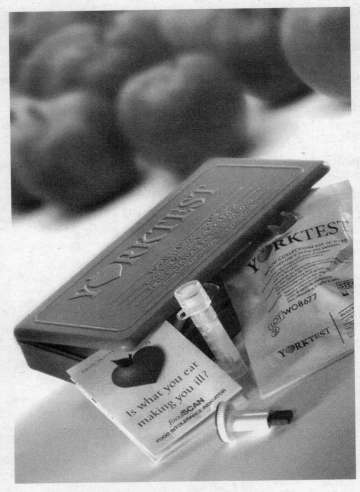

YorkTest food-intolerance testing. Clinically proven test kit for simple blood collection at home; laboratory analysis, results sent straight to you. For details or to order, call Health Products for Life on +44 (0)20 8874 8038 or visit www.healthproductsforlife.com.

Homocysteine test

YorkTest Laboratories produce a home test kit whereby you can take your own pinprick blood sample and return it to the lab for analysis. Full instructions are provided to help you reduce your homocysteine level if it is high. At the time of going to press, the test costs £75. To order, call Health Products for Life on +44 (0)20 8874 8038 or visit www.healthproductsforlife.com. See www.thehfactor.com to order *The H Factor* (see Recommended Reading).

Insulin Resistance

Individual Wellbeing Diagnostic Laboratories (IWDL) offer a test for Insulin Resistance. This requires a blood sample. Call IWDL to arrange the test on +44 (0)20 8836 7750 or visit www.iwdl.net.

Supplement, remedy and supplier directory

Finding your own perfect supplement programme can be confusing, but my website, www.patrickholford.com, offers useful guidance.

Remember, the backbone of a good supplement programme is:

- a high-strength multivitamin;

- additional vitamin C;

- an all-round antioxidant complex; and

- an essential-fat supplement containing omega-3 and omega-6 oils.

Supplement resources

The following companies produce good-quality supplements that are widely available in the UK.

Health Products for Life. It is the best e-health-food shop that stocks all the products I recommend, from supplements to water filters. Their product range includes Get Up & Go, Essential Balance, xylitol, Serotone, multivitamin/minerals, vitamin C, HCA and chromium. You can order by phone on +44 (0)20 8874 8038 or visit www.healthproductsforlife.com.

Higher Nature produce an extensive range of vitamin, mineral and herbal supplements, available in all good health-food shops. They also supply Get Up & Go, Essential Balance, HCA, chromium and Serotone (5-HTP). Phone 0845 3300012 for your nearest stockist or visit www.higher-nature.co.uk.

Health Plus sell konjac fibre, a source of glucomannan. Health Plus Ltd, Dolphin House, 27 Cradle Hill Industrial Estate, Seaford, BN25 3JE. Phone +44 (0)1323 872277.

And in other regions ...

Australia. Solgar supplements are available in Australia. Contact Solgar on 1800 029 871 (free call) for your nearest supplier, or visit www.solgar.com.au. Another good brand is Blackmores.

New Zealand. Higher Nature products are available in New Zealand. Contact Aurora Natural Therapies, 4 La Trobe Track, KareKare, Waitakere City, Auckland 1232, New Zealand, or visit www.aurora.org.nz.

Singapore. Higher Nature and Solgar products are available in Singapore. Contact Essential Living on 6276 1380 for your nearest supplier or visit www.essliv.com.

South Africa. Bioharmony produce a wide range of products in South Africa and other African countries. For details of your nearest supplier contact 0860 888 339 or visit www.bioharmony.co.za.

Index

Note: page numbers in **bold** refer to diagrams. Page numbers in italics refer to information contained in tables.

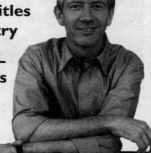

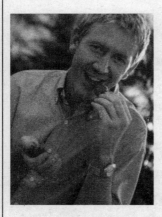